D1825058

# THE **SIX KEYS** TO OPTIMAL HEALTH

# THE **SIX KEYS** TO **OPTIMAL HEALTH**

*Achieving and Maintaining Wellness in the Twenty-first Century*

Dr. Nicolas Campos

Copyright © 2008 by Dr. Nicolas Campos.

Library of Congress Control Number:          2007903155
ISBN:          Hardcover          978-1-4257-7921-4
               Softcover          978-1-4257-7884-2

All rights reserved. No part of this book may be reproduced or transmitted in any form or by any means, electronic or mechanical, including photocopying, recording, or by any information storage and retrieval system, without permission in writing from the copyright owner.

This book was printed in the United States of America.

**To order additional copies of this book, contact:**
Xlibris Corporation
1-888-795-4274
www.Xlibris.com
Orders@Xlibris.com
39110

# CONTENTS

This book is dedicated to my loving and devoted mother, Ingard, who has been my greatest inspiration and one of my wisest teachers. Mam, I would never have been able to do any of this without your incredible guidance, your Job-like patience, and, yes, your "intuitive" understanding. Thank God your skin is thicker than a rhinoceros's. Thank you for introducing me to chiropractic, to nutrition, to spiritual thought, to visualization, to the Church of Religious Science, and to all the other crazy, progressive, and innovative stuff you've turned me on to, *and* continue to turn me on to now and in the future. You're the greatest, Mam! I love you.

# FOREWORD

*Cook a meal for a person, he will not be hungry on that day, but, teach him how to cook, and he will never remain hungry throughout his life.*

THE MOTTO OF writing a professional book always entails providing an insight to a person's own philosophy and understanding of the subject matter. When I was approached to read the manuscript, I was simply told to read the chapters and come up with any suggestions that I may have on the contents of the book.

It took me a while in order to read the first few pages due to my heavy workload with teaching, laboratories, and consultations. But after I had finished reading the first few pages of this book, my curiosity to this self-motivational approach to understanding health took me to a point where I could not stop reading, but finishing to its entirety. Every free minute I had, I kept on reading and trying to follow what the writer is conveying. I could not leave until I had finished the entire book. The dilemma became clearer when I was asked whether I would like to write a foreword for this book. It is not that I found it complex to write, but on the contrary, I found it an honor to digest the concepts of the book and convey the message that the author is propounding. So here I am, in the midst of writing about a self-guided, health-related, conceptual program, which, if followed continuously and correctly, would decrease the incidence of an ailment and bring a meaningful, optimal lifestyle with good health.

Dr. Campos has provided meaningful advice on a complex subject involving a self-directed health program. He has tried to inculcate the concept of optimal health in those who want to control their own healthy lifestyle. Actually, it is an opportune time to have a good book on this subject owing to our becoming health conscious globally. At an international level, World Health Organization (WHO) has launched the theme of "Health for All by Year 2010." Most of the countries are at a threshold of having their inhabitants embrace the concept as well as working toward achieving a healthy lifestyle.

I am delighted to see that all chapters in this book are devoted to various aspects of health-promotion programs, each adding and complementing the others, pertaining to the thoughts contained therein. Furthermore, it provides the reader an opportunity to select the programs for good and healthy living. It has eight chapters. In each chapter, the author goes through ministries to emphasize the point that he is trying to convey. The first chapter discusses the concept of cellular intelligence, thereby providing the reader a conceptual, perpetrating understanding as to the modalities to which a cell continually modulates, transforms, and adjusts. It includes discussions on the supply of proper amounts and quality of the raw materials for these building blocks of the body and the attainment of most favorable health.

Chapters 2 through 7 take the reader through several crucial guidelines that one must follow to develop and maintain a good effective program for prolonged vigor and vitality. Chapter 2 describes the importance of diet and takes the reader through a series of nutritious and healthy programs where a person can eat good foods, decrease the deleterious effects of free radical induced injuries, and simultaneously enjoy great health. Reading through chapter 1 can develop his or her own optimal diet program. Chapter 3 describes in detail the role of physical activity in maintaining muscle tone and strength. The author goes in depth about the physiological aspects of the pillars of exercise, including the benefits to overall health and fitness. In addition, he goes over, in detail, the various limbs of yoga, endurance training, and breathing exercises. Chapter 4 goes into detail on the ways to maintain a great neuromusculoskeletal balance, including massage and trigger-point therapies. Chapter 5 goes in depth about sleep and sleep disorders. It deals with the different stages of sleep and the burnout effect for those who continue to perform without proper rest and sleep. The author talks about perils of sleep deprivation in detail. Practical advice is offered to the extent of rest a person must have for proper body functions. Dr. Campos seems to have taken a great philosophical approach to talk about mind, body, and soul in chapter 6. He talks about biological and psychological models of mental illness and goes in depth to describe depression. Various modalities of treatment of depressive conditions have been described in detail. I find this book to be exceptionally eloquent in providing insights on balancing one's perceptions to a nicely articulated, fully balanced health program. A unison of body, mind, and soul is the key to a fruitful, happy, and healthy journey to aging. Significant and salient points on meditation are also included in this chapter. The author has included a timely subject on various drug interactions and exposure to toxic chemicals in chapter 7. In our society today, we do not seem to tolerate a slight discomfort to the body but combat it with an appropriate medication. The author points out several possibilities of drug-to-drug interactions if a person takes a number of these simultaneously. Exposure to pesticides, toxic fumes in the atmosphere, and contaminations in the water have been appropriately discussed in this chapter. Last but not the least, the author has combined all the six key elements discussed in this book to synergistically provide optimal health. He has provided a logistic approach to the reader to circumvent the pitfalls in today's living and control his or her own health. The inclusion of citations to the narratives has provided a meaningful and authoritative documentation to the statements.

The author has presented the material in the form of an advice to all those who could follow a guided formula to achieve health with routine yet minimal efforts. I find this book to be particularly eloquent and helpful in guiding and inducing the reader to design a well-balanced workable program, which, when put to proper use, will lead to a lifetime of healthy body and mind. Although there are many books on the subjects of nutrition and health, this book is unique in bringing various facets of our lifestyle together and preparing the reader to utilize those in a proportionate manner so that they could be assimilated easily in a person's perspective of healthy living.

Therefore, at a glance, it is an enlightening and creative book, which should prove invaluable to most of us who crave for a healthy lifestyle.

Gyan Khare, PhD
Director
Heligen Laboratories Inc.
Professor, Cleveland Chiropractic College, Los Angeles

# ACKNOWLEDGMENT

WITH DEEP GRATITUDE, I wish to acknowledge and honor some of my teachers throughout the years:

Dr. John F. Demartini, thank you for teaching me the universal truths as they relate to health and life. *You are a genius, and I am inspired by your wisdom.*

Dr. Gyan Khare, thank you for your collaboration on this book and for your very useful suggestions.

Dr. Joe Kurnik, Dr. Clarence Franklin, Dr. Gary Vitullo, Dr. Antonio Gonsalves, and Dr. Bradley Ping, thank you for teaching me how to adjust the spine.

Dr. Rick Morris, Dr. Brendan Murray, and Dr. Jerry Hyman, thank you for getting me excited about sports rehabilitation.

Dr. Patrick Defazio, many thanks for teaching me the ins and outs of the biz. Thank you for your continued guidance and friendship.

Anthony Benenati, Naime Jezzeny, and Arun Deva, thank you for teaching me the wonders of yoga. Namaste.

Dr. David Walker, Rabbi Eitan Yardini, and Rev. Pam Macgregor, thank you for your spiritual guidance.

Dr. Michael N. Brown, thank you for teaching me all about the feet and orthotic support. You're a master.

Dr. Assibi Abudu, thank you for helping me keep faith in the medical profession; you're one of a kind. They should all learn from you.

Dr. Peter C. Vollhardt and Dr. Mike West, thank you for helping me fall in love with organic chemistry.

Dr. Ruth Logan, thank you for turning me on to molecular biology—never thought I'd go in that direction!

My beautiful wife, Erika, thank you for teaching me that it's not all about me. I love you.

Troy Gagliano, thank you for reminding me that only scientists write in the passive voice. Yech! I cherish our friendship.

My family—Constantino (Pap), Tino, and Ingrid—thank you for teaching me that you gotta kick a little butt sometimes to make it in this world. I love you all unconditionally.

# Unlocking the Doors to Your Untapped Potential

*It is health that is real wealth and not pieces of gold and silver.*
—Mahatma Gandhi

HAVE YOU EVER considered what it might feel like to enjoy radiant health? Maybe you have wondered what life might be like if you had more energy to do the things you love doing. Or maybe you suffer from chronic pain. Do you ever wonder what it would be like to live pain free?

If so, then you are no different from the millions of others who have not only pondered these questions but are doing the things necessary to ensure incredible results. These are the pioneers of a new generation, the *healthy* generation, breaking ground in all areas of life, mainly because they have the energy and the drive to do so. It is your choice whether you want to be a part of this exciting revolution, and your success is inevitable since wellness is your birthright.

Imagine a life where you have an abundance of energy—enough to work, play, and spend quality time with your children, your spouse, and your friends. Imagine a life free from chronic pain, one where you actually feel your age or *younger*—not older due to hobbling and debilitating injuries. Imagine clear eyes, clear skin, and a rosy complexion. Imagine an increase in mental clarity and creativity, improved athletic performance, and improved sexual performance, endurance, and satisfaction. Imagine being told you look younger than your years and that you appear vibrant and full of life.

This is not some far-fetched fantasy or a reality reserved for the genetically gifted. It is a genuine probability for anyone who can follow a few basic principles. Without a doubt, it is for anyone who wants to give it their time and effort. Like any realistic and worthwhile endeavor, there is work involved, but the rewards are achievable and plentiful. Life cannot only be extended through applying these principles, but the quality of life can be improved as well.

What is this miraculous secret that greatly enhances the life experience for so many? It is the natural gift of health, and it is inherent in all of us. This gift was bestowed upon us at birth, but many have lost it by failing to grasp its preciousness.

This gift is powerful yet fleeting, and it will elude us if we do not treat it with the utmost gratitude. Sadly, many people today see their health literally drained away from them as they have forgotten to nurture and care for it properly.

What is more important than health? Money? Material possessions? Relationships? The truth is that none of these things can be appreciated nor enjoyed to the fullest without one's health. Just ask anyone suffering from chronic disease. I am sure that anyone suffering a severe illness, regardless of their material wealth, would trade every penny to regain their health. Even the great baseball legend Mickey Mantle, who drank himself to a diseased liver, said while on his deathbed that if he could do it all over again, he would definitely do things differently; he would not take up the destructive habit he chose and would instead focus on his God-given talents and his *health*. And who could argue with the Mick?

Taking care of our precious health is not solely reserved for the wealthy either. On the contrary, maintaining great health costs much less than losing it. The greatest cost comes in the form of time and energy. And isn't that worth investing for a brighter future?

So let's open the doors to health, with its bountiful treasures lying untapped on the other side. The keys to these doors do exist, and they are called the *six keys to optimal health*. These keys are powerful and will unlock the hidden potential that resides in all of us. Alone, they can uncover secrets that are potent in their own right, but when used together, they will manifest such a dynamic energy that its limits will seem boundless.

Many people already use one or more of these keys in their lives every day. Some have even put the puzzle together and are using all the *six keys* completely to harness their full potential. But now, this miraculous power is available to all of us. Because of the pioneering work of professionals in such diverse areas as nutrition, physical fitness, chiropractic, physics, medicine, and many other fields, we have all the tools necessary to unlock the doors and harness this untapped potential.

Enjoy the journey as we reveal each key one by one. You will find that you have had this knowledge within you all along; it has merely been tucked away and forgotten. The *six keys to optimal health* will open the window to your soul—that place in you that knows everything there is to know within the universe. Other truths will likely be revealed to you as well and, hopefully, will both excite and inspire you.

Once you have successfully integrated the six keys to optimal health into your life, you will not be able to keep them to yourself. You will naturally want to share them with others. This is the most moving consequence of unlocking the doors to optimal health. It will be like a snowball rolling down a hillside, the momentum increasing as the snowball grows larger and larger, with more and more people being affected over time. Ultimately, this will lead to a new way of thinking, where great health is no longer the exception but instead the norm.

Come join us on this fascinating and invigorating voyage through health and wellness. You will be sure to walk away from it, more informed and enlightened, and your current views on health will either expand or change completely. Without a doubt, you will find yourself more enthused about your health and the many ways in which it can enhance your life, and you will certainly want to learn more. Let us proceed to this next phase of your life, to a new level of understanding. Let us move onward to an age of optimal health.

# CHAPTER 1

# The State of Health in the United States Today

*The problems that exist in the world today cannot be solved by the level of thinking that created them.*

—Albert Einstein

## What Is Health?

IF ASKED TO list the things in life more important than health, how would you answer? Would you mention material possessions like money, clothing, or cars? Or maybe you might point out something more intangible, like friendship or love. But can you really think of anything more important than your health and well-being? In truth, without your health, it would be pretty difficult to enjoy very much at all.

How you answered the above question has a lot to do with your current set of values. Values shape our thoughts, dreams, and desires. They also form our beliefs, opinions, and behaviors. When considering values, what comes to mind for most are things like freedom, independence, and the pursuit of happiness. Justice, equality, and the right to self-expression may also come to mind. But what about health? How come we rarely talk about *that* as something we should value? When thinking about it, shouldn't health be placed at the very top of the list?

The reality is that health has actually been *devalued* in modern society. This becomes more evident when we consider some of the practices adopted by government, business, and private citizens in recent history. Each has shown a disregard for human health by taking part in activities as varied as mass pesticide spraying, chemical dumping, drug and alcohol abuse, or the excessive consumption of junk food. Health is often pushed aside for profits or pleasure, and although both have their place, neither supersedes health.

The good news is that the tide has begun to turn. Thanks to industries like the nutritional sciences, chiropractic, and physical fitness, people now have the resources to motivate and excite them about health. As a result, health is being valued more than ever before.

Despite this recent push, the American health system still ranks very low when compared to that of other countries around the world.[1] Using death and disability rates as a measure, the World Health Organization (WHO) ranks the United States thirty-seventh out of 191 nations. Isn't it surprising that a country as wealthy and technologically advanced as the United States could rank so poorly when it comes to health?

This paradox stems from a number of complex factors, some of which we will address in this book. But just being aware of the problem is not enough—we must also ask what we can do to change things. The *Six Keys to Optimal Health* will do just that. It will attempt to shed light on these issues as well as provide the necessary tools to enjoy abundant health. By learning the principles outlined within this book—and more importantly, by applying them—you can do your part to elevate the health of the nation to its proper place in the world and put it where it belongs, at the very top.

But this book is not just for Americans. People from *every* nation can use the six keys, as these principles have no bias toward country, sex, race, religion, wealth, or social status. All people, to one degree or another, can practice these principles. And hopefully, in time, these principles will become ingrained in the global consciousness and embraced as a way of life. First, though, we must break many long-standing beliefs and create a new paradigm. Only then can we pass this new way of thinking on to future generations, as we must, for the betterment of mankind.

Fortunately, this transformation is already taking place. We see it happening all around us. With the presence of health clubs, health foods, and healthy behaviors all on the rise, people are striving for wellness more than ever before. You can feel confident in making your own changes by adopting the simple yet powerful practices found in this book. To be sure, there are many other resources available for you to collect this information, yet never before has it been integrated into one easy-to-read manual as it has here. Some of this information may seem complex at first, but stick with it; you will find that by the time you finish, your understanding of the human body and the way to achieve great health will be that much deeper. And please, take your time with this material—read it, understand it, and research it further. Begin putting the six keys into action. Only by doing so will you fully appreciate how profound these practices really are. The changing of old ways begins with you, and only *through* you can new ways be adopted.

Consider this then, a journey toward better health. As with any journey, there must be a starting point. With ours, it will be to ask the question: *what is health?* In order to answer, let us first look at the definition of *health* as set forth by WHO:

Health is a state of complete physical, mental and social well-being and not merely the absence of disease or infirmity.[2]

Clearly, this definition emphasizes health as more than just the freedom from illness and disease. This view drastically differs from the one we have been accustomed to. According to our current way of thinking, we assume that health is limited and that, as a part of the natural aging process, health simply diminishes over time; hence, we believe that as we get older, we eventually become sick and die. Without a doubt, we all die sooner or later (chapter 8), but the idea that we must fall victim to disease is a fallacy. Many people are living full and healthy lives well into old age, and they are doing so simply by practicing sound, healthy habits. Some experts predict that in the future, people will routinely live to be one hundred years or older.[3] One must ask oneself, then, if reaching one hundred years old were in fact possible, wouldn't it be better to live those years in vibrant health?

The World Health Organization recognized as early as 1948 that we needed a new way to identify health. They understood that health is more than just the absence of symptoms but is actually determined by several things including physical, mental, social, ecological, and spiritual factors. If we are to attain true health, we must consider all these factors equally. *Wellness* means not only being free from disease but from detriments such as crime, violence, depression, addiction, poverty, and pollution. True health derives from a blend of sound mind, conditioned body, and strong spirit; and we simply cannot separate our health from the environment or from our connection to other people.

*The Six Keys to Optimal Health* strives to expand WHO's definition of health by outlining six simple principles that anyone can master. Living a healthy lifestyle has far-reaching benefits, many of which we will address in this book. For instance, healthy individuals are better equipped to carry out actions that bring about social, ecological, and planetary changes. These changes can in turn lead to even greater degrees of wellness, making this information even more vital.

For centuries, mystics, philosophers, and theologians have spoken of an *interconnectedness* of all things; and modern science has now uncovered evidence to support their claims.[4] We, therefore, have a responsibility to choose health as a way of life, as health is contagious and influences everything around us—our family, our friends, and our community. When health becomes our reality, then we will naturally gravitate toward it in our relationships, in our living conditions, and, ultimately, in our environment. When put in these terms, doesn't it make sense for health to become one of our highest values?

# A New View of Health

Where does health come from anyway? The answer to this depends on our perception of the universe and how we view life. Some people believe that our experiences are essentially a random series of events, chance occurrences over which we have very little control. If this happens to be your opinion, then practicing the six keys to optimal health might seem futile to you since you probably consider health to be predetermined by genetics or, quite possibly, chance. But if you believe that all living things are interconnected and if you also believe that you have some control over your experiences, then the ideas outlined in this book will not only make sense to you, but will also have tremendous value.

By using the philosophical construct that there exists a greater power in the universe—be it God, Allah, Buddha, Universal Mind, or whatever—and that this power brings order and harmony to a seemingly chaotic world, then we can deduce that everything that has been bestowed upon us, including our health, comes from this infinite source of power. To borrow a phrase from the chiropractic profession, "The power that made the body heals the body." And this power supplies us with all the health that we need, provided we care for it properly.

If you could accept even the slightest validity to this idea, you might appreciate that all people are born with an abundance of health. This is true for everyone, including those born with a genetic defect. When babies are born with a so-called defect, they too have an abundance of health. Their particular circumstances may be distinct and their health expressed in a different way, but these children still have health—it simply is unique to them. It serves no beneficial purpose, then, to compare these people to what we currently consider "normal." Although some children are born with different needs, the principles outlined in this book still apply. Take, for example, a child born with a heart murmur. This child can enjoy health to the limits of his or her capacity, but all the same, this child must still be taught healthy lifestyle habits. As for limits, well, we all have limits. The point is that a child with a heart murmur is not any less viable than any other child, and this child too can reach his or her greatest potential of health, even if it is a little different from the norm.

It is said that the universe is maintained by a *Universal Intelligence*, the great organizing power that connects all things. In the words of Albert Einstein:

> Everything is determined, the beginning as well as the end, by forces over which we have no control. It is determined for the insects as well as for the stars. Human beings, vegetables, or cosmic dust, we all dance to a mysterious tune, intoned in the distance by an invisible piper.

The organization and function of the human body is maintained by the body's own unique portion of Universal Intelligence called *Innate Intelligence.*[5] While Universal Intelligence organizes matter at the atomic and subatomic levels, Innate Intelligence organizes it at the cellular level, which is the smallest unit of life. Innate Intelligence is the organizing power for *all* living systems. A belief in this greater power, one that affords us Innate Intelligence, is known as *vitalism.*

Every cell in the human body has its own form of Innate Intelligence called cellular intelligence. Cellular intelligence allows a cell to carry out its functions in a specific and organized fashion. Every cell must interact with other cells, some similar to itself and others different. Similar cells combine to make up specific tissue—heart tissue, lung tissue, muscle tissue, and so forth—and these must communicate with one another to carry out the tissue's function (contraction, transport, etc.). Cells must also communicate with dissimilar cells; so muscle cells must communicate with blood cells, blood cells with brain cells, and so on. Rarely do cells work independently from one another; they form *symbiotic relationships* where a cell's function and survival depends on all the other cells around it. The ability to recognize, communicate, and work together in a detailed and organized fashion is attributable to Innate Intelligence. Without it, cells would not know what to do or when to do it; basically, they would exist in chaos. Yet we know this is not the case. Through an extraordinary feat of synchronization, all cells in the body perform their specialized functions in tandem with every other cell, and this is what allows the process of life to continue.

Innate Intelligence knows exactly what to do and when to do it. It knows how to differentiate every stem cell into its own specialized cell line; it knows when to secrete every chemical, every hormone, and every neurotransmitter; it knows when to regenerate its tissues and organs and when to defend itself against unwelcome invaders. If allowed to function unimpeded and by its own design, it will even know when to shut the body down and expire.

All living things have Innate Intelligence, from plants to animals to single-celled bacteria and fungi. Innate Intelligence is what separates living from nonliving matter. We see it at work whenever we cut ourselves; Innate Intelligence is what guides our wound healing, yet cut a cadaver and the wound never heals. This is because a body that has expired no longer has Innate Intelligence operating through it.

Remember that every cell has its own unique form of Innate Intelligence called *cellular intelligence*. This allows cells to maintain life outside of the body for a brief period, that is, as long as they are kept in a proper medium. Because of cellular intelligence, doctors can transplant organs from one body to another. However, an organ transplant may fail if the host's immune system identifies the donor organ as foreign and will attack it. This, incidentally, is also due to Innate Intelligence.

A competing theory on human existence, especially with regard to the physical body, says that human beings are merely a conglomeration of biochemical processes. According to this theory, health is limited, and only through the intervention of drugs and surgery can we preserve life. It rejects the concept of Innate Intelligence and instead maintains that life is controlled by the genetic code in a basically random fashion. This theory leads us to believe that health is merely "the luck of the draw" and simply comes down to the genes we have inherited. Proponents focus less on how to influence health through the body's inborn intelligence and more on the complex mechanisms of disease. They rarely concern themselves with the ways that an organism *knows* to carry out its functions. If they would, they would probably find less need for outside interventions and have more trust in the body's own incredible intelligence.

The belief that human beings are nothing more than complex machines, and that life is completely explainable by chemical and physical laws, is called *mechanism*. Mechanism has been en vogue since the Age of Enlightenment when it came about as a backlash against the repression of the Catholic Church. The patriarchs of mechanism included the great thinkers René Descartes and Sir Isaac Newton, both of whom, ironically, had a strong belief in God.[6]

A special branch of mechanism evolved during the twentieth century called *scientism*. This philosophy has a large following in the Western world today. It sees the scientific method as the only viable means to access the truth; and thus, if something cannot be observed by the physical senses, it must not exist, or at least we cannot reach any definitive conclusions on the matter. We will try to dispel this belief in chapter 8; however, at this time, both mechanistic thinkers and those that subscribe to scientism would staunchly reject the concept of Innate Intelligence.

Scientism developed into the conventional wisdom of the twentieth century. The remarkable successes realized by modern medicine, as well as the rapid progression of technology by midcentury, led to an even greater belief that science was the ultimate answer to all of man's problems. This way of thinking has helped to shape the belief that health is purely a symptom-free state. Modern medicine has therefore placed the bulk of its energy toward developing drugs and surgical procedures meant to treat symptoms and diseases. Let it be said that this paradigm has definitely served its purpose; in fact, in many instances, it has led to miraculous recoveries and has saved numerous lives. When taken as a whole, though, at least with regard to public health, this narrow focus has helped contribute to the poor health we see in this country today. It is my goal to help you appreciate the power of your Innate Intelligence. By understanding, trusting, and honoring it, you will have the foundation necessary to nurture your body and your health. When you have the right amount and quality of raw materials and you know how to properly care for your body, your body will respond with excellent health. It will do so because it knows exactly what to do and when to do it, especially if given what it needs before disease starts. And it accomplishes all this through Innate Intelligence. On that note, let us take a closer look at some of the factors that have helped shape the state of American health today.

## The State of American Health in the New Millennium

Now that we have a working definition of health, let us try to understand the state of American health at the turn of the twenty-first century. Most organizations that analyze these things all agree: the United States falls somewhat low on the health status list for a wealthy, industrialized nation. This fact becomes even more alarming when we consider that the United States spends more money on health care than any other nation in the world.[7]

How can it be possible for America to spend over five thousand dollars per person annually on health care—which, incidentally, is the most advanced system in the world—and yet still rank below such countries as Colombia, Morocco, and Israel when it comes to health? No offense to these great countries, but as far as I know, they still have to deal with an inordinate amount of life-threatening circumstances like terrorism, drug wars, and extreme poverty. These threats have both direct and indirect effects on a country's health status. Additionally, people from third world countries, like Morocco and Columbia, must struggle with infectious diseases like typhoid and yellow fever, which have long since been eradicated in the United States. True, Americans have to deal with their fair share of crime and violence too, and this of course affects their overall health status. However, when heart disease and cancer are still the leading causes of death in the United States, both of which are preventable, we have to ask ourselves what we are doing or not doing to perpetuate this scenario.

Aside from heart disease and cancer, another menace taking place with such regularity that it claims the lives of an estimated 250,000 Americans every year is medical mistakes.[8, 9] Medical mistakes have been identified as the third leading cause of death in the United States. Some experts now believe that the numbers have actually been underestimated and that medical mistakes may actually be the leading cause of death in this country.[10] They include a failure to diagnose and treat in time, unnecessary surgeries, medication errors in hospitals, infections in hospitals, and non-error negative effects of drugs.[11] What can we conclude from these harrowing statistics? That there are serious risks involved when receiving modern medical care.

Please let me acknowledge that this is a sensitive subject among medical professionals and is also very touchy for people who have had their lives saved by medical interventions. Many might see this as an unfair attack on a profession whose sole motivation is to care for the sick and to save lives. But let me state for the record that this is not an attempt to bring scorn upon this admirable and important profession. On the contrary, the practice of medicine is valuable and, in fact, necessary in times of crisis. Medical professionals are, without a doubt, some of the most dedicated and caring members of our society. As we shall see, though, the primary problem does not lie within the medical profession itself but is instead a consequence of people's use of the medical system as a whole. Today's medical system is used for far more than crisis intervention, and for many, it is actually their sole source of health care. It is not uncommon for people to neglect their health for years and then run to their doctors hoping to find a magic bullet (chapter 7), or even a miracle, when their health finally runs out. But looking to medicine as a way to counteract the consequences of faulty lifestyle habits is foolish. We must care for our health while we still have it.

So we can all agree that medical intervention is often necessary, especially in times of crisis, but we must also remember that it comes with risks. The best way to avoid falling victim to medical mistakes is to stop using the medical system as a one-stop shop for health care. If we can, instead, care for our health in more enhancing ways, then our indiscriminate use of the medical system will surely cease as a result.

What are these mistakes that are so common that they claim lives at a rate of a quarter million people per year? The first is the failure to properly diagnose and treat in time. It is so hard to be critical here because the process of medical diagnosis is as much an art as it is a science. The art of diagnosis may be based on scientific knowledge, but any physician who spends time in a clinical setting will attest that an enormous amount of intuition is involved in the practice. People are not textbooks, and therefore, memorized facts are just not enough to understand human complexity. A patient's social and cultural environment must also be considered during the evaluation, as should his or her psychological state of mind. The more experienced a doctor is, the better he or she is able to see what lies beyond the surface of the problem. This allows the doctor to more accurately diagnose the toughest and most confusing presentations.

So why are so many medical mistakes a result of improper diagnosis? One reason is that medical schools emphasize and show a preference for students who excel in the hard sciences like chemistry and biology. Although important, premed students tend to major in these subjects in college; and as a result, they may have too narrow an education than necessary to understand the broader scope of human beings. Does an education in classical literature lend itself to more well-rounded and better doctors? You bet it does. The study of humanities helps develop the creative and artistic aspects of the brain—what we would typically consider left-brained skills—that are so necessary in medical diagnosis. A narrow emphasis on the hard sciences only develops right-brained skills, like rational and linear thought. We can all agree that human beings are more than just rational beings, and therefore, a balanced approach to caring for them—one that blends all intricacies of their being—would be superior to treating them simply as textbook cases.

To the credit of the medical school system, policies are now in place to increase the emphasis on a broader education. Some U.S. medical schools have already attempted to change their curriculum to a more integrative, patient-focused system, as opposed to a subdivisional one. That is, they are moving away from focusing on just isolated parts of the body like the cardiac system, the digestive system, or the immune system and are gearing their instructions toward treating patients as whole beings since none of these systems can operate independently from the whole. Bravo to these institutions for seeing the need for change and addressing it.

How can you minimize your own risk of falling victim to improper diagnosis? You can do it by practicing the six keys to optimal health. By attending to your health as your most valuable asset, you will decrease the probability of needing a doctor. In the event that you do, though, you will help yourself enormously by getting to know your body as intimately as possible. When you are in tune with your body, you are better able to help your doctor locate the problem, thereby reducing the chance of a wrong diagnosis.

Another form of medical mistake on the rise is unnecessary surgeries. An article published in the *Journal of the American Medical Association* (JAMA) estimates that twelve thousand unnecessary surgeries leading to death are performed in this country each year.[12] These numbers only reflect those surgeries causing fatalities and do not include the thousands of others that result in removed organs, lost limbs, or detached genitals. Unnecessary hysterectomies, coronary bypass surgeries, and cesarean sections are some of the most common surgeries performed today; and some clinics have even hired "marketers" to oversee the recruitment of people who have private health insurance and are willing to undergo routine but unnecessary surgical procedures in exchange for cash or discounted cosmetic surgery.[13] Another operation carried out far too frequently is low back surgery. A number of patients undergoing this procedure reexperience their low back pain shortly following the procedure. This might lead one to ask what the point of this surgery is exactly. Simply put, this operation is easy to perform, is relatively harmless, and is financially lucrative. Many of these operations can be avoided by treating the patient with conservative and rehabilitative care, but unfortunately, these alternatives are often overlooked for the more profitable surgical options.

Once again, we should not lay fault solely with the medical profession. When the public relies on medical interventions for practically every ailment, no matter how small, they are just as much to blame. By taking the initiative to practice the six keys to optimal health, you will decrease any chance of receiving a surgical procedure you do not need. The predominance of needless surgeries merely illustrates the need for a greater cooperation among specialists including medical doctors, chiropractors, and acupuncturists to name just a few.

The next type of medical mistake contributing to the elevated death toll is medication errors in a hospital setting. These account for seven thousand deaths annually and are more than the number of deaths resulting from workplace injuries. These deaths are most commonly attributed to what is called a *systems failure* and happen in cases when a physician orders a drug but a nurse administers it.[14] As with any procedure, the more people involved, the greater the likelihood of a mistake happening. Mistakes can include any of the following: wrong patient receiving the drug, wrong drug or dosage administered, wrong route of administration, or wrong time. One solution to this problem is already in the works and that is to computerize the entire process. No doubt, this will reduce the number of deaths related to the issue, but it's probably better to stay out of the system altogether by practicing the healthy habits outlined in this book.

Another problem occurring in hospitals is a high incidence of *nosocomial infections*, which are infections acquired in the hospital itself. Around 10 percent of all hospitalized patients, or 2 million per year, pick up one of these infections.[15] Why is this happening with such regularity? It is because hospitals are breeding grounds for opportunistic organisms like bacteria. Hospital wards are filled with sick and immunocompromised people who are susceptible to all kinds of infections, particularly those that healthy individuals fight off with ease. As the organisms breed, they get stronger and often develop a resistance to antibiotics (chapter 7). This frightening and dangerous scenario can be life threatening, so why take chances? Practice the six keys to optimal health and you won't have to.

A final type of medical mistake is adverse drug reactions to prescription drugs. The cause is usually an allergic reaction and signifies that a person is either hypersensitive to that drug or took the wrong dose, or an unfavorable reaction took place between two or more drugs, which was precisely what happened with Anna Nicole Smith that eventually led to her death. This is a very special type of medical mistake, which we talk about in depth in chapter 7. Suffice it to say, adverse drug reactions cause 106,000 deaths per year, making it the most prevalent form of medical mistake there is. Even more tragic, though, is that it's also the most preventable.[16]

The reality is that each time we receive a medical procedure, we are vulnerable to medical mistakes. We tend to think of certain surgeries as "routine," or certain medications as "safe"; however, we should be aware that all treatments come with a certain amount of risk attached to them. Risks increase with each successive level of invasiveness, so medications are riskier than therapy, and surgeries are riskier yet. But by knowing the prevalence of medical mistakes, you might think twice before choosing a medical procedure as your first option. As we have said before, the medical system should be used primarily for crisis care and not as a substitute for healthy behaviors. Therefore, by doing the things that keep us healthy, we will be able to significantly decrease our chances of falling victim to medical errors.

## Lifestyle Choices Dictate Health

Clearly, medical mistakes are not the only things causing Americans to have poor health. Other reasons abound, and most of them relate to faulty lifestyle choices.[17] Heart disease, cancer, stroke, pulmonary disease, accidents, pneumonia, influenza, diabetes, and suicide are all linked to behavioral choices and/or living conditions. The Institute of Medicine states that diet, smoking, alcohol, and sedentary lifestyle all contribute to the excess burden of cancer on our society, and cancer is responsible for approximately half the deaths in this country each year.[18]

One of the most tragic consequences that results from faulty lifestyle habits has been the obesity epidemic in America. This is not purely an American phenomenon as waistlines have been expanding at record rates all around the globe.[19] In 2004, the Centers for Disease Control and Prevention reported that the average weight of Americans has gone up twenty-five pounds since 1960.[20] Twenty-five pounds! You can get a better idea of this by adding twenty-five pounds to your current weight. Scary, isn't it? But this is exactly what's happening in America today; we are simply blowing up beyond comprehension. And before you think it's just the adults, think again. American children are, on average, eleven pounds heavier today than they were in 1960. This increase is not due to children getting taller, either; the average height for children has only increased by one inch during that same period—not a healthy ratio.

How is America becoming a nation overwhelmed by obesity? There are several reasons, but one is that Americans are completely addicted to junk food. Some of the largest companies in America manufacture and sell junk food—McDonald's, Coca-Cola, and Hershey's are all household names—and they now operate in almost every country in the world. Add to this that many Americans still refuse to exercise, and it is no wonder that 65 percent of the population is either overweight or obese.[21] However, just as we should not lay blame for the high rate of medical errors exclusively on the medical profession, junk food manufacturers should not be held liable for people's poor dietary choices—they merely provide the public a product it wants. So I have no intentions of condemning the junk food industry for distributing their goods—we all know it's junk, right? What I would like to point out instead is that, as far as America's low ranking in health is concerned, the public's obsession with fast food is as much to blame as anything else.

I am sure that by now you get the point: the state of American health is a direct consequence of faulty lifestyle choices. All our choices are determined and influenced by our philosophy on health. If we love junk food, liquor, and cigarettes so much that we cannot live without them, if we cannot find the time to exercise regularly, if we look to the medical industry to provide us with magic bullets to fix the damage caused by a life of excess, what else are we to expect other than poor health?

The bottom line is that everyone needs to take responsibility for his or her own well-being. Due to a deep and often misguided reliance on medical technology and because of a cultural ideology that views illness as inevitable, many people have refused to take responsibility for their own health. Many of us have been living in denial of what we can do to nurture and enhance our bodies and maintain health through our own accord. This denial, as well as a deep-seated fear that many of us have regarding illness and death, has led to the growth of an industry so powerful, yet so unconstrained, that it now influences a large majority of our health decisions; and that industry is health insurance.

The major problem with health insurance is not that it is inaccessible to so many people—which may actually be a blessing in disguise—but that those who have it tend to think of it as a medical expense account. Some use it indiscriminately to address everything from regular checkups to occasional hypochondriasis to pampering even the most minor blemishes (hives, pimples?); the rationale being, I pay my insurance premiums, why not use it? Unfortunately, this way of thinking causes two major dilemmas; one, it perpetuates a reliance on medical care while at the same time enabling people to disregard health maintenance; and two, it keeps people in the frame of mind that their health is not their financial responsibility. This outlook is dangerous because the belief that you should not need to pay for your own health may prevent you from doing the things necessary to keep it flowing. And who do you think is responsible for your health, anyway? If you won't pay for your health, why should anybody else? The rationalization that someone else should be at least partially responsible for your health is precisely what keeps people from joining health clubs, visiting dentists, and visiting chiropractic offices in the first place; and sometimes, it even prevents people from seeing a medical doctor until it is too late. The reality is that you cannot afford *not* to invest in your health. If people would just spend the time and money caring for their health while they still have it, then they would actually save money since it is much cheaper to maintain health than to fix it when it fails.

Although unhealthy choices, medical mistakes, and the failure to invest in one's health have all contributed to America's low ranking, a greater reason for it may be that people do not yet value health as much as they should. Since values influence our behaviors, we prioritize our actions based on their importance to us. If health falls low on our list of values and we place a greater importance on, let's say, material wealth, then we will tend to make decisions based primarily on financial considerations. If this is the case, then we might choose only to do what makes the most economic sense to us, even if it's not what's best for our health at the time. This is exactly why supersizing junk food has been so popular in this country. It gives consumers more bang for their buck and is attractive to anyone who likes a "good deal," even if that means getting more calories, more salt, and more fat in the process.

An obsession with physical perfection also influences the health decisions of many Americans. The number of plastic surgeries in this country has risen 444 percent since 1997.[22] Not only does this say a lot about the negative self-image pervasive in our culture, but also illustrates how some people will go to any length to "achieve perfection," even if it means undergoing potentially risky procedures. This obsession has led to the rampant abuse of anabolic steroids by professional athletes, amateur bodybuilders, and nonathletes who just want to "look good." Think about this for a moment: regular people taking synthetic drugs and jeopardizing their health just to look better. It's pure and simple insanity!

Sadly enough, eating disorders like anorexia and bulimia are also epidemic in this country (chapter 2). Many young women fall victim to these disorders in an attempt to keep up with the images that saturate our popular media. Hollywood and the fashion industry obviously perpetuate this tragedy by using wafer-thin actresses and supermodels in their films or ads. They put forth the message that "thin is in," and that a skinny body is the only type desirable. Women who buy into this illusion often neglect or abuse their bodies to achieve this unrealistic ideal. They may overtrain, binge and purge, or consume harmful substances like ephedra or diet pills in order to obtain the "perfect" body. Many of these women do not realize that these same benefits, or better, can be had naturally through adopting healthy lifestyle habits. Working on one's self-esteem and self-perception is the first step to overcoming these disorders (chapter 5), and by practicing the principles outlined in *The Six Keys to Optimal Health*, these women will stand a greater chance of leading normal and healthy lives in the future.

Not only do many individuals value finances over health, but institutions do as well. Insurance companies have a vested interest in keeping medical costs down, and although necessary, cost cutting often happens at the expense of patient care. Coverage is limited to medically necessary procedures, which are based primarily on the presence of symptoms; and health-enhancing measures, like gym memberships or massage therapy, are almost never covered.

Profits are also the major goal of the pharmaceutical industry. We have seen a recent flood of drugs pulled off the market or given black box warnings because they posed a risk to the public's health. One must question how these drugs ever made it to the market in the first place, seeing that they were hazardous enough to elicit such strong warnings. Whether the drugs were released too early—before they could be adequately tested—or the data was simply ignored, it is evident that drug manufacturers sometimes chose quick profits over public health and safety. Unfortunately, this practice is fairly common—the business of pharmaceuticals is competitive, and research and development costly, so drug manufacturers have great incentives to put their products out quickly. Put simply, the buyer must beware since it does not appear that this practice will end any time soon.

Once again, all aforementioned scenarios—medical mistakes, the public obsession with junk food, corporate profiteering on poorly tested and risky drugs, and so forth—could never take place if health was more valued in this country. We allow this to be the norm because of the way we currently view health. If we were to change our way of thinking—that is, change our paradigm—then this change would carry over into other areas of health care. For instance, we might find more financial support from insurance companies to practice healthy lifestyle habits and not just help us when we are ill. Insurance companies would likely see their costs decrease by putting more money into *health* care and not just *sick* care. If they were to cover services and products that help us remain healthy, they could reduce what they spend on more pricey medical procedures. And if people just took better care of themselves all around, they would not need to take chances and risk their health by taking newer and more dangerous drugs.

Am I alone in finding this a superior way to approach health? I doubt it. That's why I wrote *The Six Keys to Optimal Health*. This book is for people wanting to take control of their health, to recover from illness or addiction, or to improve the quality of their life in general. It is for anyone wishing to ensure oneself great health, even into old age. I know that many people are moving in this direction already, with the numbers growing daily. If you want to stop placing your life in the hands of others and instead take care of the health you have today, then you will find this book tremendously useful. This is your guide toward achieving and maintaining the type of health you have been looking for—it will help keep you strong, vibrant, and happy for years to come.

We no longer have the option of neglecting something as basic as our health and well-being. We can never hope to elicit change politically, socially, or ecologically if we do not first care for that which we have a direct influence over. By caring for our bodies and respecting our health conscientiously, it will be impossible for health not to carry over into all other areas of our lives. When we recognize health as our greatest asset, we will have the motivation to practice the lifestyle behaviors necessary to maintain our bodies' own natural vibrancy.

Let us now begin our journey. It involves six key areas that, if addressed regularly, will all but guarantee an improvement in our health. Although this book is not intended to be a guide for curing any particular disease, people suffering from ill health can still benefit from these practices. The six keys will be discussed at length in each successive chapter; they include diet and nutrition, physical fitness, bodywork, sleep, mental and emotional health, and toxin avoidance. Once you finish reading this book and you start putting the six keys into practice, you will find that all the pleasures accompanying great health will be yours for the taking. This is the power of optimal health.

# CHAPTER 2

# The Importance of a Healthy Diet

*To eat is a necessity, but to eat intelligently is an art.*
—François La Rochefoucauld

WOULDN'T IT BE great if there were one basic diet that could guarantee perfect weight, perfect nutrition, and perfect health? Wouldn't it be wonderful if we could finally find that *one way* of eating—you know, the one that would rid the world of malnutrition, obesity, and chronic disease? Well, if we are to believe the endless assortment of experts cropping up every year who try to sell us one miracle system after another, then that diet does indeed exist. But which one is *the one*? Some say the answer is low carb, others high carb. Some swear by vegetarianism, others by food combining. Some say it depends on our blood type, others our body type. Whatever the specifics, though, each new diet only seems to add to the confusion.

The truth is that no fad diet can guarantee everything from good digestion to optimal energy to proper weight control for *all* people. The reason is that, for the most part, human beings are diverse. We have different metabolisms, different chemistries, and different responses to food. The ancient Roman philosopher Lucretius put it best when he said, "What is food to one man may be fierce poison to another." The truth of this statement becomes evident when we consider that some people suffer from food sensitivities like *lactose intolerance*. People with this disorder lack the enzymes necessary to digest dairy products and become severely bloated if they ingest even the slightest amount of milk. Cheese and ice cream are also off-limits as these foods can easily turn a moment's enjoyment into hours of discomfort. As you will see later, many other foods besides dairy can be a source of food sensitivities. So any expert who touts a one-diet-fits-all system is simply ignoring an obvious fact: we are all different.

Instead of hoping for a new diet to emerge that might be the answer to all of man's woes, we should take comfort in knowing that there are sound principles—based on science and thousands of years of evolution[23]—that we can live by. These principles, when adhered to, can provide everything we need from a wholesome and nutritious dietary regimen. A few of today's fad diets already use some of these principles. In fact, many of them *do* work for some people. Yet principles are not hard and fast rules, and therefore they may vary. For example, a low-carb diet may be an excellent way for an obese individual to lose weight but may not be so good for someone who regularly participates in intense mental activity. As you can see, one must consider several factors when choosing one's diet. We will address many of these in detail in this chapter.

So let us begin on our journey toward optimal health by investigating this first and crucial key element, diet and nutrition. We are starting with this key not because it is the most important one, but because it is possibly the most primal and basic. Food and water along with breathing (chapter 3) are essential to life. All three determine not only how well we function, but whether we will function at all. What we put into our bodies for fuel and hydration, along with what we breathe, are the substances most immediately necessary to maintain life.

## You Are What You Eat

The relationship we have with food and the role it plays in our lives is largely shaped by cultural and environmental influences. How we have been raised and the social climate in which we live contribute to the role food plays in our lives. For some, food merely serves as sustenance, while for others it acts as a way to tickle the senses.

In most cultures, mealtimes are the most important moments of the day. The dining area is where people interact with their families. It is often the social, cultural, and intellectual center of the unit. It is a place where children learn their most valuable life lessons and where parents dole out love along with delicious food. It is no surprise, then, that so many emotional memories, both positive and negative, are tied to people's dining rituals.

It is unfortunate that the custom of gathering together for meals has declined in American society. Our highly productive and fast-paced lives have led us to push aside home-cooked meals and opt for quicker and more convenient alternatives. This has resulted in an explosion of fast-food restaurants, take-out meals, and microwavable dinners that have had subtle yet dramatic effects on the state of our overall health.

As we touched upon in chapter 1, obesity has become one of the greatest health concerns of the twenty-first century, and it has not shown any signs of slowing down. Today, more than two-thirds of the population is considered overweight or obese.[24] It has reached such epidemic proportions that—get this—McDonald's has committed to providing a more healthful menu for people to enjoy,[25] or at least that has been their latest marketing gimmick. The nutritional information on their Web site, though, speaks a bit differently: a quarter pounder with cheese, small fries, and small Coke provide 69 percent of the daily fat allowance set forth by the RDA.[26] It also supplies a whopping 80 percent of saturated fat (isn't that supposed to be the bad stuff?). And to make matters worse, how many people actually order the *small* fries or Coke? My guess is that most people go for the bigger sizes, making these aforementioned numbers even higher. With McDonald's boasting 46 million customers per day alone, we can see how obesity has become an American epidemic.

So getting back to an earlier point: exactly what part of the McDonald's menu should we consider healthy? I guess their commitment to phasing out supersized meals is a good start,[27] but their idea of healthful choices is still somewhat suspect. For example, they now offer salads and a delicious fruit and yogurt parfait as alternatives. However, no matter how you shake 'em, they're still fast-food items. The salad dressings they use are high in fat, and their produce is undoubtedly processed for it to remain so well preserved. How else could 46 million people across the globe be served so efficiently? Not with *fresh* fruits and vegetables, that's for sure. By virtue of being fast food, it must be prepared to feed the masses quickly. It must therefore be subjected to the latest and most up-to-date preservation techniques, which usually include dehydrating the lettuce and adding both sugar and chemicals to the fruit to keep them consumable. Dehydrated lettuce requires more of the high-fat dressing to keep it edible, and excessive sugar consumption is dangerous—as you will see later in the chapter, particularly as we discuss diabetes.

And how about their new apple dipper dessert item, which is sold as an alternative to the hot fudge sundae? Should we make a switch to the fruit dessert because somehow it's a healthier option? A dessert is not necessarily healthier just because it contains fruit. The amount of sugar in an item is what really matters, and if you check the ingredients of the apple dippers, you will see that it has a large amount of the sweet stuff in it.[28] Without sugar, would the new dessert even sell? Probably not. Fast-food restaurants are in the "tasting good" business, and let's face it, sugar tastes good. High sugar and high fat—sounds like the same old menu with a new coat of paint. Well, I'm sure we can all appreciate the effort anyway.

Let me say very adamantly that I do not believe we should hold McDonald's or any other fast-food restaurant responsible for the American obesity epidemic. On the contrary, we all have choices when it comes to food, and along with these choices comes the responsibility of deciding which foods to include in our regular diet. Fast-food companies merely provide a product that satisfies public demand; and judging by the numbers, Americans love their burgers, fries, and shakes.

Are people who regularly consume fast food in denial? Do they not know that their choices will eventually catch up with them? Perhaps, or maybe they do not fully understand the risks of eating large quantities of this stuff.

Common sense dictates that eating fast food multiple times per week is excessive. Without a doubt, some people—usually adolescents and young adults—may get away with it for a while, but it is impossible to eat this way for a very long time without causing severe stress and strain on your body. The long-term consequences of this diet usually come in the form of malnutrition and severe weight gain. Remaining ignorant of these facts or choosing to deny them will only leave you at the losing end of a very hopeless battle.

Fast food is not the only junk Americans devour in large quantities. They consume enough soda pop to make all their other indulgences seem moderate by comparison. It is almost as if people believe that soft drinks are a dietary essential. In one year, soda manufacturers net sixty-four billion dollars on U.S. sales alone, with Americans consuming on average 2.5 sodas per day or 55.4 gallons per year.[29, 30] That's more than one gallon per week! And since some people never drink this stuff at all while others do so only on occasion, then it stands to reason that many people are drinking up to three or more cans daily.

Why is this so shocking? Each can of soda contains ten teaspoons of sugar—that equates to approximately 316 calories (16-20 percent of the healthy caloric intake for a male) coming from *high-fructose corn syrup* (HFCS) per day. HFCS is used to sweeten every sugary product sold in the United States today including baked goods, jams and jellies, and especially sodas.[31] For those people drinking two or three cans of soda a day, that's a mind-blowing 948 calories (48-60 percent healthy male intake) coming from nutritionally inert "liquid sugar." These facts become even more daunting when one considers that in 2003 the World Health Organization (WHO) recommended limiting sugar to no more than 10 percent of one's daily calories.[32] With zero nutritional value in HFCS, a heavy soda drinker would need to consume even more calories through their food to satisfy his or her nutrient needs (i.e., essential vitamins and minerals) for normal daily function. That turns out to be far more calories than the human body can use no matter what the activity level. The average sedentary person would find it impossible to burn that many calories in a day, so his or her body will basically do what it knows to do best—convert the excess calories to fat. Let me explain a basic fact relating to the energy consumption of the human body: it takes what you give it, uses what it needs, and saves the rest for later—just like a perfectly efficient little squirrel hoarding its spoils for the oncoming winter. So it is no surprise that a culture that chooses soda as its beverage of choice will have to deal with an ensuing obesity epidemic.

Despite the obvious correlation between obesity and soda consumption, there have been vehement denials from soft drink manufacturers and the Corn Refiners Association (CRA), the makers of HFCS, of an actual link. Current studies, though, suggest otherwise.[33] One study showed HFCS to be metabolized differently than sucrose (table sugar), leading to greater fat synthesis.[34] This occurs as a result of fructose's inability to stimulate insulin release. Insulin indirectly acts as a food-intake inhibitor by stimulating secretion of the hormone *leptin*. Leptin is a well-known regulator of body weight as it controls feelings of hunger and increases metabolism. HFCS stunts this important mechanism and can therefore lead to weight gain when consumed excessively.

HFCS has also been shown to raise triglyceride levels (the precursors to heart disease?[35]), increase the risk of type 2 diabetes, and weaken the bones in both children and adults.[36] We just cannot overlook these facts, especially in light of the recent and rapid rise in childhood ailments like attention deficit and hyperactivity disorder (ADHD). The unacceptable amount of soda consumed by our children is enough to unravel even the most focused of them. Instead of doing the obvious though, like cutting out some of their daily sugar intake, we have taken to feeding them dangerous drugs like Ritalin. We just might be able to reduce the incidence of ADHD by removing the ten teaspoonfuls or more of sugar a day that children consume in each can of soda.

Despite these unsettling facts, soft drinks remain America's beverage of choice. Aggressive advertising has definitely played its part in our obsession with liquid sugar, but ultimately, it is our responsibility to know better. How on earth can anyone rationalize drinking a six-pack of soda on a daily basis? Are people really unaware of the health consequences involved in this habit? And how does one rationalize putting Coke or any other soda into their baby's bottle? As far as I can tell, that's damn near child endangerment. Yet people do it anyway. In a 2001 study conducted by the American Dietetic Association (ADA), researchers found that children as young as seven months old regularly drink soda and that 44 percent of all two-year-olds drink at least one soft drink per day.[37] Even more disturbing is that they found that the most commonly consumed "vegetables" by toddlers as young as fifteen months of age were—french fries. These facts may help to explain why we have seen a tenfold increase in childhood type 2 diabetes when at one time it was nothing more than a rare occurrence.

But once again, I want to emphasize that blaming McDonald's, Coca-Cola, or any other junk food manufacturer is pointless. It is *our* responsibility to choose the foods we eat, and up until now, we have been overwhelmingly choosing junk. These billion-dollar corporations only provide the public with products it wants. Take McDonald's "healthy" menu and Coke's bottled water (Dasani) as a testament to this fact. These companies have kept abreast of the current health trends and have simply followed suit. Consumers' dollars are what determines which types of products are put onto the market, and when we stop making fast foods and soft drinks our dietary staples, then our options are bound to change.

I am sure that anyone reading this is aware of the fact that fast foods and sodas are not the healthiest choices available. But what may not be as immediately apparent is that many of the "regular" foods found in grocery stores are not always so healthy either. Take a trip down any shopping aisle and you will see shelf after shelf of processed, refined, and chemically altered foods. These are not just your cookies, cakes, and snack foods—which of course are riddled with sugar, fat, and food additives—but are also canned foods, microwavable meals, and genetically altered fruits and vegetable (see chapter 7). What is especially worrying is that many people are simply uninformed about the dangers inherent in these types of foods. Many believe that as long as a food item is sold by a reputable grocery chain, then it must be wholesome. Why else would people buy processed and prepackaged cold cuts and cracker lunches for their children? How about greasy potato chips or even soupy noodles in Styrofoam cups? If one were to just read the labels on any these items, it would become clear that many of these products contain dangerous chemicals like monosodium glutamate (MSG), nitrates, and transfatty acids. Just because these products look like food, smell like food, and even sometimes remotely taste like food does not mean that that is what they actually are.

Everywhere we turn, we are bombarded with slick advertising, cute and gimmicky toys, and "experts" giving us twisted half truths regarding the nature of their food products. What are we to do when our choices seem to be so severely limited? The truth is that healthy alternatives are available, and I will discuss many of them here in this chapter. The secret is to understand the basics. By following the sound principles contained in these pages, you are sure to get the most out of your diet; and this, of course, is the first key to optimal health. Read on, and you will become an expert at recognizing healthy and wholesome foods that both taste good and are good for you.

## Defying the Law of Thermodynamics

Before we turn you into a nutritional powerhouse, it is important that you first understand the physiological function of food and how the process of eating, digesting, and assimilating nutrients occurs in the body. First, let's understand why we even need food in the first place.

Food provides us with the energy we need to carry out all our bodily functions. Not only do we need energy to perform our voluntary actions (like walking, thinking, speaking, etc.), but we also need it for the involuntary ones (like metabolic processes, heartbeat, respiration, blood formation, maintenance of our cells and tissues, etc.).

There is a physical law called the *second law of thermodynamics*. It states that all things in the universe have a tendency to move toward chaos. That is, energy (everything in the universe is energy as you will see in chapter 6) spontaneously tends to flow from a concentrated state to a diffused or dispersed state; in other words, it spreads out. To better understand this law, think of dropping a sugar cube into a glass of water. What will happen? The energy holding the grains of sugar together will dissipate, and the cube will dissolve. This happens to all things unless there is some form of energy present to prevent or counteract this tendency to disperse. In fact, the *only* way in which life can sustain itself is by receiving a constant supply of energy that will prevent its own decomposition.

The second law of thermodynamics explains precisely why dead things eventually decay and rot. Living things prevent this from happening by obtaining energy from food. The energy derived from food is measured in calories. Bundles of energy come in calories just like bundles of money come in dollars and cents. Without food, we lose the energy needed to function, and thus, we cease to exist. That is why visions of starving people or anorexics are so frightening because we see these people literally wasting away in front of our eyes. Obviously, food is a requirement for all life.

Now that we understand the basic function of food, let us talk about how we extract energy from every bite we take. When we understand the physiology behind the eating process, it becomes more apparent why our dietary choices are so vital. So let us proceed to discuss this amazing process we call *digestion* in order to gain a greater appreciation of its benefit.

## The Long and Winding Road of Digestion

When we eat a meal, a number of processes occur that assure us of drawing out the maximal energy and nutrients from each and every bite. Highly efficient, the human body makes sure to store away enough energy for times when food may not be so readily available. If we were to follow a bite of food along its entire passage through the body, we would see some truly amazing things.

The digestive process begins in the mouth. Chewing breaks up solid matter into smaller particles, which will be easier to digest later on. Our saliva contains enzymes, which help to break down some of the larger molecules; and it also contains a mucus film, which makes it easier for the food to slide through the alimentary canal (our entire digestive tract). The partially digested food is now called a *bolus*, and it passes through the esophagus to the stomach by a process called *peristalsis*. This process is basically a constricting or squeezing of the smooth muscle in the digestive tract, and its function is to push the bolus toward the rectum (the eliminatory end of the body).

In the acidic environment of the stomach, enzymes are activated that work to break down proteins. The stomach also acts as a large mixing bowl, churning the food over and over again and breaking it into a liquid mush. The only molecules absorbed in the stomach are alcohol and drugs. With alcohol providing about seven calories per gram, one might mistake it for a great energy source. However, alcohol is metabolized far too slowly for it to be an efficient fuel; and therefore, it is simply converted to fat and stored. Alcohol is also very high in calories compared to carbohydrates and proteins (four calories per gram apiece), which makes it nothing more than an excellent source of weight gain. Unfortunately, alcohol has no nutritional value whatsoever—no vitamins, no minerals, nothing—so the pounds it provides come without the added benefits found in food. I'm not preaching prohibition here—alcohol can be fun if used responsibly—but as a dietary staple, alcohol provides little by way of nutrition.

Now back to digestion. The liquid produced by the churning of the stomach is eventually passed into the small intestines. Carbohydrates and fats (nine calories per gram) are broken down and absorbed here. Proteins, which have already been digested in the stomach, also get absorbed in the small intestines. Nutrients that are water soluble, such as carbohydrates, proteins, and the B and C vitamins, are absorbed into the bloodstream and taken to the liver for further processing and storage. Fats, on the other hand, must first be dissolved by bile acids, which are secreted by the liver, before they can be transported in the blood. Any fat-soluble nutrient, like vitamins A and D, are absorbed directly into the lymphatic system. The various nutrients, then, are shuttled off to any and all cells that need them. Any undigested or unabsorbed portion of the food passes through the small intestines and on to the colon or large intestines. Here, water and electrolytes, mostly sodium and chloride, are absorbed; and feces is formed. Waste products, of course, make their way out of the body within a couple of days.

As one can see, digestion is an amazing and complex operation. It involves a large number of organs that contribute mechanical, chemical, and hormonal actions. Many things can disrupt the natural flow of this process like excessive eating, consuming processed foods, and food sensitivities, which in turn can create distress. But this need not be the case for you. By following a few simple rules, you can be sure that your digestion will always work as smoothly as possible. As a result, your body will take in all the nutrients and energy it needs to function at an optimal level.

# Ten Simple Rules for Nutritious Noshing

Now that we have discussed the function of food and how the digestive process works, we can focus on the basics of eating a healthy diet. When you turn the behaviors outlined in this chapter into habits, it will be nearly impossible for you not to enjoy increased vigor and vitality. Becoming a master of your nutritional status is easy; there are just ten simple rules to follow. That's it! Ten rules to live by, and optimal health is all but guaranteed. Most fad diets are consistent to some degree with these rules. That's why every one of them works to some extent for some people. But the important thing to understand here is that these rules are merely the basics. If interested, one can take their nutritional regimen to a much deeper level; however, it still starts with these basic principles. By following this very simple and effective way to address your diet, you can virtually ensure yourself great digestion, proper nutrition and, of course, optimal health.

## Rule 1: Eat whole, natural foods

This one may seem obvious, but surprisingly, many people are simply out of touch with this concept. Whole, natural foods were, at one time, living matter. Whether animal, vegetable, or fungi—at one time minute strands in the intricate web of life—each contains the necessary resources to sustain life. The axiom "life begets life" is in full congruence with the fact that we must obtain all of our raw materials from other living things.

There must be a general misconception, though, of what constitutes real food. I say this only because I sometimes wonder how anyone could buy some of the garbage they sell at grocery stores. I understand that some of it might *resemble* food, but I wouldn't go so far as to call it such. It is not until you eat whole, natural foods regularly that you will be able to understand fully what I am talking about. As your palate becomes more and more attuned to organic and natural tastes, pseudofoods will soon lose their appeal—they just will not taste as good anymore. This is precisely because we are meant to eat real food.

Fresh produce, fresh meats, and real dairy products are always better than their canned, frozen, or processed counterparts. Whole, natural, and fresh foods have the perfect combinations of vitamins, minerals, and calories for each particular variety; and none have lost their nutrients because of processing. Also, certified organic produce and hormone-free meats generally have less added chemicals (chapter 7). One must only think back to the concept of Innate Intelligence (chapter 1) to understand how perfect living foods really are. Whole foods may contain elements that have yet to be uncovered, and these in turn may provide us with even more benefits than we have previously thought. Take, for instance, bioflavonoids; they were discovered by chance in the white rind of citrus fruits, and we now know how vital these nutrients actually are. By eating a diet rich in whole nuts, whole grains, fresh fruits, fresh vegetables, and unprocessed meats and dairy, you will receive a multitude of the components necessary for good health.

Many government officials and food industry "experts" claim that all nutrients are the same, whether made naturally or manufactured in a laboratory. Yet no respectable authority would ever claim that processed foods are better than whole foods, that's for sure, because you can never replace real food as a primary source of nourishment. The truth is that when the choice is available, nothing beats the real deal.

It is really very simple to prove to yourself that whole foods are superior in taste and nutritional value. Buy a couple of whole avocados; mash them up with fresh onions, fresh cilantro, fresh lime, and a little bit of salt; and taste it. Now go to your local grocery store and buy a jar of the most fluorescent green guacamole sitting on the shelf and taste that. I am completely confident that once you do, you will understand exactly what I'm talking about. I just cannot believe that anyone would honestly say that processed foods taste better—no way, no how.

So much for the taste test. But how about comparing the health benefits of natural foods to their processed counterparts? Numerous studies show the health benefits of whole foods, but to see the effects of processed foods, all we have to do is take a look around—America's obsession with junk food is starting to show in its waistlines. The number of overweight and obese people seems to increase daily, and who can deny the role processed foods play in this equation? *Men's Fitness* magazine uses the concentration of a city's fast-food restaurants as one of their criteria to evaluate the survey America's Fattest Cities. And if you haven't yet seen the brilliant but disturbing documentary *Super Size Me*, please do yourself a favor and catch it soon—it will scare you right into your local health food grocery store.

Unfortunately, at this time, the United States epitomizes what author Eric Schlosser calls the "fast-food nation."[38] To understand this, we need only look at our most significant cultural contribution to our neighbors around the world—the love of junk food. The United States is a world leader in both exporting and importing processed foods;[39] in fact, many of the first American businesses to open in former Communist countries were fast-food burger joints. The point here is that, in this country, we have lost our connection to real food; and it is high time we got it back. Whole, natural foods taste better and are just plain better for you. Everyday evidence surfaces to support this fact. Man cannot make it better than Mother Nature—not now, not ever.

The beauty of this principle is that you can easily prove it to yourself. Start today on a diet of whole, natural foods. Not only will you find that you feel much better, but you will also lose any cravings for processed and fast foods that you may have developed. Most importantly, though, if you start your children on natural foods early on, they will surely grow to love them. I was lucky enough to have my parents impress upon me the delights of natural foods at a very young age. My mother made sure to feed us only the best whole, natural foods, and as a result, I developed a taste for them. I cannot stress the importance of this principle enough. Give your children fruits instead of sweets and juice instead of soda. Feed them home-cooked meals regularly and only have fast food on occasion—it's that simple. What you feed your children today, as well as the habits you help them develop, will impact their lives forever. Give your children the greatest gift you possibly can by teaching them the wonders of whole, natural foods. They will thank you for it and reward you with a lifetime of excellent health.

## Rule 2: Eat different types of foods for different activities

Remember that we extract energy from the foods we eat. We require energy for all our activities, yet we need different types and different amounts for various actions. Carbohydrates, proteins, and fats are the substances that provide us with energy. The most readily available form comes from carbohydrates. Carbohydrate molecules (carbs) are needed for quick bursts of energy and are the only fuel source our brain utilizes. When we engage in strenuous mental activity, we need to make sure we eat plenty of carbohydrates to keep our minds sharp. Carbs can be stored in the liver and muscles as the complex molecule *glycogen*, but the capacity to do so is limited. Therefore, if we eat carbs to excess, especially when our activity levels are low, we will end up storing them as fat. Be careful, then, not to overdo it with foods that are high in carbohydrates.

Many of the snack foods we like are high in carbs as are most processed foods. Ironically, fat-free foods are loaded with carbs, and this leads to greater fat storage than with foods actually containing fat. This is because fats digest at a slower rate than carbs do, and they make you feel full sooner. Carbs digest quickly and are used for the body's immediate energy needs; therefore, they delay feelings of fullness. Most everyone is aware of the cliché associated with eating Chinese food—you are always hungry one hour afterward. There is truth to this as what we get in Chinese restaurants tends to be carbohydrate heavy. So if you are not a very physical person and your diet is high in carbohydrates, then you are likely to gain weight. If you are a moderately active person or are engaged in strenuous mental activities (studying, creating, picking the over/under), then what you will want to eat more of is carbs. Whatever the case, carbohydrates are important, and they should always be part of a well-balanced diet. Just be sure that the kind you get comes mainly from whole grains, fresh fruits, and vegetables and not junk food.

Protein, on the other hand, is necessary for tissue growth and maintenance. You must consume plenty of it if you exercise regularly; gym rats who do not get enough risk falling victim to burnout. Growing children also need lots of protein, as does anyone recovering from injury. Protein supplies the basic building blocks for all tissue growth in the form of *amino acids* and is therefore necessary for our vital repair functions. Like fats, protein is digested a bit more slowly than carbohydrates; so a diet rich in protein will make you feel full faster, which ultimately will prevent overeating. Meat, fish, eggs, and dairy products are excellent sources of protein.

The third and final source of energy is *fat*. Fats are a necessary component to so many different processes that it's a shame they have been removed from many people's diets. Fats are an excellent source of energy. They are particularly useful when we need large quantities, like when doing physical labor. This is especially true if your next meal is a long way off. Fats can also be burned to produce heat, an absolute godsend when living in a cold climate. They cushion the internal organs and make up the protective membrane for our cells. Fats make up the structural component of our brains, so we surely cannot live without them. They are also precursors to many hormones, like testosterone and estrogen; and when adolescent girls get insufficient amounts of fat in their diets, it can delay puberty and cause *amenorrhea* (the absence of menstruation). As we have said before, fats are digested *slowly*. That means they help one gain a feeling of fullness, preventing overeating. They are also necessary for absorbing fat-soluble vitamins like A, D, E, and K. Finally, for anyone wanting healthier-looking skin, fats are absolutely essential—they give skin its soft and pliable appearance. Fats should come from natural sources like meats, dairy, and fish. Seeds, vegetables, and avocados are also great sources. Whatever you do, do not avoid fats, and do not replace them with carbohydrates either. Fat-free products are neither better tasting nor better for you; in reality, they may actually be hazardous to your health. So eat fats—you cannot live a healthy life without them.

When it comes to eating, it is important to have a balanced diet that consists of all three energy sources: carbohydrates, proteins, and fats. In addition, some general precautions are necessary:

- Reduce your carbohydrate intake if you are not going to be very active for some time. Try to get carbs mainly from whole grains, fresh fruits, and vegetables and not from sweets or processed foods.

- Eat plenty of protein when exercising regularly, while pregnant, while healing from an injury, or during the formative years of child development. Also, a diet rich in protein will help to prevent overeating.
- Keep fats in your diet, but be moderate and consistent. A small amount of daily fat intake is healthy. Whole, natural foods by default have better fat than processed ones, that is, they have no transfatty acids (see below). "Low fat" products are usually high in sugar, which eventually leads to greater fat deposition.

Just remember that by eating a healthy diet balanced by all three energy sources, you will receive the vital ingredients needed for all bodily processes. By following rule number 1 (Eat whole, natural foods), you will more than likely fulfill rule number 2 since it will be virtually impossible to eat natural foods without getting all of these essential nutrients. Nevertheless, make sure to include a variety of foods in your diet so that there is never a question of whether you are getting a proper balance of nutrients or not.

**Rule 3: Eat in peace**

There is no doubt that the typical American's schedule is hectic. Between work and personal chores, much of our time is taken up by our activities. Sometimes the effort to complete them is so great that finding the time to eat can be a task in itself. Many of us even feel proud when we squeeze in a meal "on the go"—a true feat of multitasking.

Fast-food restaurants have become a huge success by accommodating this aspect of our lifestyle. Yet in this demanding age of hyperproduction and high-speed exchange, it is important to try and find the time to calmly sit and eat a nutritious meal. In order to do this, we must first become aware of how slowing down might help us. With this knowledge, we can set aside more time and eat our meals in an unhurried and peaceful manner.

To begin with, let's look at how slowing down can actually affect our digestion. By sitting down to eat a meal, our bodies become calm and physically relaxed. This is because the body does not have to split its energy between fueling the muscles and digesting. The digestive process is controlled by the parasympathetic nervous system and requires a large amount of blood to pass through the gut and intestines. Muscular action, on the other hand, particularly when under stress, is controlled by the sympathetic nervous system and also requires blood for its function. Make note that these processes are entirely opposite, so when they occur together, they tend to disrupt each other and can ultimately cause fatigue.

The longer one can sit, relax, and let the digestive system do its thing, the more completely this function can be carried out. As a result, less energy is wasted. This becomes even more important when one's general pace is intense; we just should not have to be slowed down by things like gas, an upset stomach, or heartburn. But this is exactly what we risk every time we gulp down our food; poorly chewed food leads to poor digestion. These types of digestive distresses can really slow us down, so wouldn't it be better to slow ourselves down first?

Aside from the physiological impact, there are emotional reasons to slow down too. Emotions influence our physiological functions, including digestion. Stress is related to the sympathetic nervous system, and the stress of feeling in a rush will stimulate this system to act. Recall that this process shunts blood away from the digestive system and over to the muscles. Eating in a state of stress, then, is counterproductive to its own function. To enhance digestion, it is advantageous to close your eyes and meditate or to be still for a few minutes to let your energy recoup. This often brings about calmness and can even set the pace for the entire day. If this seems impractical, just realize that we are only talking about two or three minutes here, something we can all afford to invest.

Emotional stressors like fighting, worrying, or hostile and self-defeating thoughts can also have subtle effects on the digestive process. I am not going to insult your intelligence by suggesting that as you eat, you should merely "think positively," but it cannot hurt to clear your mind a little before eating. Literally take a minute just prior to your first bite and breathe deeply ten times. Think about nothing but your breath here. On the next breath, think briefly about the digestive process as I have described it. Think about the function of food as a source of energy and how it travels through the alimentary canal to be processed. Think about each step briefly but thoroughly, and it will help neurologically to stimulate the production of enzymes and other substances that are involved in the digestive process. This works in much the same way as ringing a bell did for Pavlov's dog. The beauty is that the more you practice, the easier it becomes; and more importantly, it's the way habits develop. You will find that the habit of slowing down will greatly improve your digestion and make you feel better. This, in turn, will give you the energy you need for all your tasks, even on the most frenzied of days.

## Rule 4: Eat at home as much as possible

Consistent with the last rule, there is no better place to relax and bring calm to one's mealtime than in one's own home. Home is where people feel the most comfortable and where they actually *know* the person preparing the food. The greatest benefit of eating at home, though, is that you are in complete control of the foods you eat. Why is this important? Because you can both customize your diet to exactly fit your needs as well as assure yourself that you are always getting the highest quality of food available.

Regardless of how healthy a restaurant's menu might be, dining at home is always superior to eating out. When dining out, you sit in a room full of strangers and often with a large amount of background noise; therefore, it can never be as peaceful as when dining at home. We often dine out with friends or business associates. The conversation is usually made up of small talk or business matters, and there is no connection whatsoever to the people cooking and serving the food. We can never reap the same benefits of the eating experience in this type of situation. This is not only true on a nutritional level (based on the quality of the food), but on a mental (based on the environment) and spiritual one too (based on a connection to the people preparing the food).

This last point is important to elaborate on. The idea that there must be a connection to the person preparing the food is very important. It has to do with the concept of energy exchange. Since all things in the universe are energetic (chapter 6) and this energy is exchanged constantly, then the person preparing our food and under which conditions really do make a difference to our mental and spiritual states. When food is prepared by someone who loves you and is brought to the table surrounded by that same loving energy, then I strongly believe that this energy is transferred over to the food. If this is true, then it has to have some sort of impact on us. Emotionally and spiritually, this energy permeates all of our cells and tissues and enhances the digestive and absorptive processes. I grant you that this is an abstract concept, and Lord knows it's certainly not provable. However, there is no doubt that all humans need the energy of love to survive. Keep someone isolated from human contact and they will surely perish.[40] It stands to reason, then, that food served with love is merely a corollary to this law. Food prepared with the energy of love serves the vital functions of both nourishing the body and nourishing the soul.

Even if this concept is too esoteric for you, there are other more concrete benefits to eating at home. As I previously mentioned, food prepared at home will always be healthier, especially if it's of high quality. You can never vouch for the quality of your meals unless you make them yourself. According to the Center for Science in the Public Interest:

> Food eaten outside the home, on average, is higher in fat and lower in micronutrients than food prepared at home. Many popular table-service restaurant meals—lunch or dinner—provide 1000 to 2000 kcal each, amounts

equivalent to 35 percent to 100 percent of a full day's energy requirement for most adults.[41]

So even if you cannot appreciate the energetic theory of eating at home, the decreased nutritional level of foods served at public eateries should be enough to keep you dining in. This is not to suggest that people should stop eating at restaurants altogether. Dining out is very enjoyable and quite possibly one of the finest ways to spend an evening with friends. Yet the idea here is to keep the dining-out experience as a special occasion—a way to enjoy oneself or a way to celebrate. When eating away from home is no longer the exception but instead the norm, your health will suffer as a result.

On a final note, if you are in a situation at home that is very stressful, then either dine at the home of a friend or find a serene restaurant where you can spend an hour or two eating in calm and peace. Both of these options are better than eating in an environment that is taxing on you—and definitely better than eating food on the go. Whichever way you work it, never disregard the importance of calming your mind before and during each meal.

## Rule 5: Vitamins should be supplemented

In today's large-scale agricultural operations, the soil is tilled in such a way that has led to a severe depletion of nutrients so necessary for our health and functioning.[42] Although alternative methods of farming are currently being used—like organic farming (see chapter 7), which is soil enhancing—it is still imperative in today's environment to supplement our diets with vitamins and minerals. Vitamin supplementation is the only way to ensure that we get all our vital nutrients. Additionally, people rarely eat enough of the required foods to meet the RDA levels for each nutrient. Throw in restrictive diets, vegetarianism, and the fact that stress and exercise both deplete vitamins and it is easy to see how important supplementing with vitamins really is.

Vitamins were first discovered in the early part of the twentieth century. At that time, they were pretty much seen as substances that could prevent and cure common illnesses such as scurvy, beriberi, and pellagra. As scientists studied vitamins further, it became evident that they were also necessary for physiological functions like respiration, tissue development, and blood clotting, as well as many others. Illnesses due to nutritional deficiencies are rare but can still occur if one does not get the proper amount of vitamins and minerals on a daily basis. For the most part, though, people today supplement to optimize their health.

When I was a university student, I remember one professor asking the question, "Which nutrient is most important?"

Immediately, the class began shouting its answers, "Vitamin C . . . no—B . . . protein . . . no—chocolate!" None of these was the right answer though. So which nutrient *is* the most important one? C'mon, it's easy. The most important nutrient is *the one that's missing.*

Depending on one's dietary habits, everyone has their own unique needs with respect to the vitamins they require. The following is some very basic information on vitamins that everyone can benefit from. Please understand that the subject of nutrition is complex and would take a whole other book to cover all its intricate details. I repeat, what I present here are merely the basics—those nutrients that are absolutely essential to supplement in every diet.

## Multivitamins

The supplement I most often recommend to my clients is a good high-quality multivitamin. Multivitamins are a blend of all the essential vitamins and minerals necessary for basic nutrition. There are many excellent brands on the market today, so the one you choose is between you and your health care advisor. I definitely have my preference, but for the most part, I feel it is merely a matter of taste.

The bottom line is that if you take nothing else, a good multivitamin will give you a nice balance of most everything you need. It is a good starting point for people who have never taken a supplement before or for those who do not take them very often. By taking a multivitamin, you will be in the best position to satisfy my college professor's requirement for replacing the "missing" nutrient. The best part here is that you will not have to spend an arm and a leg to test your vitamin levels in order to determine which nutrients you might be deficient in. Testing can end up being very costly and time consuming in the long run. Taking a multivitamin solves this problem.

Here are a few things for you to think about:

- I generally prefer capsules to pills. Pills are held together by gums and other substances, and how well the vitamin breaks apart depends on the substances used. It is the degree to which the pill dissolves that determines how much of the vitamins you will actually absorb and utilize. You really won't have this worry with capsules. The only problem with capsules is that they tend to be bigger, or you have to take more of them because the vitamin molecules are not as tightly pressed as they are in a pill. This becomes difficult for people who have an aversion to swallowing pills. If this happens to be the case for you, go ahead and take the pill form. Some brands dissolve excellently (you will just have to find which ones work best for you); and even if they do not completely dissolve in your gut, in this case, something is definitely better than nothing.

- Take your vitamins with meals. Vitamins cannot be digested very well without food; and some, especially the B vitamins, can upset your stomach. Furthermore, vitamins are not food, so you cannot use them as a replacement for food and think you are still getting what you need. Remember, vitamins supplement food, not substitute for it.

- Drink vitamins down with lots of water. Take my word for it—nothing is worse than swallowing a capsule full of powdered vitamins and having them stick in your throat. It is especially bad when the capsules dissolve in your gullet (after only a few seconds) and you have to taste the bitterness of the vitamin for the next several hours.

## B Complex

The B complex is a group of eight vitamins including thiamin (B1), riboflavin (B2), niacin (B3), pyridoxine (B6), folic acid (B9), cyanocobalamin (B12), pantothenic acid (B5), and biotin (B7). Although the B vitamins have many functions, I like to think of them as the "energy vitamins" since they are involved in the production of *adenosine triphosphate* (ATP), our energy molecules which we will talk more about in chapter 3.

Although a good multivitamin will have all the Bs in it, I find that they do not always have enough in dosage, so supplementing with a B complex in addition to a multivitamin is generally a good practice. As the B vitamins work together synergistically, it is best to take them as a complex. You will want to take the B vitamins with food as taking them on an empty stomach may cause nausea. The B complex, like all vitamins, can be easily depleted by stress, drugs and medications, excessive use of alcohol, malnutrition, weight-loss diets, and excessive vomiting.

A deficiency in these essential nutrients can lead to disorders like anemia, paralysis, muscular atrophy, severe muscle spasms, fatigue, lack of coordination, loss of memory, cracked lips, dermatitis, sensitivity to light, inflammation of the tongue, painful lesions in the mouth, diarrhea, and mental illness. Many more conditions can result, but I'm sure you get the point—you need this stuff!

What are the benefits provided by regular B vitamin supplementation? To begin with, they are necessary for adrenal function, which is important in regulating stress. They also play a role in immunity by producing vital antibodies. The nervous system depends on B vitamins to produce neurotransmitters (chapter 4), and as we have mentioned earlier, B vitamins are essential for energy production. When deficient, one may feel severely fatigued and lethargic.

B vitamins also play a role in red blood cell formation, which is vital for circulation and respiration by facilitating oxygen uptake. The health of the skin, mouth, and digestive tract all rely on proper levels of B vitamins while memory and learning are also supported by a proper supply. Supplementing with these vitamins has been shown to help with depression and anxiety too, and the list of benefits goes on and on and on.

An important characteristic of the B vitamins is that they are *water soluble*—they easily dissolve in $H_2O$. What this means is that you can pretty much take as large a dose as you want without overdosing. Your body will absorb only what it needs, and remove the rest in the urine. Therefore, the worst thing that can happen is that you release very expensive fluorescent green urine, which, unfortunately, is not very valuable at this time.

Although everybody should take a B complex regularly, folic acid is especially important for women planning to have children. Taking folic acid is absolutely vital *before* conception as well as early in the pregnancy to prevent neural defects of the fetus. A *neural defect* is the incomplete development of the brain and spinal cord. This tragic situation is completely preventable by simply taking four hundred micrograms per day. A good B complex should easily supply this amount.

And finally, those who like to party also have an increased need for vitamin B. All aspects of the party life—drug and alcohol use, lack of sleep, and a high consumption of fast foods—require it. If this is the life you currently live, then for God's sake, man, take your B vitamins!

## Essential Fatty Acids

Over the last two decades, there has been a dietary movement in this country to rid our diets of fat. An influx of "fat-free" foods now lines the shelves of most grocery stores and is evidence of this trend. Although there is truth to the principle that fat intake should be moderated, many food manufacturers—primarily of snack foods—have irresponsibly misused this fact to help sell their products. Under the illusion that fat-free foods do not add on weight, people have wrongly overindulged in them—consequently avoiding a group of nutrients, the beneficial fats, so vital to the proper functioning of the human body. Let me say this loud and clear: fats are absolutely essential to our overall health and well-being!

But wait—didn't I say earlier to be moderate with your fat intake? Yes, be careful with saturated fats found in animal meats (i.e., don't eat loads of it every day). Also, the fats found in shortening and margarine are not very healthy since they are often loaded with dangerous transfatty acids (these increase the risk of cancer and heart disease). Polyunsaturated and natural fats, on the other hand, are vital—that is why they are called *essential fatty acids* (EFAs). These compounds cannot be formed in the body and must therefore be obtained in the diet. Furthermore, a deficiency in these essential fats can lead to numerous disorders.

EFAs are found in high concentrations in fish oils, seeds like flax and borage seeds, and the evening primrose plant. There are two families of EFAs—the omega-3s and the omega-6s. The omega-3 fatty acids are *eicosapentaenoic acid* (EPA) and *docosahexaenoic acid* (DHA). These are mostly found in the oils of cold-water fish. They significantly lower cholesterol and triglyceride levels—*even in the presence of high-saturated fats* (animal meats, dairy products, and other tasty stuff).[43] They also act as a natural blood thinner, which is critical for those at high risk for heart disease or those with blood-clotting disorders. One could extrapolate, then, that omega-3 fatty acids are a great preventative measure against the country's number 1 killer—heart disease.

Omega-6 fatty acids tend to be more prevalent in the typical American diet as they are a constituent of vegetable oils, breads, grains, eggs, and poultry—stuff that we tend to eat lots of. For the most part, then, we get enough of this fatty acid in our regular diets. In fact, most people tend to get substantially more of the omega-6s than the omega-3s, typically at 20:1 (omega-6:omega-3). Unfortunately, this is not a very healthy ratio. An unbalanced fatty acid intake of this magnitude is a very strong precursor of heart disease.

It is therefore important to balance the types of fatty acids in one's usual diet. Studies show that to gain the greatest benefit from EFAs, one must ingest them at a ratio of 2:1 (omega-3:omega-6). This can be done by increasing the intake of fish while lowering the intake of omega-6-containing foods. You might find this difficult to do, especially if you are like me and do not really care for fish. A much better way to increase your intake of omega-3 fatty acids is to supplement them daily with fish oils. These can be taken in liquid form or in capsules. Since I can barely stomach the taste of fish, I tend to prefer the capsules over the liquid, but the liquid form is definitely more potent since it is absorbed more completely by the body. Another way to receive a proper amount of omega-3 fatty acids is with flax seed oil. This oil has a lower concentration of EFAs than fish oil, but it is still a decent source of omega-3s and is a great alternative for anyone who can't take the taste of fish. Whole flax seeds are also wonderful when ground up and added to delicious fruit smoothies.

As I said earlier, most people receive enough omega-6 fatty acids in their diet, and therefore, they do not usually need to be supplemented. There is one type of omega-6 that should be taken as a supplement, though, and that is *gamma-linolenic acid* (GLA). This omega-6 fatty acid is found in borage or evening primrose oil. It has anti-inflammatory properties and can help prevent heart disease and other degenerative disorders.

The benefits of proper EFA intake are many,[44] and they include

- Lowered cholesterol
- Lowered blood pressure
- Decreased risk of heart attack and stroke
- Prevention of blood clots*
- Lowered risk associated with diabetes (not always true with the type of EFAs found in flax oil)
- Controlled blood sugar levels
- Decreased symptoms associated with arthritis
- Decreased bone loss associated with osteoporosis
- Decreased risk of depression; helps regulates mood swings
- Decreased risk of macular degeneration (a serious age-related eye disease that can lead to blindness)
- Decreased menstrual pain
- Decreased risk of breast cancer in women and prostate cancer in men
- Decreased symptoms associated with skin disorders like psoriasis, dermatitis, eczema, and acne

As you can see, getting the right amount of EFAs has enormous benefits to human health. People who are deficient in the omega-3s may experience depression, weight gain, allergies, violence, memory problems, inflammatory diseases, and dry skin.[45] On a personal note, I can tell you that I suffered from eczema for many years. Anyone who has had this or a similar disorder can tell you that it is an absolutely miserable condition. The pain and itching associated with eczema is enough to drive you mad. When I made omega-3 fatty acids a regular part of my supplementation program, the eczema miraculously disappeared. Along with drinking plenty of water, supplementing with EFAs are the secret to soft, supple, and pliable skin. Skin creams and facials are important too (I do both regularly), but the reality is, to have the healthiest and most glowing skin possible, you will need to supplement with this essential nutrient. Along with all

---

\*    Anyone currently taking blood thinners like Coumadin (warfarin) should first consult with their doctor so they can discuss lowering the medication dosage.

the other benefits EFAs provide, you would be foolish not to incorporate them into your daily regimen.

A final and important point must be made about EFAs: they must be kept refrigerated at all times otherwise they can turn rancid. Because of their chemical makeup—they are polyunsaturated—they oxidize easily. Oxidation leads to rancidity and, in turn, can create free radicals in the body. Free radicals can damage DNA and cause cancer. It is, therefore, not only important to refrigerate these supplements, but also to take a good antioxidant along with them. This leads us to our next topic.

## Antioxidants

As we mentioned in the last section, free radicals are substances that can damage the DNA of our cells. These harmful molecules can lead to degenerative disorders like cancer and may even speed up the aging process. Free radicals are formed naturally in the body during certain metabolic processes as well as by cells of the immune system to fight infections. They can also be formed by outside agents like cigarette smoke, pollution, and radiation.

Antioxidants are vitamins, minerals, and enzymes that neutralize free radicals. They prevent cell and tissue damage by acting as scavengers. They help defend against heart disease by preventing the oxidation of fat molecules, which can lead to atherosclerotic plaques. Vitamins and minerals that act as antioxidants can be easily remembered by the mnemonic: ACES. Those letters stand for the vitamins A, C, and E while the S stands for the mineral selenium. All of these can be found in a good multivitamin.

While I highly recommend taking a little extra vitamin C, outside of what you get in a good multivitamin, I do not advise this with the other three antioxidants. Vitamin A is fat soluble and can therefore accumulate in the lipid membranes of cells. Too much A can cause toxicity and can be detrimental to your health. In pregnant women, it can lead to birth defects. It is much better to take vitamin A as its precursor beta-carotene, and most commercial brands provide it in this form. Beta-carotene is converted to A in the body but will not proceed if A is already in ample supply. Thus, beta-carotene is a safe alternative to taking pure vitamin A.

Vitamin E is also a fat-soluble vitamin, but toxicity is very rare. It is a potent antioxidant that owes its effectiveness to the tocopherol molecules (alpha, beta, gamma, and delta). The alpha-tocopherol variety is the most powerful antioxidant, but gamma-tocopherol has been shown to fight the effects of many degenerative diseases.[46] If you can find a supplement that has both isomers of the vitamin E molecule, you will be getting the greatest benefits possible.

Selenium is a mineral that is an important constituent of the antioxidant enzyme *glutathione peroxidase*. This enzyme may protect against cancer and may even have beneficial effects in preventing heart disease and arthritis. Selenium itself is necessary for proper immune function, and studies have shown it to slow down the progression of AIDS and viral hepatitis.[47] Because this is a mineral, it is important to monitor intake: two hundred micrograms or less is considered safe. Check the amount in your multivitamin. It should probably be enough.

Now that we have discussed the basic antioxidants, I would like to talk about two other sources that I find especially useful. The first is the natural form of antioxidants, fruits and vegetables. Anything found in the produce section will generally be a great source. That is why experts recommend eating so many servings. Everything from garlic to onions to broccoli is rich in these vital nutrients. My three favorite sources are blueberries, blackberries, and pomegranates. Is it really possible to derive so much benefit from such delicious foods? You bet, and I personally eat them by the handfuls. Pomegranate juice has recently become fashionable, and although I tend to avoid trends, I endorse this juice anyway. It beats liquid sugar, that's for sure. Get plenty of these fruits in your diet. They're tasty, they're fun, and they just can't be topped for nutritional value.

The next source of antioxidants is alpha-lipoic acid. Not only is alpha-lipoic acid a powerful antioxidant, but it also plays a vital role in energy production. Its value as a supplement cannot be rivaled. Alpha-lipoic acid has the ability to work in both fat—and water-soluble tissues. It is the only antioxidant with this ability, so it is often called the universal antioxidant.[48] Many prominent researchers believe this molecule has a great ability to prevent many of today's degenerative diseases like diabetes and heart disease. Because of its ability to cross the blood-brain barrier, alpha-lipoic acid may be useful in preventing damage from stroke. It has also been shown to slow down the replication of HIV and other viruses.[49] As an added benefit, studies at the University of California-Berkeley have shown this antioxidant to improve brain function—like memory, especially in the elderly—and it may even protect against Alzheimer's disease.[50] You can see that this nutrient has broad effects and, in my opinion, should be taken as a daily supplement, especially if you are a smoker or live in a smoggy city. It is even important for those who exercise regularly as physical activity leads to the formation of free radicals.

**Rule 6: Don't overeat—less is often more**

Part of the obesity problem we see in Western society is simply due to overeating despite a popular theory circulating within the health community that genes, single or multiple, are responsible for obesity.[51] Indeed, a gene *has* been isolated, which may increase the chances of becoming obese; however, it would still require the inheritor to overeat regularly and/or neglect exercise for obesity to set in. Can you see my point here? Gene or no gene, overeating is still part of the obesity equation.

The unfortunate consequence of pushing the genetic predisposition theory is that it almost always absolves the person battling the problem from any responsibility. It's just too easy to say, "Well, my genetics prevent me from losing weight, so what's the use? I may as well eat what I want to." Sadly, this way of thinking removes any freedom of choice. The person subscribing to this theory may end up feeling hopeless and kill any further efforts.

The fact is that no matter how you slice it, when trying to lose weight, the body must use more calories than it consumes. Period! This is true for everyone, regardless of genetics. Additionally, we know that obesity increases the risks of many fatal disorders, one being heart disease. So genetically speaking, very few benefits can be attributed to this so-called risky gene. Doesn't it stand to reason, then, that if obesity is, for the most part, detrimental and unfavorable traits are diminished, if not outright eliminated during the evolutionary process, then the numbers of obese individuals should decline or stay constant at the very least?

Yet we know this is not the case. Obesity is on the rise and increasing at a rapid rate. The genetic theory, then, does not seem plausible, especially in a country like the United States where food is so plentiful. There is simply no biological advantage to storing excess fat in our current environment. Excess fat storage is only an advantage when the food supply is low. My point is that from a purely biological standpoint, there just is no genetic advantage for the trait of obesity.

Here is the grim reality: obesity is due, in part, to the consistent intake of excess calories, or, simply, by eating too much. The answer to our severe weight problem, then, is to eat less and exercise more. I believe that Americans really started to overeat following the Great Depression. The decades following World War II were so prosperous that Americans celebrated by eating large and extravagant meals. Just watch any rerun of the 1950s sitcom *Leave It to Beaver* and you will see exactly what I am talking about. A huge roast served with all the fixings was very much the norm, and piling it high was done as an emotional response to the harsh realities of a previous era. The memory of standing in breadlines, feeling lucky to be eating at all, was not so far removed from the collective psyche. Then along came fast foods and the popular value meals—the bigger the portions, the better the deal—and this is how the obesity epidemic began. Add to this the advent of processed foods and liquid sugar, and it is no surprise that America's waistlines have been expanding ever since.

Looking again at the digestive process, we find neurological mechanisms in place to tell us when we have eaten enough for our energetic and nutritional needs. One major apparatus exists in the stomach itself. Remember that the stomach, along with its churning and digestive properties, is also a storage bag for chewed-up food (bolus). The food slowly leaks into the small intestine for further digestion and absorption into the body. When the stomach is stretched, nerves lining the gut wall are stimulated, sending impulses back to the brain saying, "OK enough . . . I'm satiated." But along with our incessant desire to get the best value, we have also cultivated a society where productivity far outweighs slowing down to eat a meal. As a result, most people have developed the habit of underchewing their food and gulping it down quickly. This leads to inefficient digestion since a poorly chewed bolus will not be absorbed completely in the small intestine. When food is not digested properly and the body fails to get the nutrients it needs, it will naturally delay the feelings of satiation. Neurologically, the stretch response of the stomach has less time to kick in, leaving the eater with the illusion of still feeling hungry despite having plenty of food in the stomach already. We have all felt the effects of this at one time or another, maybe at Thanksgiving or another time when we ate too much. We may have gulped down our food without letting this mechanism kick in, and what happened? We ended up feeling bloated, unable to move and ready to explode.

The unfortunate consequence of repeatedly gulping down our meals is that the body quickly gets used to the excessive intake of food. The stomach becomes desensitized, and it takes a little longer for the stretch mechanism to kick in. The feelings of satiety are therefore delayed, and as a result, the stomach becomes larger—just as any muscle would with regular exercise. Furthermore, the digestive process becomes more efficient. As the digestive system soon learns, food comes through rapidly and is passed through more quickly. Only the outer surface of the bolus is digested, and the body requires more food than normal to receive all its nutrients.

This scenario is not a fantasy. It is exactly why a five-foot-eight man like myself could eventually eat two double-double cheeseburgers, large fries, and a milk shake and blow up to 165 lbs. Been there, done that. It's called extreme gluttony, and it's one of the worst things you can do to yourself. But there is good news: just as this process moves in one direction, it can move in the opposite one as well. Like most things, controlling one's appetite is a process, but it works. It just requires patience and diligence. Both come easier though with a little understanding of how it all unfolds.

By decreasing the amount of food we ingest, there may initially be feelings of intense hunger. This is due to several factors, some psychological but many physiological, and they are related to the appetite control mechanisms inherent in our bodies. We have already discussed one type, the stretch response in the gut and small intestine; but there are hormonal and oral regulators too, which are stimulated by the chewing and salivating processes. These short-term appetite regulators help decrease our feelings of hunger over time.

As we mentioned earlier, an adequate supply of nutrients in the body acts as a long-term regulatory mechanism for the appetite. That is, when the body is sufficiently nourished, it shuts off the hunger response. These mechanisms, unfortunately, can get thrown out of whack when one overeats and becomes obese.[52] This is one reason why obese people have intense feelings of hunger despite having an excess of nutrients. What this means for people embarking on the practice of food restriction is that initially the long-term regulation mechanism will function improperly. This, of course, will lead to feelings of hunger. But over a short period, the other three mechanisms (stretch receptors, hormones, and oral regulators) will eventually kick in and normalize the appetite.

This lesson in physiology emphasizes that many people eat way too much. The body often fools the brain into thinking it needs more food, which only perpetuates the cycle. By decreasing the portions of food we eat consistently, the regulatory mechanisms of appetite balance out—leading to weight loss, increased energy, and optimal function.

I would now like to suggest an exercise that can be done by anyone. At your next meal, decrease the portions by one-third to one-half of what you would normally eat. Eat slowly and chew meticulously, then wait between ten minutes and one-half hour before eating any more. If you feel hungry—just wait! I promise that you will feel satiated within one-half hour. If not, then go ahead and eat the rest. It may just be that you need the extra energy at this time, especially if you are in a healthy weight range for your height or you are highly active. But don't fool yourself. If you are overweight, you probably have enough energy stored to take care of your immediate needs. Any feelings of hunger in this case are most likely due to your long-term regulatory mechanisms being unbalanced. But these feelings will pass. It just takes time. By the way, this exercise definitely works. It is not the sole answer to losing weight, but it is a step in the right direction.

I would like to conclude this section by mentioning that there is a movement in the antiaging sciences looking at *caloric restriction without malnutrition*, and they have found some fascinating results.[53] Research data has shown that reducing calories, yet still obtaining an adequate supply of vital nutrients, can lead to decreased effects of aging, especially on the brain, and may even prevent neurodegenerative disorders like Alzheimer's disease.[54] Not only do we know that overeating and obesity can actually speed up the aging process and lead to the development of degenerative diseases, but also that undereating or caloric restriction may have a hand in slowing down aging significantly, thereby preventing disease. These findings make a very strong case for limiting processed foods (rule 7 below) since they are generally high in calories and low in nutritional value and also for taking nutritional supplements or vitamins (rule 5 above). Please remember, though, that we are talking about *restriction without malnutrition*, so undereating to a point of anorexia or bulimia is still detrimental to your health. We will take a look at these eating disorders in further detail later.

## Rule 7: Minimize the intake of processed foods

In the last rule, we talked in detail about being overweight. We discussed decreasing caloric intake while continuing a program of optimal nutrition. In this vein, it is also important to point out that consuming processed foods regularly violates both rules severely. The bottom line is that processed foods—fast foods, cakes, candies, french fries, and sodas—are all very low in nutritional value and high in calories. This is also true, my liquor-imbibing friends, of alcoholic beverages. It is not that people should stop eating or drinking these products altogether as they can definitely be enjoyable, but it would be wiser to make them occasional indulgences as opposed to dietary staples.

Aside from the two facts I have just mentioned, many processed foods are high in sugar and transfatty acids. Transfatty acids can increase the risk of heart disease and should obviously be avoided. Likewise, you should refrain from eating too much sugar as it can lead to various disorders including[55]

- Decreased insulin sensitivity causing abnormally high insulin levels and eventually diabetes
- Suppression of the immune system
- A rapid rise of adrenaline, hyperactivity, anxiety, difficulty concentrating, and crankiness in children
- A significant rise in total cholesterol, triglycerides, and bad cholesterol, and a decrease in good cholesterol
- Loss of tissue elasticity and function
- Increased fasting levels of glucose and can cause reactive hypoglycemia
- Weakened eyesight
- Premature aging
- Tooth decay and periodontal disease
- Obesity

- Autoimmune diseases such as arthritis, asthma, and multiple sclerosis
- Hemorrhoids
- Varicose veins
- Elevated glucose and insulin responses in oral contraceptive users
- Lowered vitamin E levels
- Increased systolic blood pressure
- Atherosclerosis and cardiovascular disease
- Skin aging by changing the structure of collagen
- Increased formation of kidney stones
- Headaches including migraines
- Depression
- Increased free radicals and oxidative stress
- Promotion of excessive food intake in obese people
- Slowed ability of the adrenal glands to function
- High blood pressure in obese people

I think I have sufficiently made my point here—a high consumption of processed foods can severely diminish one's health. In my opinion, the worst products on the market today are *sodas, artificial sweeteners, fast foods, and canned or frozen foods* (especially when they contain MSG). Limit these to occasional indulgences only, or even better, abstain from them completely and your health will respond in a dramatic way.

## Rule 8: Keep a rhythm in your eating schedule

As we will discuss in greater detail in chapter 6, everything in the universe follows a rhythmic pattern. Whether it is the rising and setting of the sun (planetary revolution), the ebb and flow of the tides, or the change of the seasons, the universe tends to follow a pattern of oscillation. Electrons oscillate as they spin around an atomic nucleus; our biological clock oscillates too, at least when it is working properly. For this reason, it is helpful to maintain a rhythm to your eating schedule as much as possible.

Eating at approximately the same time every day maintains this rhythm. No, you do not have to be accurate by the minute; but if you eat three major meals a day, then you should try sticking to an approximate time for each one. You should also try to not skip any meals throughout the day because it can lead to low blood sugar, which might leave you feeling fatigued, shaky, irritable, dizzy, or confused. If you allow your blood sugar to get too low too often, it can also leave you susceptible to accidents or cognitive and mental impairment.[56]

Keeping a rhythm will not only prevent your blood sugar from getting low but will also ensure optimal digestion, absorption, utilization of nutrients, and defecation. Changing your eating pattern in any way can disrupt these functions in much the same way jet lag does, which ultimately can leave you feeling drained. Obviously, it is not *always* practical to eat at the same time every day, but consistency definitely makes a difference.

On a final note, some people—especially those who are highly active—may feel the need to eat smaller meals or snacks in between their major ones. Some people actually feel better by eating only a few small meals throughout the day instead of three larger ones. Each person must figure out for herself if this is the best way to go. In any case, make sure that the foods you choose are the most nutritious available, and also make sure you slow down to eat. You see, all the rules of diet fit perfectly together, just like the pieces of a puzzle.

**Rule 9: Listen to your body at all times**

We have already discussed some of the ways your body conveys messages to you. Stretch receptors in the digestive tract, when stimulated, let you know you are full. Hormonal signals can also indicate feelings of fullness as well as let you know when you are tired, stressed out, or in need of a good vacation. Some of the other ways the body communicates with you include rhythmic contractions of the stomach, or hunger pangs, that tell you when you are hungry, feelings of drowsiness that tell you when you need rest, pain that tells you when there is a dysfunction or imbalance in the body, and even feelings of uneasiness that warn you of impending danger.

Unfortunately, many people do not understand or are unaware of these vital warning signs, and even worse, some people ignore them and push themselves to the limit. To be in touch with your body and listen to its various signals is not only essential to maintaining good health, but also ensures your very survival. I would, therefore, like to discuss some more ways in which our bodies communicate with us.

One method the body uses is to drum up feelings of discomfort. Some of the more common sensations include nausea, bloating, gas, diarrhea, heartburn, and constipation. Any of these may occur immediately following a meal or even several hours afterward. It is important to understand that these feelings are not normal in any way. Commercials that advertise over-the-counter (OTC) medications may try to convince us that they are and that by merely taking their products can we combat these problems in an oh-so-normal way. But don't buy it for a minute—these symptoms are actually the body's way of alerting us that something is not quite right and that you have probably ingested something your body does not tolerate very well.

"But wait," you might ask, "food is food, isn't it? Why shouldn't my body be able to handle whatever I give it?" The reason is that everybody is different. We have different makeups, different chemistries, and different needs. We may be sensitive to certain foods, even some that medical science does not yet recognize as causing adverse reactions. It is precisely because everybody is so different that some foods might bother you and not others. And the foods that do bother you must be uncovered through a process of trial and error.

Sometimes this task will be simple, and sometimes it will not; but it is certainly worth investigating. Some of the foods that I have found to bother me are chocolate, caffeine, mint, basil, cilantro, and pork. Sounds crazy, right? But they do. I love eating each one of these foods, but my body isn't very happy when I do. Each causes me to react miserably either with gas, cough, or a runny nose. I still eat these things on occasion (OK, coffee more than just occasionally), but I know that when I do, I will have to pay the price later. My symptoms are my body's way of letting me know that these foods do not agree with me. "Eat what makes me unhappy, and I'll make *you* unhappy" is what my body tells me. The key is to find out which foods bother you and either avoid them completely or simply minimize their intake. By listening to your body, you will always be led in the right direction.

Another way your body communicates with you is through cravings, which we all have from time to time—be it for greens, fruits, or protein (meat or otherwise). Listen to these signs and eat those foods accordingly. It is important to be careful, though. When unbalanced, our bodies might also crave things that are not so good for us like sugar, alcohol, or even chemical additives. I find this to be especially true with foods that we are sensitive to—just another reason to identify them. When you consistently avoid these items, your body will rebalance itself and eventually stop the cravings. It takes time, but recognition is the first step. Again, be sure to listen to your body.

Not only does your body tell you what to avoid, but as you become more in tune with its messages, you'll find that it also tells you what it likes. You'll begin to recognize which foods, and even which activities, make you feel alive and energetic. For instance, your body will tell you how many hours of sleep you need to feel properly rested. You will also recognize when your body feels out of whack, when you need to visit a chiropractor, when you need to stretch, or when you just need to move in general. This is the beauty of connecting to your body and being aware of the many messages it sends you on a daily basis. Do not ignore them. Listen, and your body will guide you wisely.

As you get even better at recognizing these physical messages, you will also start to develop a greater understanding of your intuitive senses. Intuitive messages come from a much deeper place than the conscious mind and can tell you if you are in danger, when a situation is in your best interest, or even if a relationship is taking you down the right or wrong path. All these things are communicated to you through intuition. Like any skill, it must be nurtured and developed, and a good place to start is by recognizing the basic messages your body sends you after you eat. Have fun and pay close attention to what your body tells you.

### Rule 10: Take it easy—don't be too strict with yourself

Ahhh . . . This rule is so important. I find that when some make the commitment to change, they may actually become fanatical. Some people do this to keep themselves on track; however, they may become so strict that they lose the flexibility to adapt to an ever-changing environment.

This, my friends, is a big mistake. It is the surest way to trash the entire effort toward change. Being hard on oneself only creates unnecessary feelings of anger and guilt that can lead one to give up or become bitter, depressed, or an all-around drag to be around.

Why put yourself through that hardship? It's not worth it. Instead, be realistic about your health, your goals, and your routine. If you slip, slip! It's no big deal. But you must also be honest with yourself. Do you slip only once in a while, or do you find yourself making a lot of excuses? You know the truth. Whatever the case may be, just know that indulging occasionally in the things you like is sometimes good for the psyche.

If you find that you crave a food that bothers you, say chocolate for instance, then eat it once in a while. My God, life is worth living after all, even if it is with a little bit of recklessness now and again. And don't guilt-trip yourself either. Enjoy it. Once in a blue moon ain't gonna kill you. But if chocolate makes you break out into hives or pork causes you to have a three-day bout of diarrhea, then you'll have to ask yourself if it is actually worth it. If, however, you only have minor discomfort from these foods, then by all means, indulge in them periodically.

What, then, should we consider "periodically"? Again, you have to be honest with yourself and judge wisely. Do you smoke an occasional cigar? Eat a piece of cheesecake once in a while? Have a few drinks on Friday night with the boys? Don't sweat it. Really, life is meant to be enjoyed. Occasionally indulging in the things you enjoy but which may not always agree with you can be as important to your health as mostly avoiding them. This is very different from indulging in foods or behaviors excessively—smoking a pack of cigarettes a day, eating a bag of cookies every night, or drinking till you drop—as they will ultimately lead to poor health.

The bottom line here and actually one of the running themes of this book is to understand that consistency is the key. Occasional indulgences make us happy and give us a chance to be carefree. It is only when our indulgences become habits that they present a problem. This is precisely what is wrong with smoking in general (chapter 7). Cigarettes are so highly addictive that attempting to smoke only on occasion is futile. True, some people can take it or leave it, but I bet you know very few who demonstrate this type of discipline. The large majority of us who pick up the smoking pastime actually become addicted. And guess what? At this point, we can no longer consider it an occasional indulgence. Occasional indulgences often become habits; and these, in turn, can quickly turn into addictions. If you can live without some of the more highly addictive substances like nicotine, alcohol, sugar, or diet soda, then by all mean do. Otherwise, know the risks and moderate yourself. But don't be fanatical, either—at least not if you wish to maintain your good senses. Your sanity depends on it.

## Water: The Importance of Staying Hydrated

Our bodies are comprised mostly of water, 55 percent in females and 60 percent in males to be exact.[57] Because of water's ability to dissolve so many substances, it is known as the universal solvent. Water is the medium for all biochemical processes and is also the major component of body fluids like blood, digestive juices, and saliva to name just a few. It has a role in nutrient transport and waste elimination from the body. So put very simply, water is essential to all life. Without it, we would die.

Humans have no long-term storage system for water; therefore, we must replenish stores daily. Neglecting this may lead to dehydration. Dehydration is not a condition to be taken lightly. Losing 10 percent of our body water can kill us while losing as little as 1 to 2 percent can cause any number of complications.[58] As a point of reference, it is possible to live without food for several weeks, but without water, an adult will die within ten days. Children can last for only five days without water. The bottom line: drinking water is as important to life as breathing itself.

It is amazing how many people ignore this important fact. I ask all my incoming patients about their water consumption. Many say, "I don't like water" or "I drink lots of juice or tea." Sorry, guys, it's just not the same thing. Others say, "I know I should drink water, but I just can't bring myself to do it." Well, you'd better. If you don't, you'll end up paying the price later. Losing as little as 1 percent can cause weakness, dizziness, or fatigue. I call this state *subclinical dehydration* (a.k.a. hypohydration). I use this term to indicate that a person has not yet become clinically dehydrated—a medical emergency—but has lost enough water to affect them physiologically. The signs and symptoms of subclinical dehydration are dry mouth, dizziness, weakness, fatigue, confusion, constipation, heart palpitations, increased body temperature, and a low output of dark and concentrated urine. When subclinical dehydration becomes chronic, it can affect all body processes and organs including the heart, muscles, blood vessels, digestive tract, immune system, kidneys, temperature regulation system, and the brain. Each one of these becomes compromised when water levels get too low.

Clinical dehydration, as I have said before, is a medical emergency. People who allow themselves to get this depleted of water can actually go into shock. Every year, thousands are hospitalized for symptoms related to dehydration; and it is, in fact, one of the most common causes of hospitalization of elderly people. Dehydration can lead to heat cramps, heat exhaustion, and heatstroke. In 2001, NFL lineman Korey Stringer died from complications related to heatstroke.

Dehydration occurs when a person's water intake is less than that lost through sweat, breath, urine, and defecation. Although an internal thirst mechanism alerts us to our hydration needs, it does not always function properly, and sometimes people can misunderstand the signals. For instance, humid conditions retard the thirst mechanism while hot and dry conditions rapidly evaporate sweat, leading people to miscalculate how much fluid they have actually lost.[59] The solution is to always replenish your internal water supply by drinking plenty throughout the day *before* you get thirsty. Always keep a water bottle handy—in your car, in your office, and when you work out—making it an accessory. We sweat even more on hot days, particularly when active. During these times, it is especially necessary to keep a bottle of water around for replenishment. Please note that when your urine volume is low and dark in color, dehydration is not far off. When this is the case, start the hydration process immediately. During dehydration, the rate that water leaves the stomach and enters the intestines for absorption slows down, making replenishment that much harder. It is therefore crucial to be conscious of your water intake at all times, even more so if you drink alcohol or caffeine. These substances are diuretics; that is, they make you urinate. So drinking them will cause you to lose more water than usual. Drink at least one glass of water for each dehydrating beverage you have. It's a good rule to live by.

Another good hydrating habit is to drink at least two liters of water per day, *every day*. Drink as much as you comfortably can. Then after several days of doing so, make it a habit to drink three sips of water every half hour. Drink a glass of water upon awaking first thing in the morning and drink plenty when you work out. The more water you drink, the more you'll become conscious of your hydration needs; and eventually, you'll have no problem providing your body with exactly the amount of water it needs.

Being properly hydrated not only assures you of functioning optimally but has cosmetic effects as well. For instance, sufficient hydration leads to soft and supple skin. Anything that increases dehydration leads to wrinkling and includes many medications, recreational drugs, alcohol, and even cigarettes. Although kicking these habits is by far the best remedy, simply increasing your water intake will counterbalance the ill effects caused by these toxic and dehydrating substances.

Another benefit to being properly hydrated is that it might actually help people lose weight. By drinking plenty of water, we feel full longer. Some people may even overeat because of not being sufficiently hydrated. Experts believe that subclinical dehydration leads to hunger pangs *before* the thirst mechanism kicks in, fooling some people to believe that they are hungry when, in fact, what they really need is water. A recent study suggests that sufficient hydration may increase one's metabolic rate, leading to an increased burning of calories. This is exciting news for anyone trying to lose weight. By combining adequate water intake with eating smaller portions and exercising regularly, you may find that you are losing more weight than ever before.

Drinking sports replacement drinks (chapter 3), by the way, is not a substitute for drinking water. Although they are great for replenishing electrolytes (sodium, potassium, and chloride) that are lost through sweat, they are not meant to be consumed during times of inactivity. Sports drinks are preferable for athletes *during* their athletic activity (especially if greater than one hour in length) or afterward, but not before a workout or sporting event as they may affect performance by causing premature fatigue.[60] Drinking a sports replacement drink when you are not exercising is only slightly better than drinking a soda since it is high in sugar and can lead to weight gain. Obviously, the added electrolytes make it preferable to soda, but I would not recommend it as beverage of choice during leisure times. For that, you will be better off drinking water.

When we are properly hydrated, we are in metabolic balance. When we become water deficient, all of our organs and tissues become stressed, even down to the cellular level and, as a result, cannot function to their full capacity. By maintaining our water balance at all times, we guarantee optimal performance from every one of our systems. Drinking enough water may seem hard initially, but I guarantee it will feel as natural as breathing once you make it a regular and daily habit.

## Preventing Some of Today's Most Prevalent Disorders

Now that we have discussed ten simple rules of diet that will virtually guarantee optimal nutrition when followed diligently, let us look at some of today's most prevalent dietary disorders so that we may better understand them, combat them, and, hopefully, even reverse them. The three disorders we will investigate are obesity, diabetes, and eating disorders like anorexia and bulimia.

## Obesity

Obesity, as we have already pointed out, is epidemic in this country. Two-thirds of the population is considered overweight or obese. A 2003 report from the RAND Corporation uncovered an even more disturbing fact: one in every fifty American adults is now "extremely obese" or greater than one hundred pounds overweight![61] This form of *severe obesity* is increasing at a much faster rate than obesity itself. The report's author accurately predicts that extreme obesity will become more prevalent at its current rate and will further tax an already strained medical system.

All analysts can agree on one thing: obesity is due, in part, to the excessive intake of calories, or, simply, overeating. Another major contributing factor is a lack of *regular* exercise. The principle is basic: if you take in more calories than you use, you gain weight. But I would like to offer a third factor that I believe plays a large part in excessive weight gain—one that is perhaps not addressed often enough, if at all—and that is the psychological component of obesity.

Weight problems, especially extreme ones, are almost never purely physical. Emotional aspects are often involved and may be so strong that they act as an obstacle to successful weight loss. I have observed many patients battling obesity who had serious self-esteem issues underlying their problem. Whether they felt self-loathing or guilt or even suffered emotional abuse at the hands of a loved-one, these people struggle in one way or another with severe emotional issues. We all have insecurities, but obese individuals tend to comfort themselves by overindulging in food and/or drinks. Whatever the cause of their pain, their basic need is to feel loved (true for all of us), but love has to start from within. The best thing one can do to help these people is to be supportive, show no disappointment if they relapse, and let them know they are loved no matter what.

For obese people, it is important that they love themselves first regardless of their circumstances. I realize this may be easier said than done, but recovery begins here. This is true with any addiction—be it with food, drugs, or sex. It means loving yourself regardless of your shape or size and accepting yourself at this present moment. If you need support, please hire a therapist or join a support group. However, I urge you to keep away from anyone or any group that enables you to continue on a path of self-destruction by advocating the idea that you are not in control of the situation. This is the biggest lie that can ever be fed to you and is perhaps the biggest obstacle you will ever face.

Accept the responsibility of your condition completely, that is *you are where you have allowed yourself to go, and you are equally capable of going in the opposite direction at any given time.* By loving yourself, the energetic composition of your body will ultimately change (chapter 6), allowing your physical efforts to take over. Even Oprah Winfrey has said that she was only able to lose her weight once she accepted herself exactly as she was. When you can achieve this mental state, you will naturally be drawn to doing things that are good for you, like exercising and eating right. Just follow the ten simple rules of eating as previously outlined, and the weight will shed naturally. It is simply impossible not to lose weight if you burn more calories than you take in—*absolutely impossible.* So for those of you who seem to respond poorly to eating less and exercising more, practice self-love and self-acceptance immediately. Do not allow the state you are in to dictate how you feel about yourself. Start loving yourself now, and your body will reshape into its most natural and healthful form.

## Diabetes

Another common dietary disorder is the devastating disease known as *diabetes.* This is a very serious condition characterized by a defect in carbohydrate metabolism. There are different types of diabetes, but they all have two things in common: glucose intolerance and high blood sugar. Glucose intolerance can be due either to the inability to properly produce insulin (insulin is necessary to bring glucose or sugar into cells), or to insulin resistance. Glucose is a carbohydrate and, as we have said before, is needed for energy production. When deficient in glucose, cells waste away, breaking down their own protein for fuel. High concentrations of sugar in the blood cause long-term damage in virtually every organ and tissue in the body, including the heart, blood vessels, kidneys, eyes, nerves, and skin. Along with cigarette smoking and chronic alcohol abuse, diabetes is one of the most extensively damaging disorders to the human body. Some of the more common complications associated with diabetes are heart disease, blindness, neuropathy, skin ulcers, lowered immunity, and depression. Diabetes is also the most common cause of limb amputation in adults.

Type 1 diabetes is the inability to produce insulin. People who have type 1 diabetes are born with it, and they must administer insulin through regular injections. The form I wish to focus on here, though, is type 2 diabetes. It is also called *noninsulin-dependent diabetes mellitus* (NIDDM) since the body produces adequate amounts of insulin but has a problem responding to it. It is not completely understood how this dysfunction sets in. But one theory is that the insulin receptors become "desensitized," or that the cells stop placing receptors on their surface; and without surface receptors, insulin cannot "open the gate" for glucose to enter the cell. No glucose, no energy; and even worse, glucose accumulates in the blood.

A couple of disturbing facts remain regarding type 2 diabetes:

1.   It represents 90 percent of all diabetes cases.
2.   Is strongly associated with obesity.

The easiest way to prevent type 2 diabetes is to control one's weight. If all the other devastating health consequences associated with obesity are not enough to scare you, then the details of diabetes certainly should. Some things you can do to prevent this disorder are to reduce food portions, minimize soda consumption, and reduce or completely discontinue eating processed foods. Additionally, remember to balance your diet with an adequate amount of fats and proteins since type 2 diabetes is a disease of sugar (carbohydrate) imbalance.

## Eating Disorders

Finally, I would like to discuss a couple of eating disorders currently devastating scores of young women and men in our society, anorexia and bulimia. These are the two most common eating disorders afflicting people today. Both are very complicated, and I do not wish to trivialize them here with an oversimplification of the facts. However, discussing them in detail would take us away from the scope of this book, so all I wish to do here is discuss them with respect to their psychological aspect regarding food.

Both of these eating disorders have to do with issues relating to body image. What this means is that people who suffer from these disorders have a convoluted perception of what their bodies should look like. In general, they are afraid of looking fat. This is quite possibly one of the saddest situations we have to deal with in Western society. In our culture, we are perpetually inundated with images of ultrathin women (and men, but particularly women) in films, television, and on the covers of popular fashion magazines. As a result, thin has become our societal ideal of beauty. This is an especially tragic situation for our youth as children and adolescents are so impressionable, particularly when it comes to looks. By being constantly reminded that thin is beautiful, it almost guarantees a flirtation with an eating disorder. When celebrities become "too thin," the media glorifies them by pasting them on the cover of every major tabloid sold in the country. What else are children to think when an emaciated celebrity gets so much media attention and adoration?

The reality is that eating disorders are a result of nonacceptance of one's body type and shape. There is no easy answer to this problem other than to teach your children that skinny is not necessarily beautiful, but *healthy* is. When they understand this and they have great role models at home (another reason for parents to follow the *six keys to optimal health*), then their chances of developing an eating disorder decrease exponentially. Show them images of healthy-looking people and rave over them. Most importantly, teach them early on about health and get healthy yourself. Naturally healthy people develop their normal body shapes and sizes. In my opinion, there is nothing more beautiful than a natural-looking body. You can bet my children will be raised with this notion too. As far as society's obsession with thinness is concerned, the changes must start with us foremost. Stop buying magazines that promote this absurdity, and maybe their editors will find different images to entertain us with. This is not going to happen overnight, but it has to start somewhere.

This concludes our chapter on the first key to optimal health. The take-home lesson is that diet is a dynamic process and needs to be modified periodically. It is better to adhere to a sound set of principles based on what we *know* about digestion than to follow the often limited and unproven ones set forth by a number of today's more popular fad diets. These principles must be flexible enough to allow for variance among human beings while taking into account their changing needs shaped by an ever-changing environment. Fad diets usually incorporate into their programs only one or two of the principles we have discussed here but often neglect many of the others that are essential for a complete nutritional regimen. None of the principles discussed in this chapter can be ignored; not if you wish to maintain your health, that is.

What I have presented here is not a diet per se, but tools with which to guide your eating habits. Nothing is set in stone—just use common sense and a bit of moderation. A balanced diet of whole foods is generally the best, and it helps to supplement with vitamins. If you are someone who requires proof, then do the research yourself. The information is available to anyone who wants it through books, magazines, and the Internet. Sure, you might have to sift through a plethora of conflicting information; but by investigating this subject yourself, you will see that the advice I have given is based on sound science. It is true that some of my points may seem abstract, but a different way of thinking is exactly what is in order to make the changes so desperately needed. Too many people are overweight and malnourished. Too many of our children despise their bodies. And fad diets have yet to provide a solution. The best proof comes from trying something yourself. Commit to following these principles for six months, and I promise you will be sold. Fad diets may promise miracles, but the only miracle I promise is an advancement toward your most natural state of being—one of fantastic health.

# Chapter 2 Summary

## Key Number 1: Diet and Nutrition

- Eat whole, natural foods as much as possible.
- Make sure to match your diet with your current activity level (e.g., times of high mental activity require carbohydrates; wound healing, pregnancy, and child growth require protein). Low activity levels call for lower carbohydrate intake.
- Make sure to get plenty of fats in your diet, especially the omega-3s found in fish and seeds.
- Eat in peace.
- Chew your food adequately. Slow down.
- Eat at home. Go grocery shopping, buy a bunch of food for the week, and eat in.
- Take your vitamins. Take them at least twice a day, morning and evening.
- Don't overeat. Slow down and listen to your body.
- Minimize processed foods. Here's a short list: soda, chips, fries, corn dogs, cakes, candy, frozen foods, and microwavable foods.
- Reduce intake of high-fructose corn syrup (HFCS). The list is the same as above. Also, reduce artificial sweeteners.
- Eat at about the same time every day. Don't skip meals.
- Listen to your body's messages. Gas, heartburn, and feelings of overfullness are all warning signals.
- Indulge at least once a week (sometimes more).
- Drink two liters of water every day.

# CHAPTER 3

# Movement: The Lifestyle of Fitness

*All parts of the body which have a function, if used in moderation and exercised in labours in which each is accustomed, become thereby healthy, well-developed and age more slowly, but if unused and left idle they become liable to disease, defective in growth, and age quickly.*
—Hippocrates, the Father of Medicine (460-377 BC)

*Lack of activity destroys the good condition of every human being, while movement and methodical physical exercise save it and preserve it.*
—Plato

MOVEMENT AND FITNESS have been an integral part of man since he first started walking upright. A sturdy body allowed man to adapt to a constantly changing environment while giving him the strength and endurance to successfully perform his daily activities. Whether catching food, escaping predators, or toiling the fields, a well-conditioned body offered man a distinct advantage over his surroundings and his competition. For the most part, man conditioned himself through his work, but he eventually figured out that physical training could make him even better at carrying out his endeavors.

Although the Chinese practiced some version of physical fitness as early as 2600 BC and yoga has been said to have originated over seven thousand years ago, it is the method devised by the ancient Greeks that most closely resembles what we do today. The idea of working out at a gym actually originated in ancient Greece around 460 BC. Young men there went to the *gymnasium* to receive a formal education, and the curriculum always included some type of physical training. Even children were routinely educated on the importance of regular exercise. In some ways, the Greek form of exercise differed greatly from our own. For example, they often exercised in the nude. This is because the gymnasium—a word that has its origin in the root *gymnazein*, meaning "naked"—was also the public bathhouse. They knew very well back then the importance of combining bodywork (chapter 4) with physical activity, and so they made sure that every health club had its own spa.

As for the Greek method of exercise, it was not really that much different from what we do today. The Greeks developed upper body strength by sparring with heavy objects like swords and shields, and they developed powerful legs by lifting or wrestling. For endurance, they would run or swim. Although the Greeks may not have known every scientific detail behind their fitness practices, they certainly knew how to take full advantage of the benefits.

It was not until the early twentieth century that the science behind exercise physiology really took off. In 1920, Danish scientist August Krogh won the Nobel Prize for discovering that blood vessels increase their capillary surfaces during exercise, allowing the body to take in more oxygen. He also uncovered the body's ability to use fat as a fuel for exercising muscles. Otto Meyerhoff and A. V. Hill won the Nobel Prize for discovering a relationship between oxygen uptake and lactic acid metabolism (anaerobic respiration).

In 1927, the Harvard Fatigue Laboratory was created.[62] This was the first institution developed for the sole purpose of studying human health and fitness. Scientists there studied things like exercising at high altitudes, exercising in hot climates, and the effects of exercise on aging. They were also one of the first groups to quantify measurements like maximal heart rate and maximal oxygen uptake. Much of our earliest knowledge on human health and fitness originated from the work carried out at this lab, and many experts in the field today regard this institution as the birthplace of exercise physiology.

Although a scientific understanding of physical fitness was under way, there were still a number of misconceptions regarding exercise at that time. For instance, it was a common belief that weight training would ruin an athlete. Coaches felt that this type of exercise would bulk athletes up and ultimately slow them down. Weight lifting was therefore shunned as a viable means of training. Endurance training was also looked upon unfavorably. It was considered too strenuous for the heart, and people were strongly discouraged from doing it. Women and older people could pretty much forget physical fitness altogether as it was considered dangerous for either one of these more "fragile" groups to partake in exercise.[63] Fortunately, the work of the Harvard Fatigue Laboratory and other pioneers led to the dismantling of those outdated theories.

The field of exercise physiology saw great advances during the second half of the twentieth century. The National Athletic Trainer's Association (NATA) became an official organization in 1950 while the American College of Sports Medicine (ACSM) followed suit in 1954. These organizations were among the first to specialize in training and caring for athletes, and they added a sense of legitimacy to the exercise sciences. Through modern research practices, scientists began to understand the physiology behind weight training and its effects on muscle tissue. Studies confirmed that stressing muscles through exercise (including the heart) could lead to great gains in strength and performance. This was known as the *overload principle*, and it has become the basis for all forms of exercise done today.

It was also during the 1950s that a pioneering star in the world of fitness began to rise—his name was Jack La Lanne. *The Jack La Lanne Show* enjoyed a popular run on television, spanning several decades. He instructed people on the ins and outs of aerobic exercise, water aerobics, and resistance training. Jack La Lanne is considered the Godfather of Instructional Fitness, and he paved the way for such icons as Jane Fonda, Richard Simmons, and Susan Powter. We attribute La Lanne with the introduction of many pieces of exercise equipment including the cable pulley, leg extension machine, and Smith machine—a safety system for doing squats and other exercises. We can even thank him for teaching us the simple yet effective movement known as the *jumping jack*.[64] This man was a forward thinker in the truest sense of the word, and his philosophy on health, fitness, and prevention were definitely ahead of its time. We owe much to him for bringing the concept of "exercise as lifestyle" back into modern thinking.

While Jack La Lanne was bringing exercise into the homes of millions of Americans, the sport of bodybuilding was playing its part in glamorizing physical fitness. Bodybuilding was first recognized as a commercial sport in the early twentieth century. It had its fair share of stars like the chiseled Charles Atlas. Who can forget those ads of his: Skinny wimp gets sand kicked in his face by the arrogant bully and loses the girl. Wimp embarks on bodybuilding program, gains size and confidence, and ultimately wins back his girl—all by knocking out the now-smaller bully. That ad inspired many young men to exercise, and as a result, dumbbell sales skyrocketed in the 1920s.

The sport of bodybuilding worked hard to distinguish itself from traditional weight lifting. With the latter, the goal was to lift the heaviest weight possible whereas with bodybuilding, it was all about physical development. Bodybuilding not only motivated people to improve their looks, but also to maintain health through regular resistance exercises. Men like Joe Gold (founder of Gold's Gyms), Harold Zinkin (inventor of the Universal Gym Machine), George Reeves (Superman), Joe Weider (*Men's Fitness* magazine), and Arnold Schwarzenegger made bodybuilding and, consequently, resistance training the worldwide phenomena they are today. We owe a great deal to these men for increasing our awareness of this very valuable form of fitness.

The 1950s were a busy time for the health and fitness industry. With the advancement of scientific knowledge, as well as the development of athletic organizations, the federal government enacted its first policies on physical fitness. In response to America's poor performance in the "Minimum Muscular Fitness Tests," President Dwight D. Eisenhower formed the President's Council on Youth Fitness.[65] Along with the American Medical Association (AMA), the American Health Association, and the American Physical Education Association (APEA), the president's council sought to educate the public on the dangers of being physically out of shape. The government recognized that a country is only as strong as its fittest citizens and therefore pursued the campaign vigorously. The result was an increased national awareness, and it became a huge factor in legitimizing the fitness movement.

Despite the recognition, not all Americans caught on. Fitness levels remained substandard. Experts took the cue and began studying the health risks associated with poor physical conditioning. In the 1960s, evidence surfaced implicating the lack of exercise as a risk factor in the development of numerous degenerative disorders, most notably ischemic heart disease.[66] This prompted President John F. Kennedy to revamp Eisenhower's fitness council, renaming it the President's Council on Physical Fitness. In an article he wrote for *Sports Illustrated* magazine titled "The Soft American," Kennedy pointed out the need for Americans to seriously improve their condition. He noted that "Physical fitness is the basis for all other forms of excellence," and he pushed the federal government to pursue an even greater role to ensure its end.

Over the last thirty years, the public's participation in fitness for health has heightened, leading to an unprecedented explosion in the health club industry. Gyms are now a staple in every American city, with numbers reaching a record seventeen thousand in the United States alone.[67] Yoga and Pilates studios also enjoy increased memberships as people seek alternative ways to improve their health through exercise. Studies are finally being carried out to look at the effects of exercise on women and older adults. And the federal government continues to play its part in advocating fitness as lifestyle with their Healthy People 2000 and 2010 campaigns. The goals of these programs are to "increase life expectancy and improve [the] quality of life" for people of all ages and "to eliminate health disparities among different segments of the population."[68]

Many Americans have clearly taken the exercise-regularly campaign to heart, yet in spite of this, the percentage of the population exercising consistently is still only 55 percent.[69] According to a 2000 poll by Maritz Research, people who do not exercise cite "lack of time" as the most common reason they keep from doing it. We can certainly acknowledge that today's high-paced lifestyle makes it increasingly difficult to find the time to work out. However, people must simply *make* the time for exercise just as they make time to eat, rest, or to have a social life. Regular physical fitness is nothing less than a matter of life or death. No exaggeration here. Read on, and you will see that without regular exercise, your body will deteriorate and age rapidly. On the other hand, by exercising regularly, not only can you add years to your life, but you can definitely improve the quality of your life as well.

Unfortunately, too many people see exercise solely as a means to an end. If asked, many people will admit that they work out mainly to improve their looks. While nothing is wrong with this desire per se, it is simply not enough to keep one motivated for very long. This approach can also lead to unrealistic expectations (like trying to lose a large amount of weight in an unreasonable amount of time) and, when not immediately realized, might cause some people to feel discouraged and give up their efforts altogether. This is especially true in today's push-button culture where people have been conditioned to seek instant gratification. Many people give up when faced with challenges and tend to shift to more comfortable behaviors. To foster long-term motivation, something more than physical appearance is needed to keep one's interest sustained. That "something" is a new way of looking at exercise in general. It is having an intellectual understanding of all the benefits related to physical activity, many of which go well beyond just looking good. The goal of this chapter is to help you achieve a deeper understanding of the advantages that make exercise a necessary component of every health regimen.

If you can shift your view of exercise to fit this context, it will help you from feeling any unnecessary guilt when you miss a few sessions. A well-known disorder afflicting many people (mostly men) who lift weights regularly is *muscle dysmorphia*. This condition causes people to obsess about their muscularity, feeling small despite having normal or large muscle mass. Another name for this psychological disorder is *bigorexia*, and it is estimated to affect up to 10 percent of all male bodybuilders.[70] I believe that even more people suffer from a slightly lessened version of this disorder, which manifests itself as guilt when that person misses an exercise session. They have an irrational fear of "losing it" if they do not work out continuously, and some may even use it to push themselves to the brink of exhaustion. Anyone who works out regularly will know exactly what I'm talking about as we have all experienced it to some degree or another. But please understand that this is only a mind game. You simply do not lose muscle mass that quickly. A one- or two-month hiatus is a different story as *atrophy* (decreased muscle mass) sets in over this length of time. But you certainly won't lose muscle in a day or two. By breaking the habit of exercising only for the sake of looks, you will prevent yourself from falling victim to lost motivation or to the little tricks your mind might play on you.

## Physiological Effects of Exercise

Putting exercise into a new perspective starts first by understanding how it affects your body physiologically. Exercise puts stress on the body, especially the heart and skeletal muscle, and forces it to adjust, bringing itself back into balance. This process is known as *homeostasis*. Basically, this is the body's ability to withstand stress by creating internal changes, which allow it to adapt to its environment. The function of homeostasis is vital to ensure the survivability of an organism. With regard to exercise, homeostasis allows us to change physically in order to better accommodate outside stressors.

An immediate physical change that occurs during exercise, like increased heart rate, is known as a *response* while long-term ones, like muscle growth, are known as *adaptation*.[71] Adaptation occurs as a result of repeated stress and generally involves the production or degradation of cellular proteins. *Overload* is the method of progressively increasing the intensity, duration, or frequency of exercise to continue the body's adaptive process. The overload principle is the basis of all successful exercise programs.

To fully understand the benefits of exercise, though, one must understand the physiological processes that occur in the muscle cells themselves during different types of activity. Most of the benefits associated with exercise have to do with the body's incredible ability to adapt. Three of the adaptive processes the body goes through are increased strength, increased endurance, and increased flexibility.

Strength is determined mainly by the size of a muscle. Individual muscle fibers grow in diameter in response to stress, and this increases the mass and bulk of the muscle. Although there are a few different theories available to explain this process, the most popular one relates to the tearing of muscle fibers. Torn fibers need repair, and the body does this by adding more contractile proteins, which in turn increases girth.

Endurance, on the other hand, is determined by the amount of mitochondria present in the muscle cells. *Mitochondria* are the structures of the cells (organelles) responsible for energy production—the more mitochondria available, the better able to perform aerobic respiration. In aerobic respiration, mitochondria use oxygen to produce a large amount of energy. Because of their role in energy production, mitochondria are known as the powerhouse of the cells. The more mitochondria present in the muscle tissue, the more energy available for long-term endurance activities.

The third type of adaptive process is muscle flexibility. It involves the lengthening of fibers, usually through stretching, that allows a joint to move through its full range of motion. This process actually involves a form of muscle growth that adds fibers to the ends of the muscle tissue. It increases the muscle's physical length without distorting the tissue itself. This property makes muscle tissue elastic and, much like a rubber band, allows it to retain its tautness even after being stretched. The length of any muscle fiber determines the overall force of its contraction—longer fibers generating more force than shorter ones. Flexible muscles, then, have a greater power of contraction, and this in turn increases their strength. On the flip side, muscles not stretched regularly lose fibers on their ends and become shorter over time.

At this point, it will be useful to discuss how muscles derive energy to carry out their functions. By understanding this, you will see the difference between various exercises and how they affect your body, and you will therefore be able to choose the methods that best accommodate your needs. The basic source of energy in our cells is adenosine triphosphate (ATP). Only limited amounts of ATP are actually stored in the muscle tissue—in fact, just enough for about three seconds of maximal muscle power.[72] The muscles also store another high-energy molecule called *phosphocreatine*, which is capable of producing between five to seven seconds of maximal muscle power—enough for a hundred-meter dash. *Creatine supplementation*, which has become popular with bodybuilders, increases the storage of phosphocreatine in the muscle tissue and, as a result, leads to greater power outputs. Bodybuilders taking this supplement can lift more weight, which, of course, leads to greater muscle growth. The ATP and phosphocreatine systems are what we would call *anaerobic*; that is, they work in the absence of oxygen. Anaerobic respiration is the form of energy production that predominates in quick, explosive actions like sprints or lifting heavy objects.

Another form of anaerobic energy production is the process of glycolysis. *Glycolysis* is the breakdown of sugar molecules (glucose) to form ATP (energy). The sugar comes from glycogen stores present in the muscle tissue and liver. If oxygen is in ample supply, the by-product of glycolysis, *pyruvate*, goes through a chemical reaction called *oxidative phosphorylation* to form large amounts of ATP. However, if oxygen levels are low, pyruvate is converted to lactic acid. Glycolysis manufactures ATP rapidly, and although producing only limited amounts, this quick energy can be used for intense muscle contraction like when lifting weights. The glycolytic system can provide up to a minute and a half of maximal muscle power, in addition to the other two anaerobic systems (stored muscle ATP and phosphocreatine). Because glycolysis depletes the somewhat small stores of glycogen in the muscles and liver, it is important to always replenish them during and after a workout. Any type of high-carbohydrate meal will do, but I personally prefer sports replacement drinks (Gatorade or Powerade). These are high in glucose; so they will not only restock the precious glycogen stores, but also cause us to become thirsty, which will remind us to rehydrate with water.

As I have just mentioned, when oxygen is in ample supply, the glycolytic by-product—pyruvate—goes into the mitochondria and is further metabolized to produce large quantities of ATP. This is called *aerobic respiration*, and it is oxygen dependent. Glucose is not the only molecule metabolized this way. Fatty acids, or fat, also go through oxidation. Energy obtained aerobically does not happen as quickly as anaerobically, but is produced for an unlimited amount of time—that is, as long as sufficient nutrients are available. The aerobic system, therefore, is important for activities requiring endurance as opposed to those needing a quick surge of power. It is important to note that muscles trained for endurance have higher concentrations of mitochondria than muscles trained for strength. Remember that the mitochondrion is where oxidative phosphorylation occurs (ATP produced in large quantities), and a high concentration in certain muscles is vital for carrying out endurance activities. Larger and stronger muscles actually have less mitochondria since contractile proteins occupy the majority of the muscle's volume. This is known as *mitochondrial dilution* and actually limits the endurance of the muscle involved.[73] This will be an important point for our next discussion regarding the three pillars of exercise.

## The Three Pillars of Exercise

Now that we have discussed the effects of exercise from a physiological standpoint, we can look at its three primary forms more closely. They are known as the *three pillars of exercise*, which consist of resistance, cardiovascular, and flexibility training. Each has its own distinct function and adds a different set of benefits to overall health and fitness. Athletes focusing on a particular sport may be able to concentrate on one or two of these activities solely, but for a person mostly interested in improving or maintaining health, it is of great benefit to devote time to each one of these training modalities.

### Resistance training

The first pillar of exercise is *resistance training*. Lifting weights is the most popular form, but there are several other ways to do it. Basically, any use of muscular contraction against resistance to increase mass and strength falls into this category. Power training is a subtype of this exercise and relates to the greatest amount of force produced in the shortest amount of time. Whereas power training is important for certain athletes, like football linemen or big men in basketball, *strength training* (force produced independent of time) is usually sufficient for the average person.

Resistance training not only increases strength and size but has many other benefits as well. To begin with, it increases blood flow to the areas exercised, which brings oxygen and nutrients to surrounding muscles and tissues. Tissues that are regularly perfused with blood tend to look better and give a healthier glow. Moreover, resistance training is particularly advantageous for people as they age or for people who remain mostly sedentary as they run the risk of developing blood clots from stagnating blood.

Resistance exercise also prevents muscles from atrophying (atrophy is a decrease in size). Muscles that are not used regularly tend to waste away—they degenerate or get smaller. Aside from the fact that this does not enhance one's physical appearance, it can lead to a number of various aches and pains. As a chiropractor, I see all too often the effects of muscle atrophy in people complaining of everything from back pain to shoulder pain to arm and leg pain. Many of these painful conditions can be avoided with regular resistance exercise. To make matters worse, atrophied muscles may also cause sagging skin, particularly in people who were at one time "in shape." Skin is attached to muscles through a tissue called *fascia*, and as the muscles grow, the fascia stretches and lengthens. If the muscles are allowed to atrophy, the fascia remains stretched, leaving the skin to sag. A lack of blood flow to the muscles further exacerbates atrophy. By incorporating resistance exercises regularly, not only will you enhance your health, but you will improve your looks as well.

Yet another benefit of resistance exercises is that it affects the health of the skeletal system by increasing bone density. Nineteenth-century surgeon Julius Wolff pointed out that bone forms in areas of increased stress. This is known as Wolff's law. The stress of weight resistance pulling against a bone causes its cells to deposit even more bone tissue. Hence, resistance training is absolutely imperative for anyone at risk of developing *osteoporosis*, a dangerous condition characterized by weak and brittle bones. If not prevented or if left untreated, osteoporosis can lead to broken bones. Although women and the elderly are especially at risk, men can develop it too. Just think about it: by practicing resistance exercises, one can dramatically lower the risk of developing this dreaded condition, which often causes fractures of the shoulder, hip, or spine. Osteoporosis is especially daunting since the fractures it causes often lead to severed arteries and can actually cause death.[74]

Probably the most attractive reason to take up resistance exercise, though, is that it has an unrivaled ability to burn fat. What? Burn fat? You heard me right—weight training is one of the best fat-burning activities available. How unfortunate that so many people are unaware of this fact. If they were, gym memberships would likely go through the roof. Here is how it works: Muscle tissue that has been subjected to the stress of heavy contraction tears microscopically. The metabolic cost of repairing torn muscle is large, and there is no better fuel to power the job than high-energy fatty acids. Most people will labor through extended cardiovascular workouts in an attempt to lose weight, yet they are usually working harder than they have to and getting much less for it. Although cardiovascular training is both beneficial and necessary, it does not accomplish the same fat-burning results as lifting weights does. Here's why: Whereas cardiovascular exercises actually burn more calories during the length of the activity, resistance exercises continue to burn calories long after the session is over. This is especially true when working out the larger muscles of the body, primarily the legs. The legs have the biggest muscles; therefore, they burn the most calories. I know, I know, everybody hates doing legs; however, as a way to burn fat—and eventually lose weight—there is just no better option.

So as we have said, lifting weights is the most popular form of resistance exercise, yet you do not have to limit yourself to just pumping iron. There are several other options available that will allow you to take full advantage of the benefits of resistance training. One way is through open-chained calisthenics (these happen to be my personal favorites). Open chain means that the terminal end joint remains free. It has nothing resisting it—no weight, no surface. Examples of these types of exercises are abdominal crunches, reverse crunches, and other abdominal exercises, as well as full body dips between two parallel bars and chin-ups. I like these because they are *functional* movements; that is, they simulate movements that one may actually do in the real world. Don't get me wrong. I do biceps curls too; but let's face it, other than competitive beer drinking, there aren't many activities that actually require this particular type of movement. I prefer functional movements to nonfunctional ones because they train us in a way that makes us stronger to perform our daily activities. Furthermore, these are usually compound exercises, many muscle groups working together synergistically, which maximize results.

Although I happen to love doing open-chained exercises, people most often do the closed-chained variety. With these exercises, the terminal end joint meets some sort of resistance, like a weight, which acts to prohibit free movement. Exercises that fall into this category are any that require pushing or pulling a weighted object but can also include push-ups, wall squats, or walking lunges—all of which are quite functional in their own right. The beauty of the latter exercises is that one need not belong to a gym to do them. In fact, to some degree, I think they are even better than regular weight lifting because of their functional nature and their ability to hit several muscle groups at the same time.

If you want to receive the benefits of lifting weights but do not wish to join a gym, you can just as easily work out at home. Many household items can act as a resistive force. Bags of soil, five-gallon bottles of water, bricks, or wood can be used in some way to create resistance. Even everyday chores like sweeping, raking leaves, chopping wood, digging holes, or mowing the lawn can be a good workout. Of course, practicing caution is warranted, especially if you've never exercised before, because you can still injure yourself while doing your daily household chores. Basically, for beginners, I definitely recommend joining a gym *and* perhaps even hiring a trainer. This way, you can learn the basics of exercise and ensure yourself the greatest safety when embarking on a new program.

Another way of doing resistance exercises is by using cables or rubber tubing. Both of these methods add resistance consistently throughout the entire range of motion. In contrast, when lifting weights (free weights, like dumbbells or barbells), the resistance varies at different points in the arc of contraction. The benefit of a constant resistive force is that it requires a more prolonged contraction at maximal strength than when lifting a free weight. This adds even greater stress to a muscle, thereby increasing its strength and size.

Speaking of free weights, I prefer them to machines. Most machines allow movement in only one plane (up and down or forward and backward). This has the effect of isolating muscle groups, and while not bad in and of itself, it does not allow for you to work the other supportive muscles in the region. Free weights, on the other hand, force your body to use smaller stabilizer muscles to initiate the movements of the exercise as well as to help you maintain balance. Think about it, if an unsupported weight can move in many different planes at any given time, then it will make you work harder to balance that weight. This has an overall effect of strengthening your stabilizer muscles. Balance is an important and often overlooked function, which many biomechanical processes depend on. For example, how our bodies move as we walk, run, or perform other actions depends on our balance as does our general sense of position. The ways our bodies develop physically also rely on exercising *every* muscle, and this includes our stabilizer muscles. However, machines are fine for beginners or people returning to exercise after an extended layoff. And yes, they are also good for anyone trying to boost their strength without relying on a partner for assistance.

A common experience for anyone who has ever lifted weights is the feeling of *delayed onset muscle soreness* (DOMS). This aching soreness usually follows a workout session one or two days afterward and occurs as a result of metabolic processes that accompany intense muscle contraction. Remember that resistance training is an anaerobic activity, and lactic acid is its metabolic by-product. Lactic acid increases the acidity of the muscle tissue, creating soreness. This process plays an important role in stimulating the repair process of the muscles, and therefore the "no pain, no gain" theory actually holds true. Soreness equates to muscle adaptation, which equals muscle growth. Voila! With soreness, what you have is a properly exercised muscle. If there is no soreness at all following a workout, then you did not stress the muscle enough (too little resistance), and you probably got very little from that session.

As I mentioned earlier, I am a firm believer in joining a gym and hiring a trainer. A gym provides the equipment necessary for a full body workout without making you have to get too creative in the process. I also believe that beginners should hire a trainer, even if for only a few sessions. A trainer can help you clarify your goals as well as teach you the proper way to do each exercise. I can't say this strongly enough: form is everything! Exercise done with poor form not only leads to poor development but is dangerous too. Hire a trainer, buy a book, or read exercise magazines. Do whatever it takes to learn proper form. Take my word for it. Injuries that occur as a result of weight lifting can be tough to treat, and they may even turn you off to exercise altogether. Don't do this to yourself—learn to exercise the right way. Remember, movement should be a lifestyle habit; and for this reason, you'll want to learn how to do it properly.

Let me now take a minute to say something about pushing too hard. It is completely inadvisable. When people exercise intensely but fail to allow for sufficient rest and recuperation between sessions, they run the risk of burnout. This form of burnout is a real disorder with real symptoms, and it is known as *overtraining syndrome*. The warning signs include

- Increased fatigue
- Feeling drained
- Persistent soreness
- Grumpiness or negative attitude
- Loss of appetite
- Insomnia
- Headaches
- Persistent illness, colds, sore throats
- Fidgeting or persistent twitching
- Increased body fat

Overtraining is no joke, and many people suffer from it without even knowing what it is. To avoid overtraining syndrome, you'll have to find the frequency, duration, and intensity of a workout that is suitable for you since everyone is different. Be in tune with your body at all times and don't succumb to the fallacy that "more is better" because, often, less is actually more.

On a final note, don't forget to change your diet to accommodate your exercise regimen. Increasing your intake of protein is absolutely essential. Building muscle tissue requires protein as a nutrient source, and if you fail to get enough in your diet, your body will start to feed off its own supply. Not only will this prevent muscle growth, but it is yet another cause of overtraining syndrome. Try increasing your daily protein intake by one half. So if you normally eat two eggs for breakfast, eat three instead; if you eat one chicken breast for dinner, increase it to one and a half.

Not getting an adequate amount of protein is especially problematic for vegetarians. I would like to suggest a protein replacement drink as a supplement. You should be able to find the vegetarian variety at any health food store. Drink these within one hour of your resistance training workout. For nonvegetarians who need more protein, chocolate milk is also a pretty good source; but if you are wary of the fat and sugar content, then stick to the protein powder. Also, be sure to eat solid protein (turkey, cheese, turkey meatballs, tuna, tofu, or whatever you like) within two hours of each workout session. This dietary regimen will give your body what it needs to build muscle and prevent self-digestion.

As we mentioned earlier in the chapter, you will need to replenish your glycogen stores following a workout, so eating a sports bar within the first hour of completion is a good practice. Remember that a sports replacement drink is also beneficial and can even be used during your workout, especially if you are exercising at high intensity. This will give you greater endurance and power to use throughout your session. And please, don't forget to drink plenty of water before, during, and after your workout. Sweating leads to water loss, and since we have already discussed the importance of staying properly hydrated, you'll want to make sure that you are.

Finally, you should always incorporate a strong antioxidant like alpha-lipoic acid, into your diet when exercising regularly. Remember that exercise can lead to free radical formation, particularly during anaerobic respiration, so a good antioxidant is imperative. Combining exercise with intelligent nutritional practices is a must and is also your first taste of how each key actually works synergistically with all the others. You will see how the principle of synergy works to enhance your efforts when you make it to chapter 8 (Integration: Creating Synergy with the Six Keys).

## Cardiovascular training

The second pillar of exercise is cardiovascular training. As the name implies, this type of exercise is aerobic in nature; that is, it uses oxygen to provide the high levels of energy needed to sustain its action. Cardiovascular exercise not only stresses the skeletal muscles, but the heart and lungs as well. By virtue of being an aerobic activity, it is a great way to build endurance in the body.

Any activity that sustains an increased heart rate for an extended period is cardiovascular. It would include aerobic step classes, swimming, basketball, racquetball, jogging, and a whole host of other exercises. Even walking at a moderate pace can be a cardiovascular workout for some. In fact, walking is the best exercise to begin with if you are obese, have a heart condition, or are new to exercise altogether.

As mentioned previously, cardiovascular activity can be sustained as long as there is sufficient fuel to power the body. The body burns glucose and fatty acids and sends the broken-down products into the muscle cell's mitochondria. Here it produces high levels of ATP. Lactic acid also builds during cardiovascular exercise although at a much slower rate than during resistance training. In fact, when the levels of lactic acid get too high, the body will shut down completely as we have seen happen to marathon runners and triathletes. This is called *hitting the wall* and has to do with exceeding one's *lactate threshold* (LT). The LT is the amount of lactate the body can handle before shutting down and can be increased significantly with regular cardiovascular training.

Despite a popular misconception among workout novices, cardiovascular exercises like running do very little to build strength in the legs. This is true of the popular StairMaster and elliptical machines as well. Remember, to build strength, one must continually stress the muscles with a resistant force. Therefore, you can't neglect a good leg workout with weights just because you've done thirty minutes on the StairMaster—it just doesn't work that way. Swimming, on the other hand, is a great exercise to both build strength and work your cardiovascular system because the water actually acts as a resistive force. This is also true of the popular sculpt classes, where participants use a combination of weight training and aerobic exercise to get a complete workout.

Because cardiovascular training requires so much oxygen, it naturally conditions the heart and lungs. Lungs take in oxygen for respiration while the heart pumps it to the working muscles. I cannot emphasize enough how vital cardiovascular exercise is to your health and well-being. A well-trained cardiovascular system protects us from heart disease and *hypoxia* (insufficient oxygen to the organs and tissues of the body). It also allows us to handle a greater amount of physical and mental stress. A heart that is used to pumping blood at a high rate will not shut down when encountering an unexpected high-stress situation.

A good aerobic workout increases blood flow to all the muscles of the body. The constant movement of blood ensures that the vessels will always be open and free flowing. There is an interesting phenomenon that involves the venous system, but before we discuss it, it will help to understand a little basic physiology of the vascular system. Arteries move oxygenated blood from the heart to the rest of the body, including the distal muscles in the arms and legs. Veins, on the other hand, bring deoxygenated blood back from the body to the heart and lungs. Blood moving out to the distal regions of the body is helped along by the pumping action of the heart as well as by the contraction of the arteries themselves. The veins, conversely, must rely solely on muscular contractions to pump blood back toward the heart since they have no pump of their own. It is not hard to see, then, that constant muscular contraction is vital to bringing deoxygenated blood back to the lungs where the blood will pick up more oxygen before being shuttled off to the heart. There are obvious reasons why this is important, but what may be less obvious is that blood can stagnate in the distal regions of the body like the legs, for instance. Stagnant blood has the tendency to clot and can cause a painful leg cramp called a *deep vein thrombosis*. The danger of this disorder is that the clot can dislodge, travel up the vein, and block a blood vessel in the lungs. This is called a *pulmonary embolism* and is life threatening. An embolism can obstruct blood flow to the lungs and can cause death within hours.[75] The general recommendation for prevention is—you guessed it—regular cardiovascular exercise.

Increased blood flow is not only a great preventative measure in general but has a beneficial effect on the sexual organs as well. Proper blood flow to both the female and male genitalia is absolutely vital for sexual stimulation. It is the reason why most urologists urge people to kick the smoking habit. Cigarette smoking decreases the overall blood flow in the body and can cause erectile dysfunction (ED). Medications like Viagra work precisely because they increase blood flow to the sexual organs. But why rely on medications? You can prevent ED from happening in the first place by quitting smoking and participating in regular aerobic exercise.

If cardiovascular exercises increase endurance, then it should go without saying that doing them regularly will boost your overall energy levels. To be a sexual dynamo, it takes more than just the ability to stand upright at attention. A person's cardiovascular conditioning, then, can go a long way in the bedroom and should not be overlooked.

The increased intake of oxygen is not only beneficial for your sexual organs, but for your brain and all the other organs in your body as well. Each one goes through oxidative respiration regularly, so why not do what you can to enhance their functions? Even more exciting is that regular cardiovascular exercise can help people lose weight and look better. But don't forget, resistance training is still the most effective way to lose weight. By incorporating both resistance *and* cardiovascular exercises, you will get the most out of your weight-loss regimen.

I feel compelled to address a recent news article that has warned against drinking too much water during "intense exercise."[76] This study showed that marathon runners drinking more than three liters during a race risked severe blood dilution, which can cause *cerebral edema* (water on the brain) and eventually death. The unfortunate consequence of this study is that the media, smelling an excellent opportunity to cause public paranoia, had taken it upon themselves to report that drinking water may not be as healthy as we had originally thought. Unfortunately, they failed to mention that the runners in the study drank excessive amounts of water, ran for a length of time greater than four hours, and had a low body mass index or, in other words, were very thin. They also failed to mention that running a marathon is not exactly exercise; instead, it is an intense endurance event, quite possibly the most extreme sport next to a triathlon. To extrapolate these results to the general public—that is, people who exercise for general health—is both idiotic and irresponsible. Yes, it makes a good news story, which in turn produces ratings and sells papers; however, are the conclusions accurate? The reality is that when people exercise, they sweat, losing body water in the process. Replenishing lost water is absolutely essential for the proper functioning and survivability of the human body. There is a group of scientists who would like to refute these facts; however, one need only look at the dehydration statistics of any big city hospital to recognize how important proper hydration really is. Opponents might say that there is no proof showing a causal relationship between sweating and dehydration. Yet they fail to recognize that dehydration is not a singular event, but instead a cumulative condition. Regular replenishment *prevents* dehydration just like filling you car's gas tank prevents being stalled on the side of the road. It's as simple as that. Therefore, if you drink plenty of water before, during, and after a good cardiovascular workout, you will ensure yourself a properly functioning body that feels great. Unless, of course, you decide to run 26.2 miles in four hours—then you'd better be sure to keep your water intake to less than three liters.

**Flexibility training**

The third pillar of exercise, and quite frankly the most often overlooked, is flexibility training. During flexibility training, muscles are stretched to increase their length. Muscles that are not stretched actually lose bands of fibers on their ends, causing them to shorten.[77] Stretching creates length by adding fibers to the ends of the muscles. Since muscles usually cross joints (the areas of movement in the skeletal system), tight muscles prevent a joint from moving through its full range of motion. Clearly, a joint that has restricted motion will be less able to perform its function than one with complete freedom of movement. When a joint is restricted for an extended period, a degenerative process can set in, causing arthritis (see chapter 4). One way to prevent this is to open immobile joints through chiropractic care, yet without stretching the muscles that cross the joint, mobility will not last for very long.

Stretching also helps the muscle reach its greatest potential of development by allowing it to contract through its entire range of motion. By increasing a muscle's length, its ability to contract increases too. Every muscle fiber then receives the full benefit of the contraction, thereby leading to a more fully developed physique. An axiom used in bodybuilding circles is "Partial contractions lead to partial muscles." Basically, you can't expect to look your best when you don't work your muscles throughout their entire range of motion; so a well-stretched muscle is not only a more efficient muscle, but a better-looking one as well. And speaking of looks, the hypercontracted appearance prevalent among so many amateur bodybuilders is just not very attractive. We call this a *flexure posture*; and it is characterized by hunched shoulders, turned-in arms, and a forward-drawn head. It always reminds me of Quasimodo, the Hunchback of Notre Dame. The good news is that this posture can be reversed. It might take a little chiropractic intervention and, of course, lots of stretching; but eventually, one can regain one's normal shape. No one can deny that one's looks are enhanced tremendously by great posture, and stretching will significantly improve one's appearance toward that end.

Stretching not only benefits the muscle tissue, but also affects tendons, fascia, and joint capsules—all of which are intimately tied to joints. Each one can develop restrictions, which would limit a joint's overall range of motion. Moreover, stretch receptors called *muscle spindles*, which lay alongside the muscle fibers and communicate with the central nervous system (CNS), also respond favorably to stretching. The job of the muscle spindles is to monitor the amount of stretch occurring in a muscle by sending signals to the spinal cord. The spinal cord, in turn, protects the muscle from lengthening excessively by causing a counteractive contraction (a reflex) within that same muscle. Assisting this process is another group of receptors called the *golgi tendon organs*. These receptors allow muscle tissue to relax during a stretch, thereby protecting the surrounding connective tissues from injury. When one adheres to a regular flexibility practice, muscle spindles and golgi tendon organs adapt, allowing muscles to maintain their new length.

This adaptation is especially effective when one holds a stretch for a prolonged period, since it allows for greater lengthening of the muscle. A great saying and also a good rule to live by is "It's not how far you stretch a muscle that matters, but how long you hold the stretch." The reality is that many people do not hold their stretches long enough for positive effects to take place. Holding a stretch for at least thirty seconds allows for the addition of new muscle fibers, thereby creating length. It is also advisable to increase the degree of a stretch moderately each session or, in other words, push yourself a little further each time. Just be careful not to overstretch as this can cause injury and pain. There is a distinct difference between the "good pain" associated with a healthy stretch and the "unusual pain" associated with tearing connective tissue. Once again, being in tune with your body is invaluable here, so challenge yourself but know when enough is enough.

Another great benefit to stretching is that it is an excellent way to reduce pain and tension in the body. When muscles are tight, they can create painful, burning, and aching sensations that can be more than just minor annoyances. Tight muscles are often a large factor in low back pain, neck pain, and chronic headaches. They also play a part in shoulder, hip, and knee disorders and may increase the incidence of injury to any of these areas by restricting their range of motion. Under these circumstances, everyday movements like bending forward, lifting objects, or twisting and turning can lead to sprains, strains, and muscle spasms. Isn't it a relief to know that just by making your body more flexible, you can easily dissipate tension, ultimately bringing about a greater state of all-around comfort?

Stretching also enhances circulation. When muscles are tight, they constrict blood vessels and, in turn, hamper blood flow throughout the body. We have already discussed at length the importance of proper blood flow; so obviously, regular stretching will allow this vital function to carry on unimpeded. Much less obvious, though, is how tight muscles can affect the peripheral nerves that control the muscles themselves. When muscles are chronically tight, they can cause nerve impingement, which may lead to dysfunctions like numbness, tingling, and muscular weakness. As you will see in chapter 4, these symptoms should not be taken lightly nor should they be ignored; nerve tissue is delicate, and long-standing problems can lead to permanent damage. When we lay out all the disadvantages to having chronically short and tight muscles, doesn't it make sense to do everything you can to become more flexible?

## Yoga: Bringing All Three Pillars Together

I would now like to take this time to talk about a health practice that has had such enormous impact in my life that I feel compelled to share it with you, and that is the practice of yoga. I have been practicing yoga for the last several years to augment my already-full workout regimen and was introduced to it by my mother who had been enjoying her own practice for many years. I must admit that my earliest impressions of yoga were nothing more than visions of sweaty "earth children" twisting themselves into pretzels and chanting "om" to the sweet sounds of Enya. As I fancy myself a bit more sophisticated (or self-delusional, as the case may be), I really had very little interest in trying yoga. But frankly, I was wrong. As it turns out, I not only find yoga thoroughly enjoyable, but also remarkably life altering.

Some people may think of yoga as scary, weird, or overly difficult; but really, it isn't any of those things. In actuality, yoga is a way of opening oneself up, physically and mentally, to such a degree that permanent changes can take place. To understand what I mean, let us take a look at what yoga is and where it comes from.

When most people speak of yoga, they naturally think of the practice of doing postures, but yoga is actually a way of bringing together the mind, body, and spirit "to enhance the higher forces within us."[78] *Yoga* literally means "to yoke" or to bring together—a union, if you will. The origins of yoga are "shrouded in the mist of time," but there are accounts of it dating back as far as seven thousand years while the oldest archeological evidence dates back to about 3000 BC. It was supposedly Patanjali who compiled the *Yoga Sutra* around AD 200, a major work containing practical and philosophical wisdom regarding the practice of yoga. The *Yoga Sutra* is a guidebook that outlines the practice of yoga as we know it today and presents the first written account of the eight limbs of yoga.[79] The eight limbs are the steps to living an ethical and meaningful life and are defined as

1. *yama*: personal code of conduct
2. *niyama*: moral code of conduct
3. *asana*: practice of posture
4. *pranayama*: practice of breath control
5. *pratyahara*: withdrawal of the senses
6. *dharana*: concentration or focus
7. *dhyana*: meditation
8. *samadhi*: absorption into a state of stillness

Today, most people who practice yoga, especially in Western society, focus mainly on the third limb, or *asana*. As discussing all eight limbs would require a separate book altogether, we will concentrate solely on the practice of postures here, although I encourage you to investigate the full practice further on your own. You will find that there are plentiful sources on the subject like books, magazines, instructors, and Web sites, which will help broaden your knowledge if you wish.

Let us discuss, then, how yoga, when used for purposes of physical fitness, can offer a broad and well-balanced program to addresses all three pillars of exercise concurrently. Many people have the misconception that yoga is a passive form of stretching and meditation. In reality, yoga uses an effective combination of both stretches and contractions to bring about strength, flexibility, and balance to the body.

Yoga is far from being passive—in fact, doing yoga passively is probably one of the surest ways to hurt oneself. Instead, when doing yoga, one should be actively engaged at all times, both physically and mentally. In each pose, one set of muscles contracts while another set relaxes. Sometimes the only muscles allowed to relax are the ones in the face, a monumental task in itself. Either way, the body is always completely engaged throughout the entire practice. Those who go into yoga thinking it will be a passive exercise soon realize their miscalculations as their bodies eventually become drenched in sweat.

While doing *asanas*, the mind never finds itself passive either. Many people mistakenly believe that by doing postures they will eventually enter a state of meditative bliss. Not so as yoga requires intense focus. Whereas meditation is the art of conscious unconsciousness (chapter 6), focus is the art of conscious consciousness. In other words, you will have to keep your mind completely present to perform each pose. Do not worry about the possibility of losing your attention while you practice. The discomfort associated with opening up areas of your body that, through years of neglect and minimal usage have become chronically restricted, will no doubt keep your head in the game. This is how yoga unites the body and the mind. At times, this may be an uncomfortable process, but yoga has a way of developing your focus to such a degree that it can be tapped into whenever you might need it. In this way, yoga helps people better handle stress. And it is precisely your ability to tap into this skill in your daily life that leads many instructors to assert that the real yoga begins the moment you leave the studio. It is also the reason why we call what we do in the studio *practicing*.

I realize that my description of yoga may sound daunting to some, but before you blow it off as too physically grueling, please let me describe some additional benefits to adopting a regular practice. Obviously, you develop flexibility; but along with it, you also receive the many benefits that come with being flexible, like reduced pain and tension, greater blood flow, and a more developed physique. Moreover, you will also develop enormous strength. A word of caution to the macho: this practice is not for wimps. If you want to see a grown man sweat, grimace, and curse, then watch a bodybuilder do yoga for the first time. Yoga takes strength and endurance together, especially since the poses are held for a long time—much longer than most weight lifters are used to. The strength the body develops through yoga is empowering; your self-confidence will soar as you master poses with formidable names like warrior, crane, and cobra. And most classes are done in a continuous flowing manner, so your cardiovascular system will not be neglected either.

Possibly, the most powerful gift you will receive through yoga, though, is a greater sense of spirit. In yoga, the body is seen as a temple, the house in which our spirit lives. By placing meticulous attention to the body—opening up closed-off areas, creating strength, and decreasing stress—we "create a comfortable house for the body to sit in."[80] Also, by uniting the body and the mind as well as connecting the breath to movements, yoga has a way of centering us. As we push through difficult postures, we improve our ability to trust ourselves, and the resulting boost in self-confidence helps to push us to even greater heights in both a mental and emotional capacity. Many people, myself included, report a greater sense of well-being as a result of practicing yoga. The way we see the world and how we ultimately relate to it often changes. Maybe it has to do with our improved ability to handle stress, or maybe it is because yoga makes us feel so good. Either way, it is something that has to be experienced to be understood.

If you are still unsure of whether yoga is right for you, just go out and try it. Find a class near home and commit to a practice for at least six months. I cannot guarantee that you will find the process fun, but you will no doubt find it rewarding. If you do yoga consistently, even if only just one time per week, then you can't help but experience all the wonderful benefits yoga has to offer. Like I said in the beginning of the section, practicing yoga is truly a life-altering experience. Give it a shot, and I am sure you will agree—it's nothing less than remarkable.

## A Few More Benefits We Should Not Forget About

So far, I have discussed how much we can improve our health with regular physical fitness. I have discussed how we can achieve great gains in strength, endurance, and flexibility as well as prevent disorders like blood clots, chronic pain, and heart disease. I have talked about the various physiological processes that are optimized like blood flow, respiration, and energy production. I have even emphasized the enhancement of looks through weight loss, muscle development, and improved posture all by embarking on a consistent exercise program. And if that's not enough, I've even gone so far as to describe how much our sex life will improve when we get into proper shape and condition. Yet there are still a few more benefits that I think we should talk about before finally putting this matter to rest.

The first has to do with a topic that is reaching new heights in the public awareness—it is called *antiaging*. In the middle part of the twentieth century, studies on exercise virtually ignored the elderly since experts felt that they should not physically exert themselves too much. However, we now know differently. Not only is exercise healthy for people of all ages but may even do wonders to extend life. There is absolutely no doubt that quality of life improves dramatically with regular exercise, but to what extent it prolongs life is the question scientists are now asking.

Obviously, by the sheer fact that physical fitness reduces the risk of heart disease, it improves one's chances of living into older age. Yet exercise also reduces the risks associated with diabetes, high cholesterol, and excessive weight gain—all of which can severely limit one's life expectancy. But there's even more. As we age, our ability to take in and use oxygen diminishes, decreasing the amount that can be distributed to our tissues over any given time. Heart rate slows down every year too. This means that the ability of the heart to pump blood to our tissues also decreases—not a good way for our bodies to function. But there's good news. We can counter these effects with regular cardiovascular training as aerobic exercise strengthens the heart and increases the ability of the muscles to utilize the oxygen they receive. Although a well-trained older person cannot utilize oxygen as efficiently as a well-trained younger person, he or she can certainly do better than an older person who is in poor physical condition. Oxygen is absolutely essential to the health and survivability of human life, so being able to distribute and utilize it effectively is crucial.

Another antiaging benefit linked to exercise is the production of *human growth hormone* (HGH). This hormone produced by the pineal gland is responsible for increases in bone density and muscle mass. HGH also speeds up fat metabolism and is therefore helpful in maintaining one's shapely figure. HGH has been shown to increase strength, exercise tolerance, and energy production as well as playing a role in immune, cardiac, and respiratory functions.[81] People who are deficient in HGH show a greater loss of bone density, loss of memory (both short- and long-term), increased stress levels, and moodiness. As one can see, low HGH levels in the body lead to degenerative changes while adequate amounts enhance the quality of life. Preliminary studies have even shown HGH to extend the life span in rats, but whether we can extrapolate these findings to humans has yet to be determined.[82]

These preliminary findings have created an enormous desire among some to jump into supplemental human growth hormone (HGH or just GH) replacement therapy. As a result, many companies have surfaced claiming miraculous results with their GH products. I strongly recommend not jumping on this bandwagon just yet. At this time (and thankfully so), HGH must be administered by a qualified physician; so purchasing pills, nasal sprays, and other products sold on the Internet can be a waste of money at best and perhaps even dangerous to your health. While HGH injections from your doctor will not come cheaply (as much as two thousand dollars a month[83]), there is a way to boost your natural hormone levels, and that's with regular anaerobic exercise. Remember, anaerobic exercise is resistance training, so lifting weights is one way to successfully increase your HGH levels. Another way to boost levels is by getting proper sleep (chapter 5). HGH is secreted while you slumber, so getting plenty of rest is a real life-enhancing practice.

There is no doubt that HGH is important to human health, and we now know that it may even slow down the aging process, but increasing it naturally is the most prudent and cost-effective way to do so. Making exercise a regular part of your lifestyle will allow you to enjoy all of HGH's benefits without risking the potential dangers associated with injecting synthetic hormones.

Another benefit of exercise that also helps to slow down aging is an increase in social interaction. We often work out with others, whether a partner, a trainer, or in a class. Social interaction does wonders to increase our relationships and keep us feeling young and vibrant. People who play sports are at a particular advantage since team sports are fun and are appealing to one's competitive nature. They also kindle group camaraderie. Even individual sports like golf or tennis provide physical conditioning while offering social interaction.

Maintaining social interactions are important to mental health (chapter 6), and most experts agree that a rich social life is instrumental in keeping a person mentally sharp.[84] Take advantage of this fact and use exercise to enhance your social circle. Work out with friends or try to meet new people. Approaching it from a social angle, you may even be lucky enough to meet that special someone. It has been said that sports clubs are today's singles bars; they are definitely less expensive than nightclubs, and think about it, you can be certain that you share something in common with every person in the gym—the desire and drive to stay physically fit. It seems a bit more substantial than what one has to sift through "in da club," does it not?

It is well documented that exercise has other measurable effects on mental health. Both anxiety and depression are reduced considerably with regular exercise.[85] The key here is *regular*. The greatest gains in reducing depression are seen in those who work out several times per week for more than nine weeks. The benefits of exercise are therefore cumulative. In fact, in his position paper for the President's Council on Physical Fitness and Sports (PCPFS), leading mental health expert Dr. David M. Landers of the University of Arizona points out that "exercise is at least as effective as more traditional therapies" and may be a viable alternative to combating depression, "especially considering the time and cost involved with treatments like psychotherapy." [86] He goes on to conclude,

> Exercise is related not only to a relief in symptoms of depression and anxiety but it also seems to be beneficial in enhancing self-esteem, producing more restful sleep, and helping people recover more quickly from psychosocial stressors . . . exercise has an important role to play in promoting sound mental health.[87]

It is pretty amazing that something like exercise can reduce feelings of depression and anxiety, improve self-esteem, and result in a more restful sleep. How can it do all that? It has to do with a compound called *phenylethylamine* (PEA). PEA is produced naturally by the body and has properties similar to amphetamines. Experts believe it works by making the body produce endorphins, our body's natural opiates. Just as the opiate morphine makes people "feel good," so do endorphins, and they are known as the "driving force behind pleasurable effects."[88] Not surprising, PEA is also found in chocolate, long thought to have special properties, and it mimics the brain chemistry of a person in love. PEA has "been shown to reduce depression in 60 percent of depressed patients."[89] A few of the many effects of PEA are mood elevation, increased energy, greater alertness, and a greater sense of well-being and contentment.[90] The exciting news is that recent studies show PEA to be produced even during moderate exercise in most people.[91] Ah yes, I do remember once hearing that exercise might be better than drugs for depression. Hmmmm . . . Maybe there's something there, what do you think?

Aside from all the physical, social, and mental benefits of exercise, there are spiritual benefits as well. Remember that in yoga the body is considered the house of the soul. It is understood, "yogically" speaking anyway, that keeping the body fit makes the house a strong yet comfortable place for the soul to exist. Along with that, physical fitness improves the mental outlook. It doesn't take a rocket scientist to figure out what this can do to your overall essence. When one feels stronger, has less pain, looks better, and has an improved mental outlook, it will be almost impossible to relate to the world in a less-than-improved fashion. The reality is that when we feel good physically, we find it much easier to maintain a healthy perspective; and we are much more inclined to practice tolerance, gratitude, and charity. True, we all have periods in life when our mental stresses may be more than we can alleviate by just "feeling good," but let's face it—knowing, feeling, and experiencing great physical health gives us more of an edge when having to face life's many challenges.

# Breathing: The Essence of Life

We have briefly touched upon the process of breathing and its importance to cellular respiration and energy production. Because we breathe without having to put too much thought into it, we sometimes take this function for granted. Yet if we could become more conscious of our day-to-day breathing, then we could actually harness the power of the breath to enhance our health and vitality.

To fully understand the nature of breath, we must first look at the physiological process of breathing. The respiratory system is comprised of our nasal passages, mouth, trachea, bronchi, and lungs. The biomechanical equipment that allows us to take in air is called the *thorax* (chest cavity). This region consists of the heart, lungs, ribs, and several muscles of the neck and thorax. At the center of the thorax lies the *diaphragm*, a dome-shaped muscle that separates the thoracic and the abdominal cavities. The apex of this muscle points toward the heart; and when it contracts, it expands the ribs, opening up the thoracic cage. The lungs are attached to the ribs through a protective sheath called the *pleura*. When the chest cavity expands, it opens the lungs so that they expand like balloons. Breath is taken into the lungs through a method called *negative pressure*. The pressure inside the lungs is less than the pressure outside of the body, and since air tends to flow from areas of high pressure to areas of low pressure, air flows inward.

Inside the lungs are little sacs called *alveoli*. Blood vessels line the alveolar walls so that gasses like oxygen (O) and carbon dioxide ($CO_2$) can be exchanged readily. The oxygenated blood that exits the lungs is shuttled to the heart for further distribution to the rest of the body. As we exhale, $CO_2$ is expelled from the lungs and is distributed freely into the atmosphere. Plants use $CO_2$ to produce glucose (sugar) in a process just the reverse of respiration called *photosynthesis*. The cellular by-product of photosynthesis is oxygen. It is released into the atmosphere and is eventually consumed by air-breathing organisms. This completes the respiratory cycle.

Remember that oxygen is distributed to all the tissues of the body and is used for aerobic respiration. Along with food, our ability to take in and utilize oxygen is essential for energy production. Breathing also removes metabolic wastes from the blood, like $CO_2$, and returns them into the atmosphere.

There is another concept or function of the breath called *pranayama*, which is taught in the yogic philosophy. It describes the air as a medium for *prana*, a life force, that permeates the universe and energizes us. This is an abstract concept, I know; but if you can make use of it, even if just for the symbolic value, it can be very advantageous to you. Here's how: We obviously need air for all the reasons we have previously mentioned. If you can actually visualize the physical nature of air, as opposed to never thinking about it at all, you will be able to breathe it in more heartily. You will also be able to visualize it revitalizing you and be less inclined to breathe polluted air when other options are available (see air purifiers in chapter 7).

The capacity for us to utilize the full benefits of oxygen is directly related to our ability to take in air efficiently. There are conditions that can hamper maximum oxygen utilization like cigarette smoking, asthma, emphysema, poor conditioning, bad posture, or spinal subluxations (chapter 4). Obviously, breathing polluted air lowers the amount of fresh oxygen we take in at any given time. Some of the obstacles we face for breathing sufficient oxygen are directly and immediately controllable by us; but others, like pollution, are a bit more complicated. I would like to take this time to teach you something that will greatly enhance your breathing capacity; it will give you all the advantages we discussed above as well as improve your posture, reduce neck pain, and minimize tension headaches. This tool is *abdominal breathing*.

Abdominal breathing is carried out through diaphragmatic contraction. The diaphragm muscle contracts in a downward fashion, expanding the belly. Diaphragmatic breathing is the most natural and efficient way to breathe, yet many of us develop the habit of chest breathing instead. Chest breathers use the accessory muscles to lift the thoracic cage upward as opposed to outward, which is less efficient. The accessory muscles are located at the front of the neck, the chest, the upper back, and the back of the neck. Chest breathing is unfavorable for two reasons: First, it does not allow as great an expansion of the chest cavity as abdominal breathing and therefore allows much less air to be taken in at any given time. Second, chest breathing can cause overuse of the accessory muscles. This can lead to neck pain, headaches, and even nerve impingement conditions like thoracic outlet syndrome (TOS). TOS is the pinching of the nerves that travel from the neck to the arms and can cause numbness and tingling of the hands and fingers, or even carpal tunnel syndrome.

As you can see, abdominal breathing provides a number of critical advantages. It allows for greater oxygen intake, which ultimately leads to an increase in energy. By increasing the *tidal volume*, the amount of air you take in on each inhalation, the heart has to work less to pump oxygen to the outlying tissues, thereby decreasing heart rate. The brain also benefits considerably from the respiratory increase since it is the largest consumer of oxygen in the body (about 20 percent). You can expect your concentration and memory to sharpen as oxygen is intimately tied to these mental functions.

One of the most rewarding benefits of abdominal breathing, though, is that it may help you during times of stress like nothing else. There is a connection—a triad, if you will—between stress levels, the breath, and heart rate. When under stress, our respiratory rate increases, becoming both rapid and shallow. Our heart rate also increases as the cardiovascular system works harder to pick up the small packets of oxygen rapidly entering the lungs. The key to maintaining our composure during high-stress situations, then, is by controlling the only facet we can—our breath. We can neither control our heart rate nor the circumstances surrounding stressful situations; therefore, controlling our breath is really our only option.

As I said earlier, chest breathing engages the accessory muscles of respiration. The true function of the accessory muscles is to increase our respiratory function when we find ourselves in stressful situations, like when being chased by the cops or if caught in a fire or any other time we may need the extra air. Unfortunately, chest breathers engage the accessory muscles regularly, and this only perpetuates the stress response, which is counterproductive when we need to calm down. Breathing abdominally, on the other hand, allows us to consciously slow down our respiratory rate. It also slows down the heart rate, which allows us to calm down just enough to evaluate the situation at hand, deal with it if possible, and, if necessary, leave.

So how do you know if you are a chest breather or an abdominal breather? The best way to find out is through simple observation. Look at yourself in the mirror: Does your chest lift up and expand on each inhalation? If so, you're a chest breather. You may also suspect chest breathing if you frequently have a sore neck (particularly in the front just above the collarbones) or if your breath tends to be short and shallow.

If you find that you are a chest breather and would like to reap the benefits of abdominal breathing, try the following exercise. First, lie down as this exercise is more comfortable in the recumbent position. Once you master the exercise, you will be able to do it anywhere, in any position, but lying down is best when starting out. Lie on your back (with a pillow under your head if you'd like), place one hand on your abdomen just above your belly button, and one hand on your breastbone. Take a deep breath in. Push your diaphragm downward so that your abdomen expands fully. Push it out so that it looks just like the belly of a very happy Buddha. Your lower hand (the one on the abdomen) should rise before the upper one does. When your lungs fill to capacity, hold your breath for one second, then release. Your lower hand should also fall before the upper one does. Repeat this several times. On each successive breath, try to push your belly out a little farther.

You might find this exercise somewhat challenging to begin with, especially if you are like most people and have been a chest breather for a long time. If this is the case, your diaphragm muscle has probably become weak and perhaps even a bit lazy. And why wouldn't it? The accessory muscles have been doing most of the work after all, and like people, muscles will not work any harder than they have to. Over time and for unknown reasons, a neurological shift takes place, leading the nervous system to accept chest breathing as normal. The nervous system then perpetuates this pattern of dysfunctional breathing by engaging the accessory muscles automatically.

By practicing abdominal breathing daily, you can slowly break the chest-breathing pattern you have developed over the years. We call this *neuromuscular reeducation* where you essentially retrain the diaphragm and nervous system to function the way it was meant during breathing. In the case of abdominal breathing, neuromuscular reeducation happens surprisingly fast. Do the exercises two times per day: once in the morning as you wake up and once at night, right before you go to bed. Do it for one minute each time. That's it—one minute, morning and night. You will find that the extra oxygen you take in each morning adds energy throughout your day; and at night, it will help you relax, bringing on a more restful sleep. You can also practice any time throughout your day whenever you might think about it, like while watching TV or when stuck in traffic. You will find that practicing this exercise during stressful situations will calm you down, making this practice essential to your mental health.

Abdominal breathing strengthens the diaphragm in much the same way resistance exercises strengthen your other muscles. It is such an effective tool that singers, actors, and professional speakers practice it regularly to make their voices sound more powerful. Practice abdominal breathing if you want to feel stronger and more energized. Practice it if you want to gain a more self-confident and commanding voice. Practice it if you want to have greater composure during times of stress. Either way, you will be sure to gain enormous benefits from doing this exercise.

This concludes the second key to optimal health. The most important thing to walk away with from this chapter is to see exercise as an integral part of your lifestyle. One should not view it as an obligation or a drag, but something that can be fun if approached with a little creativity. Physical fitness is simply a matter of life or death—there is no denying it. By getting into shape, you will not only increase your chances of living longer, you will also improve the life that you have today. The smiling and exuberant people who grace the covers of today's fitness magazines are not faking it. They exude health, wellness, and vitality from every ounce of their being. If you are not exercising now, start today. It's never too late. And if you are exercising regularly, then congratulations, and keep it up. With all your hard work, you will not want to miss the reparative, restorative, and relaxing benefits that you will find in *key number 3*.

# Chapter 3 Summary

# Key Number 2: Fitness and Exercise

- Learn basic muscle anatomy (see Suggested Reading for suggested books on this subject).
- Do resistance exercises one to three times per week.
- Work your legs and buttocks at least once per week.
- Work your abs at least once per week.
- Mix it up. Vary your workouts.
- If you've never exercised before, hire a trainer.
- Rest between workouts.
- Increase your protein intake by one-half.
- Eat a protein bar within one hour following a workout. Eat a protein meal (turkey, tuna, eggs) within two hours.
- Drink a sports replacement drink following your workout at least one time per week.
- Take a strong antioxidant like alpha-lipoic acid.
- Do thirty minutes of cardio one time per week.
- Drink lots of water (now keep it under three liters if you're to run a marathon, OK?).
- Stretch every day (OK, at least every other day).
- Take a yoga class at least twice per month (you have got to learn *how to* stretch).
- Hold your stretches for at least thirty seconds.
- Work out with others.
- Practice abdominal breathing.

# Bodywork: Maintaining Neuromusculoskeletal Balance

*The doctor of the future will give no medicine but will interest his patients in*
*the care of the human frame, in diet, and in the cause and prevention of disease.*
—Thomas Edison

H UMAN BEINGS ARE complex living systems comprised of both a physical and mental component, each inseparable from the other. No doubt that all of man's experiences, from his actions to his thoughts and feelings, impact his physical body.[92] Every activity he engages in, every emotional stress he suffers, and every tension he endures reflects itself in his musculoskeletal system. It is therefore essential for every person to receive some form of regular bodywork to keep themselves physically balanced, pain free, and functioning properly at all times.

Bodywork is the use of physical techniques to remove tension, relax the body, and restore proper function. These techniques affect either directly or indirectly joints, muscles, ligaments, nerves, blood vessels, and organs—all of which need regular stimulation for a sound operation. In fact, many of these systems may receive very little attention during a person's lifetime without the physical stimulation of regular bodywork.

Man has recognized the benefits of bodywork for thousands of years. The first written accounts dating back to 3000 BC in China where priests practiced a form of energy work called Qigong. Qigong was based on the concept of the life force *chi*, which, if imbalanced, causes illness and disease. The Chinese also developed the practice of *acupuncture*, which uses needles to stimulate or depress energy points (meridians) for various therapeutic purposes. At around 1000 BC, the Japanese expanded on the Chinese method of bodywork, using their fingers (*shi*) to exert a pressure (*atsu*) on energy points similar to those of the meridian system. This form of bodywork is known as *shiatsu*.[93]

Bodywork was not exclusive to the Far East. Indian civilization had its own form called *ayurveda*, which was complementary to the practice of yoga. Ayurveda dates back to 1700 BC, and it combines herbal remedies, dietary practices, and massage to facilitate the healing process. In the West, some Native American tribes like the Navajo and Cherokee used massage to prepare their warriors for battle; and following war, they used it to help their wounded recover.

The value of bodywork was not lost on the ancient Greeks either. They used massage in the gymnasium to condition their athletes and also as a form of relaxation. They were the first to incorporate *aromatherapy*, using essential oils to elicit various actions like stimulation or sedation. Hippocrates, the Father of Modern Medicine, was a strong advocate of regular bodywork. He wrote in the *Corpus Hippocraticum*,

> The physician must be experienced in many things but assuredly in rubbing . . . For rubbing can bind a joint that is too loose and loosen a joint that is too rigid.

The Romans too understood the benefits of therapeutic massage: Julius Caesar was said to have had his body "pinched" daily to relieve him of severe nerve pain; Pliny, the great naturalist, received regular massages to treat chronic asthma; and the physician Celsus readily used spinal manipulation and massage to relieve headaches and other physical disorders. Galen, the most famous of all Roman physicians, strongly recommended bodywork for a large number of ailments—most notably, the improvement of blood circulation.

Several of these ancient forms of bodywork are still in use today. Acupuncture and massage remain popular while newer methods like reflexology, Reiki, and craniosacral therapy have found their way into the mainstream. Although each of these techniques has great merit in its own right, I wish to address only one form of bodywork in detail here, and that is chiropractic. Chiropractic is the most comprehensive form of bodywork available, affecting more systems of the body than any of the other forms combined. And it is also the only method known to correct the vertebral subluxation, a painful and often-debilitating health hazard.

## Chiropractic: The Way to Stay Well Adjusted

*Chiropractic* is a powerful healing art. It is based on the philosophy that true health comes from within; that is, we are born with everything we need to live rich, full, and healthy lives. Chiropractors call this inborn capacity for health *Innate Intelligence*. According to the chiropractic philosophy, health only becomes compromised when an obstacle prevents the body from functioning at its full capacity. There are many things that can act as obstacles such as toxins, germs, and even malnutrition. But the obstacle that chiropractic specifically addresses is the vertebral subluxation.

A *vertebral subluxation*, or just subluxation, is often described as a misaligned bone; but more accurately, it is a joint that has lost a fraction of its normal motion or has become "stuck." Since a subluxated joint cannot move through its entire range of motion, it may leave a person susceptible to any number of problems including pain, inflammation, muscle spasms, decreased sensory function, diminished reflexes, poor circulation, and lack of movement.

The most common reason people seek out a chiropractic doctor is for pain relief. Approximately 25 percent of the population suffers from low back pain at any given time. In 1997, Americans made 192 million visits to chiropractors, with more than half of them going for the treatment of back or neck pain.[94] A large number of cases that chiropractors see are chronic conditions, ailments that a person has had for a long time. Recent findings show that chronic pain sufferers actually age faster, losing gray matter of the brain (information processing) at an equivalent of ten to twenty years of aging.[95] This alone should motivate you to seek out a solution for chronic pain, but as you shall soon see, there are many other reasons as well.

Before we get into these, it is important to discuss the vital function pain plays in our lives. Pain is necessary to let us know that something is not quite right in our body; it is a protective mechanism that alerts us to any potential dangers that may jeopardize our ability to survive. Although pain plays an important role in survival, it is of no advantage when chronic. Therefore, it is much better to address the *cause* of pain immediately than to ignore the pain itself and allow it to become long-standing.

Pain can arise from any number of sources, but chiropractic focuses specifically on those that are biomechanical or neurological in origin. Mechanical pain can come from the joints, like in the case of degenerative arthritis. Joints are structures between bones that allow movement. Arthritis literally means an inflamed joint. And the term *degenerative* refers to the wearing down of cartilage that lies on the joint surfaces. *Degenerative arthritis*, then, is the inflammation of a joint due to worn-away cartilage. This type of arthritis is a wear and tear disorder, so the risk of it developing increases exponentially with long-standing, uncorrected subluxations.

Joints are self-lubricating structures, which rely on motion to carry out their function.[96] Since subluxated joints are stuck, they lose the ability to lubricate themselves, further exacerbating their immobility. Studies show that immobilized joints suffer from degenerative changes and eventually break down.[97] *Ligaments*, the structures that attach bone to bone and act as joint stabilizers, also become weakened with decreased joint mobility.[98] This can lead to joint instability, which the body often tries to correct by fusing joints together. Joint instability, and any subsequent fusion, is the hallmark of degenerative joint disease (DJD). Chronic subluxations, then, are precursors for developing arthritis or DJD.

Arthritic pain is excruciating and debilitating. It begins as a generalized discomfort and is accompanied by decreased motion of the joint. As the disease progresses, even the slightest movements become unbearable. Arthritis can affect any joint, but it is especially devastating when it occurs in the cervical spine (the neck). With this form of arthritis, turning the head becomes a near impossibility, and people in the later stages often need to turn their entire bodies just to look over their shoulders. I see the disability and distress caused by this horrible affliction in my daily practice, and I have to say that it is the most difficult aspect of my job to witness a grown man or woman break down in tears because they can no longer take the pain. What makes this scenario even more upsetting is that arthritis can be totally prevented by including regular chiropractic care into one's health regimen early on, well before arthritis sets in.

Another way that subluxations cause pain is by affecting the adjacent yet nonsubluxated joint. Normal joints must move excessively to make up for the lack of movement by their subluxated counterparts; this, in turn, causes the nonsubluxated joint to become inflamed. In chiropractic, we see this happen often in the sacroiliac joints (SIJ), which lie between the tailbone and the pelvis. It is a common cause of low back pain and is felt just above the buttock region. Anyone who has ever experienced this type of pain knows exactly how excruciating it can be. It can make walking, sitting, or bending over quite difficult, and just touching the area of the SIJ can cause horrible pain. It is an extremely common subluxation, which can only be corrected through chiropractic care.

The other type of biomechanical pain that may wreak havoc in one's life is neurogenic pain. Neurogenic pain originates from a nerve and can occur almost anywhere in the body, like an arm or leg or tooth, wherever nerves can be irritated. Here, however, we will concentrate solely on pain generated at a nerve root, the portion of the nerve that exits the spine. This is known as *radicular pain*. Radicular pain is most often the result of a *herniated disk*, a condition where the cartilaginous disk material sitting between two spinal bones bulges out and presses against the nerve root as it exits the spine.

How does one get a herniated disk? Contrary to popular belief, it is not the result of one specific incidence, like bending over to pick up something off the ground (if it were, then we would all suffer from herniated disks). In reality, most of these injuries result from one or more factors including excess weight, poor abdominal tone, poor flexibility, and faulty biomechanical motion (subluxations).

When any of these conditions are present, the stability of the disk material and the back in general are weakened. Thus, compound movements like bending over, jumping, running, or anything else causing compression or shearing of the spine can cause herniation through the weakened disk. Basically, only dysfunctional disks become injured from these movements. Herniation is unlikely to occur in a healthy disk; normal, healthy disks can withstand these movements with ease just as they were meant to.

Radicular pain manifests itself as a sharp, burning electrical pain, usually down an arm or leg, the most common being sciatica. Sciatica feels like scalding hot water poured down the back of one's leg. If the affected area is the neck, then the same symptoms are felt down an arm instead. Radicular pain can be accompanied by numbness and tingling of the hands or feet. It can also lead to progressive muscle weakness, so that holding on to regular objects may become increasingly difficult or impossible. When a herniated disk is very large and impinges several nerve roots, it can cause urinary incontinence (difficulty holding one's urine), numbness in the "saddle" region, and loss of control of the anal sphincter. Going into detail here is not necessary; suffice it to say that this is a medical emergency.

Chronic subluxations decrease a person's ability to move freely. This may seem obvious since we are talking about stuck joints here, but it is important to note that subluxations can also cause muscle spasms, which lead to even greater stiffness and lack of movement. As the number of subluxated joints increases, so does the amount of stiffness. Lack of movement, along with pain, often prevents people from performing even the most routine tasks. Sitting, standing, walking, exercising, and getting in and out of the car can be limited because of subluxations. Even sex can be painful when subluxations are long-standing. The pain and immobility caused by subluxations can make every aspect of your life miserable and can eventually lead to depression (chapter 6).[99]

Another ill effect of chronic subluxations is that they may cause poor posture. Stuck joints can prevent you from standing upright and, over time, can lead to a hunched-over posture. Most everyone will agree that poor posture makes you appear older, but what we don't consider is that it may also make you *feel* older since poor posture often causes pain and discomfort. Over time, this can lead to arthritis, which will make you feel a lot older than you actually are. The good news is that the problems we have discussed—arthritis, herniated disks, radicular pain, sciatica, poor posture—are treatable, and, in fact, are even preventable. In preventing them, you will undoubtedly experience a better quality of life. Thankfully, by the time you finish reading this chapter, you will have all the information you need to prevent the devastating effects caused by chronic subluxations.

## Maintaining the Master Control

As we have said, most people use chiropractic care to alleviate and prevent pain. Be that as it may, the true purpose of chiropractic has always been to maintain the function of the nervous system. The nervous system is the master control of the body; it commands and coordinates all bodily processes from the beating of the heart to respiration to digestion. All systems of the body need input from the nervous system to carry out their functions. The nervous system is an electrical system, using nerve cells (or neurons) in the same way an electrical cord uses wires; yet it processes information much more quickly and efficiently than any of the world's greatest supercomputers, making it one of the most fascinating and resourceful tools known to man.

The function of the nervous system is to gather information from the external environment and relate it to the inner state of the body. It analyzes the collected information and initiates a response to satisfy certain needs, most notably survival, but can carry out any response necessary to maintain the internal balance of the body (chapter 8). The central nervous system (CNS) is made up of the brain and the spinal cord. Whereas the brain controls motor function (movements and actions), cognitive ability (problem solving, language, and memory), and emotions, the spinal cord organizes sensory input (information coming in from the outside world; our perception) and sends it to the brain for processing. The spinal cord contains hundreds of nerve tracts, which in turn contain hundreds of thousands of nerve fibers that travel down the spine and out through the spinal nerves. The spinal cord also carries motor information sent by the brain and transmits it through the spinal nerves to all our organs, tissues, and muscles.

The nervous system is the most intricate system in the body; it is so complex that there is still much about it we do not yet know—that is, many of the details of how it works, how it regenerates, and how certain neurological diseases like Alzheimer's or amyotrophic lateral sclerosis (ALS), better known as Lou Gehrig's disease. operate. It is also very delicate. In fact, nature made sure—over thousands of years of evolution—to protect the CNS by encasing it in a hard, bony shell. This shell is comprised of the skull and spinal column.

The spine is made up of twenty-six bones called *vertebrae*. It is a dynamic system, which means it moves as we move; and therefore, the spine must be flexible. Nature has provided the spine this flexibility by inserting disks between the vertebrae. The intervertebral disks are joints that allow movement between two adjacent spinal segments and are made up of fibrocartilage, making them both tough (fibrous) and spongy (cartilaginous). This dual property gives the disks flexibility, enables them to act as shock absorbers, and adds a bit of protection to the delicate spinal cord. Remember that the disks are joints, so they can become stuck, or subluxated; and this can lead to degeneration or even herniation.

But let's get back to the nervous system. Sensitive receptors placed throughout the body gather information from the environment and send it up through the spinal nerves to the spinal cord and, eventually, to the brain where it is organized, stored, and analyzed before the CNS works on delivering a response. Messages from the brain are then sent down the spinal cord and out through the spinal nerves to all the organs and tissues in the body, exciting an action.

The nervous system is made up of neural tissue, which is extremely sensitive and specialized. The cells of the neural tissue are neurons, and their function is to transmit electrical impulses from the CNS to rest of the body and vice versa. These currents travel the entire length of the neuron in an all-or-nothing fashion. That is, once a nerve fires, it fires. There is no such thing as a partially activated nerve. Eventually, the impulse reaches the end of the nerve cell where chemical neurotransmitters are released into the synapse. The *synapse* is the space between nerve cells, and neurotransmitters are responsible for communication between adjacent cells. The role of neurotransmitters is to act as a stimulator for the next cell to begin firing. The intricate process of the neural firing occurs millions of times over, every day, in every system of the body. Because of its delicacy, it can easily be disrupted.

Subluxations can compromise neural integrity by irritating the sensitive nerve tissue as it exits the spine. Because a subluxated joint does not move, pressure may build in the area of the nerve root—causing chafing, inflammation, and excruciating pain. Some subluxations are so severe that they actually cause impingement of the nerve; that is, they press directly on the nerve root, producing severe radicular pain.

More ominous, though, is that impingement can disrupt the function of the nerve. Remember, spinal nerves control the body's organs and tissues. If nerves become even slightly compromised, the operation or function of their end organs—the heart, the kidneys, muscles, etc.—may become distorted. We know that excessive nerve stimulation, as seen with subluxations, can lead to a hyperexcitability of an organ [100]. When chronic, a subluxation can predispose a person to many disorders such as hypertension, renal weakness, or hormonal imbalance.[101]

This is not to say that subluxations cause disease, per se—they do not. Instead, they cause physiological changes or dysfunctions in the tissues and organs supplied by the irritated nerves. Over time, these changes may weaken the organs and leave them susceptible to disease. What are the effects of multiple subluxations, then? Well, if one subluxation can compromise the integrity of one end organ, then several may have wider and more comprehensive effects on the entire body.

It is a very simple concept. The nervous system is the master control of the body. Its cells, the neurons, are very sensitive. They are so sensitive that evolution has found it necessary to protect the CNS with a strong bony shell. If we know that subluxations lead to dysfunction of the end organs, then logically, they must disrupt the body's overall internal balance. Think of it in the same way you would think of the electrical system of a precision automobile. Would you neglect the electronic component of a Mercedes or BMW? Not if you want it to perform at its best, you wouldn't. The bottom line is that a system with all its parts working unimpeded will last longer and perform better than one that has been neglected. Another way to think about it would be to consider the CNS like the hard drive of a computer. A body with multiple subluxations would be analogous to a computer with several corrupted files. If left in this condition, the body may work properly for a while, but it will soon malfunction; and eventually, it will break down.

## The Chiropractic Adjustment

I have spent all this time telling you how destructive subluxations can be—how they cause pain, damage nerves, and disrupt the delicate balance of the body. Without a doubt, subluxations are obstacles to health; but there is a solution: *the chiropractic adjustment.*

The adjustment is a method chiropractors use to correct subluxations; it is a gentle yet high-velocity thrust administered to a stuck spinal joint. This thrust—which is highly specific in location, direction, and force—opens up the affected joint, allowing the joint's lubricating fluids to move freely throughout its surface area and restore its normal motion. Accompanying the adjustment is a characteristic "popping" sound called a *cavitation*. Many people mistake this sound for the "cracking" of bones; however, it is actually the release of gas—nitrogen, oxygen, and carbon dioxide—which has been built up in the joint. It is very similar to the sound made when removing the top off a champagne bottle. The gas in the closed bottle builds pressure, and when the cap is removed—*pop!*

A chiropractic adjustment is usually painless although some people do report a minor discomfort when their muscles reflexively tighten or spasm. Many chiropractors have methods to reduce spasms like heat therapy or massage before they perform the adjustment, and this lessens any discomfort associated with tight muscles. Some chiropractors may even use an alternative form of adjustment that is very low in force. Either way, an adjustment usually feels quite good.

Adjustments have many positive and wide-ranging effects on the body. First and foremost is the return of normal motion to stuck joints. Remember that the spine is a dynamic system, and as a result, it engages in some sort of movement at all times. Everything from walking to exercising to working at a computer requires movement of the spine. It even moves as we sleep. For instance, we roll from side to side, flex and extend, and move our arms and legs periodically. The vertebrae also move every time we take a breath. They separate as we inhale and come back together when we exhale. As we discussed in the last chapter, breathing is essential, and we want to be able to expand our chests fully so we can take in the greatest amount of air possible. By reducing subluxations, then, the body is able to maintain its normal movements and allow many of its other vital functions, like breathing, to occur unimpeded.

The restoration of movement gives us the ability to once again perform activities that we generally take for granted—such as walking, sitting, or bending forward—things that we should be able to do pain free but sometimes can't because of subluxations. Muscle spasms often occur as a result of subluxations, and they can also make movement painful. When subluxated, the body considers itself to be in an injured state, and it creates spasms in the vicinity of the joint to prevent further insult. By correcting the faulty biomechanics of the joint—that is, lack of movement—muscle spasms are reduced.

Along with a reduction in pain, people often report feeling younger, or at least feeling their age again, when proper joint biomechanics are restored. Nothing makes one feel older than a combination of pain and restricted movement. By receiving regular chiropractic adjustments, people can live pain free and ensure that their bodies move freely, just as they are supposed to.

Another benefit of receiving regular adjustments is an increase in vascular circulation. Since blood vessels enter and exit the spine, they can become impinged just like nerves. Impinged vessels can lead to blood stagnation, which may ultimately form clots. Blood clots can dislodge and find their way into the lungs, causing a fatal disorder called a *pulmonary embolism* (chapter 3). Chiropractic adjustments allow the spinal vessels to maintain free blood flow. This is particularly important in the neck region where the vertebral arteries pass through the cervical (neck) vertebrae and travel to the brain. Although every organ needs proper blood supply for their function and survival, none needs it more than the brain. Regular adjustments ensure that the brain always receives an adequate supply of blood. Consequently, migraine and tension headaches often disappear with regular chiropractic adjustments as well.

Another wonderful benefit of the adjustment is that it alleviates pressure from the sensitive nerve tissue. Of course, this removes pain; but more importantly, it ensures that the organs and tissues receive proper innervation to carry out their functions. With regular chiropractic adjustments, the body remains balanced and functions static free, with nothing to disrupt its delicate and precise operation. Remember, the nervous system controls and coordinates every action and process in the body. By reducing subluxations, then, the immune system, hormonal system, digestive system, genitourinary system, and all other systems of the body can operate at their optimum level.

Even though chiropractic care can return the body to balance and restore optimal function, the removal of subluxations does *not* cure disease. Only the innate healing ability of the body can actually do this. Nevertheless, people with diseases definitely fare better without subluxations than they do with them; and in all cases, correcting subluxations make the body healthier and stronger. This is true because by correcting subluxations, obstacles that weaken and interfere with the body's overall functioning are removed. Thus, chiropractic adjustments are both health restoring and life enhancing.

As I present to you all the many extraordinary advantages of chiropractic care, I mustn't forget to inform you of the most obvious and gratifying benefits one receives by getting adjusted—it just plain feels good! Chiropractic adjustments remove tension, restore flexibility, and return freedom of movement, thereby invigorating and nourishing the body. Only when we lose our ability to move do we fully appreciate how much it means to us. Freedom of motion is a precious gift, and much of our existence depends on it.

I too am a regular recipient of chiropractic care. I cannot even comprehend what my life would be like without chiropractic. Every aspect of my life is physical, from my work to my leisure activities. And my lifestyle would be severely diminished if I were unable to move with ease and comfort. I count my blessings every day for the privilege of receiving regular chiropractic care. Take it from a guy who would be an invalid by now if chiropractic adjustments were not available to him.

Trust me when I say that if you try chiropractic care for at least six months, you will know exactly what I am talking about. You will experience more energy, better sleep, better sex, improved athletic performance, a healthier and more radiant glow, greater productivity, a more youthful appearance, and a greater overall enjoyment of life. And chiropractic is 100 percent natural. Don't take my word for it—try it yourself. I am certain you will find it as helpful and as pleasurable as I do.

## A Brief History of Chiropractic

Before the birth of modern chiropractic, adjustments were known as *spinal manipulations*. Manipulations were used as a form of bodywork by almost every civilization in history. The first documented case was in 2700 BC in ancient China, but there are also accounts of its use in ancient Greece, Babylonia, Egypt, and India.[102, 103] The practice of chiropractic as we know it today has its roots in nineteenth-century America. Chiropractic was discovered in Davenport, Iowa, in 1895 by Daniel David "D. D." Palmer. D. D. Palmer provided the first chiropractic adjustment to Mr. Harvey Lillard, a deaf janitor who cleaned the offices where Palmer practiced as a magnetic healer. As legend has it, by adjusting a vertebra in Mr. Lillard's thoracic spine, Palmer helped facilitate the restoration of the deaf man's hearing. Although this account may be more a product of folklore than reality, the events that transpired that day essentially led to the birth of the amazing healing art known as *chiropractic*.

Chiropractic was founded on the philosophy that subluxations disrupt the natural balance of the body, and as such, they have a negative affect on human health. During its infancy, chiropractic helped many people overcome physical disorders like hip pain, low back pain, limping, headaches, and much more. Some people even reported finding relief from ailments such as menstrual cramps, fatigue, and digestive disorders. Although the accounts of chiropractic curing nonmusculoskeletal disorders were mostly anecdotal (patient description and testimonial), they helped attract hordes of people into chiropractic offices throughout the country, many of who were unable to find relief through traditional medical care.

During the 1920s, the medical profession had concerns regarding chiropractic and its effect on public health and safety. Organized medicine, though, was ignorant of the practice and philosophy behind chiropractic and made little effort to learn more about it. There were also economic concerns: what exactly was this infant healing art that was taking people out of medical offices and . . . helping them? The American Medical Association (AMA) took the initiative to outlaw what they perceived to be competition at best, but at worst, a threat to public safety. They started a campaign against chiropractic by bringing criminal charges against a Japanese American chiropractor named Shegataro Morikubo. They charged him with practicing medicine and surgery without a license and wanted to use this rationale as a basis to outlaw all chiropractic in the country.

This landmark case began the legitimacy of chiropractic in the public health sector. Morikubo's attorneys contended that chiropractic was a practice distinctly different from medicine; it was based on its own unique philosophy that human beings are born with good health, and they can keep their health by removing obstacles (i.e., subluxations) which might prevent their bodies from functioning properly. Chiropractors could never be accused of practicing medicine, they argued, since chiropractic and medicine were two totally different systems with entirely different methodologies. As it turned out, chiropractic proved its case and won.

Many people do not realize this, but the chiropractic profession actually paved the way for all forms of alternative health care in this country including acupuncture, nutritional supplementation, and physical fitness. Each one of these healing arts might have experienced its own difficulties had it not been for chiropractic establishing the legitimacy of alternative forms of health care. Thanks to this revolutionary case, the doors were opened for all forms of bodywork to be practiced in this country.

Fast forward to the 1960s: Because of the Morikubo case, organized medicine knew that they could not eliminate chiropractic; so instead, they decided to launch a smear campaign designed to discourage the public from seeking chiropractic care. The American Medical Association (AMA) formed its Committee on Quackery whose sole purpose it was to discredit the chiropractic profession. They carried out this campaign by spreading the word that chiropractic was unsafe and that it could hurt people, maim them, and maybe even kill them. The AMA knew that the public would believe their allegations because they were the most powerful and influential health organization in the world. And that was not all—they threatened to punish any hospital or doctor that worked in conjunction with a chiropractor by removing the hospital's funding or revoking the doctor's treating privileges. This seemed a sure way to put chiropractors out of business for good.

An insider's tip led to the exposure of the scheme laid out by the AMA. It took some very brave souls in the chiropractic and legal professions to file suit against the AMA for violating U.S. antitrust laws (*Wilk v. AMA*).[104] The medical association was charged with trying to develop a monopoly within the U.S. health care system, and the case was taken all the way to the Supreme Court. In 1990, the case was decided in favor of chiropractic. Not only was this an enormous victory for the chiropractic profession, but also for every other form of "alternative" health care and bodywork in existence. The overall effect was that it allowed the public to maintain free access to a number of valuable forms of bodywork, which have been used successfully to treat people for centuries. We can all be grateful for these landmark decisions, which have given us the right to choose the natural and powerful approach of health—and life-enhancing bodywork.

## Some Common Myths Dispelled

Even though people have been using chiropractic for years to alleviate pain, restore biomechanical and neurological function, and improve health, there are still some who have yet to experience its power. Probably the most common reason people fail to try chiropractic is because they are afraid. Usually, fears are based on a handful of misconceptions: some a result of false information, and others due to ignorance. Either way, if I can dispel some of these myths by providing you with the most accurate and up-to-date information on the subject, then maybe those of you who have avoided chiropractic in the past will feel safer, and perhaps even motivated, to finally check it out.

One common misconception people have is that chiropractic treats diseases. The truth is that nothing could be further from the truth. Chiropractic detects and corrects spinal subluxations *only*. The theory behind chiropractic is that subluxations cause dysfunction to the joints as well as to the nerve tissue associated with those joints. Nerves innervate organs, so when there is an insult or irritation to the nerves, the end organs will also be affected. By removing the source of irritation (the subluxation), the balance and function of the body is restored. A well-balanced and properly functioning body is naturally better able to heal itself than an unbalanced one, and there are a number of people who, under chiropractic care, have experienced miraculous healing from various states of disease and dysfunction through their own innate reparative processes.

Another misconception is that chiropractic can harm you. This one happens to be true . . . well, somewhat. When a chiropractic adjustment is administered by an untrained individual like a personal trainer, a massage therapist, a martial arts instructor, a midwife, or anyone else who is otherwise unqualified, then it can be dangerous indeed. Adjustments can be harmful even when administered by a medical doctor or physical therapist if they have not had sufficient chiropractic training. Chiropractors spend years learning their craft, and one cannot become proficient by simply attending a weekend seminar, even if one happens to have medical training. The chiropractic adjustment must be studied and practiced for a significant length of time to be mastered, and it would be unwise to allow anyone other than a trained chiropractic professional to administer one. Unfortunately, some people do allow unqualified individuals to adjust them, and many end up paying the price for their decision. Most injuries reported as resulting from an adjustment have usually been performed by nonlicensed individuals.[105]

Chiropractic care administered by a qualified practitioner is one of the safest forms of health care available. There have been some claims that chiropractic adjustments pose a risk for causing stroke; however, according to a study conducted by the RAND Corporation, the risks are "about one in a million."[106] This fact is supported by a 1995 survey of sixty-four California neurologists who concluded that stroke was seen in only one out of five hundred thousand adjustments. According to one coinvestigator, Philip Lee, MD,

> Our intent is not to scare people away from chiropractic. Indeed, most interventions by allopathic physicians [MDs] have a higher complication rate than chiropractic interventions.[107]

These numbers should ease the minds of those avoiding chiropractic for fear of injury. When we evaluate chiropractic in context of its risk-to-benefit ratio, it is easy to see that chiropractic care is one of the safest health care modalities available.

Yet another misconception about chiropractic is that there is insufficient scientific evidence supporting it, which is also not completely true. According to the Foundation for Chiropractic Education and Research (FCER),

> Since 1980, the Foundation for Chiropractic Education and Research (FCER) has funded nearly $10 million in research. As the oldest research-funding organization for the chiropractic profession, FCER has been able to support grants, fellowships, and/or research residencies at an impressive list of colleges, universities, clinics, and institutions around the world.[108]

For sure, there is still much to know about how chiropractic works, but this is true of all medical and health science—there is still so much about the human body we do not yet understand, and we should continue to study it extensively. Many pharmaceutical drugs, for example, are placed on the market before they are completely understood despite the danger this poses to public health (see chapter 7). On the other hand, much of chiropractic's efficacy in relieving back pain and other musculoskeletal conditions *is* known and supported. Some studies have reported,

> chiropractic almost certainly confers worthwhile, long-term benefit in comparison with hospital outpatient management. The benefit is seen mainly in those with chronic or severe pain.[109]

> At three years the results confirm . . . that when chiropractic or hospital therapists treat patients with low back pain . . . those treated by chiropractic derive more benefit and long-term satisfaction than those treated by hospitals.[110]

> Patients of chiropractors were three times as likely as patients of family physicians to report that they were very satisfied with the care they received for low back pain.[111]

The lower costs . . . along with the favorable satisfaction and quality . . . suggest that chiropractic deserves careful consideration . . . to control health care spending.[112]

The reality is that many of the wide-ranging benefits that regular chiropractic patients experience are not quantifiable; they are measured, instead, on how people feel afterward (see chapter 8). While some might discount the validity of this method as a viable outcome measure, I happen to believe that it matters. The way one feels following any particular therapy is as important as what the research literature says one should experience.

We also cannot disregard the numerous accounts of people's overall health improving while under chiropractic care. We say that patient descriptions or testimonials are anecdotal and, indeed, subjective. Anecdotal reports are by no means scientific, but they still cannot be discounted as valuable pieces of information. Without a doubt, we need to continue to study the ways in which chiropractic affects healing, and the chiropractic profession is diligently working on it. However, any suggestions that chiropractic is not scientifically valid are simply absurd.

Some people have the misconception that chiropractors are not real doctors. The term *doctor* is Latin for "teacher," meaning that the true purpose of a doctor is to teach patients about their health and the ways to maintain it. In this regard, chiropractors are the quintessential doctors of the twenty-first century as they have traditionally focused on teaching their clients about health and wellness.

As far as the term *doctor* as a licensed professional is concerned, chiropractors are educated, trained, and licensed by their state board organizations. They are fully recognized by the states in which they practice, the federal government, and the U.S. Supreme Court.[113] The profession is reimbursed by Medicare and the U.S. Department of Veterans Affairs. It simply does not get any more "real" than that.

You also often hear that chiropractic is addictive. OK, this one is true—chiropractic *is* addictive. It is addictive in the same way that exercising or brushing one's teeth or breathing is. All of these things, along with regular chiropractic care, are essential; so in that sense, yes, I guess it is addictive. But chiropractic adjustments also make the body feel great, so you certainly might become addicted to feeling good and functioning better. However, unlike many of the other things people get addicted to like drugs, alcohol, or even other people, chiropractic is good for you. There is nothing wrong with that kind of addiction, now is there?

This does not mean that you will need to see a chiropractor every day just to feel good. On the contrary, once your body regains its balance, you will need only periodic checkups to detect and address any returning subluxations. When coupled with the other five keys, especially exercise, you will find that your periodic adjustments do wonders in keeping your body moving and feeling great.

The final misconception about chiropractic care is that it is inappropriate for children. Well, let's see. I received my first chiropractic adjustment as a seven-year-old, and aside from an occasional bad attitude, I have done quite well.

I treat many children and expecting mothers in my practice, including my wife when she was pregnant, and they thrive under chiropractic care. One lovely couple, in fact, brought their baby in to see me when he was just one-week-old. His name is Luca; and he is a healthy, robust, and vibrant baby who loves his adjustments. His parents are giving him the greatest gift they can, the gift of health. And I even adjusted my beautiful daughter, Delilah, when she was just hours out of the womb. Why? Because birthing can be hard work for a baby too, you know.

If you find that any of these reasons I have just discussed have been keeping you from seeing a chiropractor, please do yourself a favor and give chiropractic a try. Despite the prevalence of these misconceptions, chiropractic remains the number 1 form of alternative health care that Americans choose. Why? Because it works. Everyone from professional dancers to professional athletes to Hollywood celebrities use chiropractic to maintain their bodies and optimize their health. If these professionals trust their million-dollar bodies to chiropractic care, then so can you. Please do not hesitate to incorporate this amazing healing art into your life today. When you do, you'll understand exactly what I've been talking about; and even better, it will show in your body as vibrant health.

The following are some things people are saying about chiropractic:

- Arnold Schwarzenegger: "I am very fortunate to have, so to speak, my in-house chiropractor, Dr. Franco Colombu, as my own personal chiropractor. He adjusts my wife, my kids, me, everybody gets an adjustment. And we always feel great when Franco leaves . . . You chiropractic doctors are really miracle workers . . . Let me tell you there is no better profession than chiropractic. You really helped me. Every day you are preventing injuries; helping people. You let them walk out of your office feeling great about themselves and feeling good in their bodies, relieving pain. I can tell you this from firsthand experience."[114]
- Barry Bonds: "I think it should be mandatory for all athletes to see a chiropractor. I see [my chiropractor] about once a week, in between my

training [sessions]. By getting an adjustment once a week from him, I feel I can sustain my career a lot longer."

- Lance Armstrong: From http://www.nike.com, "After last year's Tour de France, Lance said that he could not have won without [his chiropractors] help."[115]

- Dr. Phil: "I'm a big believer in chiropractic . . . And I've got a chiropractor that I see, two or three times a week . . ."[116]

- Madonna: From http://cnn.com, "Madonna gets a chiropractic adjustment in 'Truth or Dare,' a 1991 documentary of the singer's 'Blonde Ambition' tour."[117]

- Emmitt Smith: On chiropractic, "I decided to invest in me, to keep me going . . . You can have a Ferrari body, but your wheels need balancing . . . I felt if I took care of my body, I could still function when I got older . . . Some of it may seem hokey to some people, but if you traveled where I've traveled, done what I've done and seen the results that I've been getting, then you'd understand where I'm coming from."[118]

- Tiger Woods: Rode the Alliance for Chiropractic Progress's Tournament of Roses Parade float in 1995. "Being a chiropractic patient has really helped me a lot . . . When I was in a growth spurt, my back became very sore and I was weak. My chiropractor really helped me. Not only did he adjust my spine, he also gave me strengthening exercises to do. If you are tall and gangly, like I am, or play sports, I would recommend chiropractic."[119]

- Cher: "The grind [of touring] is tough. Performing is the easy part. The hard part is going from place to place, hotel to hotel, venue to venue. This tour would kill girls half my age. It's strenuous and backbreaking, which is why I have my chiropractor on the road. I can't do things I could do 10 years ago."[120]

Other noted chiropractic clients include Mel Gibson, Evander Holyfield, Joe Montana (adjusted on national TV right before Super Bowl XXIV in 1990), Tom Brady, Jerry Rice, John Stockton, Ted Danson, Kelsey Grammer, Detroit Lions, Denver Broncos, Baltimore Ravens, Kansas City Chiefs, St. Louis Rams, Major League Baseball umpires, and the list goes on and on and on . . .

# Chapter 4 Summary

# Key Number 3: Bodywork

- See a chiropractor for a spinal checkup. Get adjusted once a month after an initial introductory balancing regimen.
- Get regular muscle work—massage, shiatsu, trigger point therapy, myofascial release—at least one time per month.
- If you have pain, see a chiropractic doctor immediately for an evaluation.
- Stretch daily.
- Have any muscular imbalances identified (yes, by a chiropractor) and ask for an exercise regimen to correct them.
- Work on your balance (standing on one leg, tree pose, etc.).
- Do abdominal exercises at least one time per week.
- Focus on posture. Some of the professionals who can help you with this are chiropractors, yoga instructors, Alexander technique trainers, pilates instructors, and drill sergeants.
- Do *not* let your personal trainer, yoga instructor, midwife, or any other untrained individual adjust you. Never. Ever. Period.

# CHAPTER 5

# Sleep: The Art of Rejuvenation

*[Sleep is] the golden chain that ties health and our bodies together.*
—Thomas Dekker

WHEN WE THINK of sleep, rarely do we consider its role in health. Just like breathing, sleep is a process we often take for granted. For the most part, it comes with very little thought or effort at all. Only when we become deprived of sleep do we ever give it much thought. Yet if we fail to respect the importance of sleep or we neglect it, then our health can become seriously compromised as a result.

Sleep is controlled by the hypothalamus region of the brain. The hypothalamus manages our *circadian rhythms*, the daily cycles of biological activity that regulate many metabolic functions. Although our circadian rhythms are usually in sync with the rising and setting of the sun, we do have an innate cycle that we call our biological clock. Heart rate, blood pressure, body temperature, hormonal secretions, and sleep are all attuned to the tempo of the biological clock. Neurons (nerve cells) in the hypothalamus have an internal timing mechanism that works alongside external factors, like daylight, to start and stop our natural rhythms. This internal mechanism of the sleep or wake cycle can also be set by outside stimuli such as an alarm clock or the timing of meals.

The hormone melatonin plays an important role in regulating sleep cycles. It acts on the area of the brain that controls our circadian rhythms and causes us to feel drowsy. During the day, when we need to be wide awake, the production of melatonin is shut off. Daylight causes photoreceptors in the retina (a tissue present in the back of the eye) to send a signal down the optic nerve, stimulating the hypothalamus to inhibit or prevent the production of melatonin from the pineal gland. As day turns to night, less and less signals are sent to the hypothalamus, allowing the pineal gland to freely secrete melatonin—this eventually leads to sleepiness. Because of its role in initiating sleep, some people find melatonin supplements useful as a natural sleep aid.

Our sleep cycles are not set in stone; that is, they can be altered or changed to suit our needs, like when we experience a change in schedule or travel to a different time zone. We may not adjust to our new sleep cycle immediately as it takes several days for our bodies to adapt. For example, when flying from the West Coast of the United States to the East Coast, we lose three hours. We might find it difficult to get up the next morning since according to our biological clock, it is three hours earlier. On the other hand, traveling in the opposite direction may cause us to wake up well before sunrise as our biological clock will be set for three hours ahead. Over time, though, our internal timing mechanism resets itself to accommodate these changes.

## Stages of Sleep

As we sleep, we pass through five different stages characterized by specific patterns of electrical activity or brain waves.[121] The first four stages are what we would call *nonrapid eye movement* sleep while the fifth stage is called *rapid eye movement*, or REM sleep. We pass through the five stages successively and then repeat the entire cycle over again at stage one. This happens repeatedly throughout sleep—with 50 percent of the time spent in stage 2, 20 percent in stage 5 (REM), and 30 percent in the other three stages.

Stage 1 is a transitional state between sleep and wakefulness. People in stage 1 can be awakened easily, and if asked, they will often deny being asleep. During this phase, it is not uncommon for people to experience a sensation of falling, followed by a sudden muscle twitch or contraction, which jars them awake. We are all familiar with this stage. Unfortunately, we're usually reminded of it at the most inopportune times, like while in class or in the middle of a staff meeting. In stage 1 sleep, which lasts for only about five minutes, our brain waves begin to change from alpha waves to slower theta waves.

In stage 2, breathing and heart rate slow down, eye movement decreases, and theta waves begin to dominate the brain wave activity. Remember that theta waves are slower than alpha waves, so this stage is characterized by a much deeper sleep than stage 1. Stages 3 and 4 have the slowest brain wave activities, with stage 3 generating both theta and delta brain waves (delta being slower than theta) and stage 4 producing only delta rhythms. It is very difficult to wake somebody while they are in stage 3 or 4 sleep. If awakened, they are often groggy. Stages 3 and 4 together are called *deep sleep*.

Stage 5 is known as rapid eye movement, or REM, sleep. During this phase, heart rate increases and breathing becomes faster and shallower. The eyes begin to dart back and forth in various directions, giving the stage its characteristic name. Although skeletal muscles experience a sort of temporary paralysis during REM sleep, penile and clitoral erections often occur. The brain waves present at this stage are mainly beta waves. These are the same rhythms present as when we are alert and conscious; however, some researchers believe that our brains may actually be working harder during this stage than when we are awake. Since this is the phase in which dreams occur, muscle paralysis prevents us from acting out our dreams, which—for many of us—is a blessing indeed.

## Functions of Deep Sleep

Each stage of sleep is responsible for carrying out one or more important physiological functions.[122] During deep sleep (non-REM stages, especially stage 4), various hormones and chemicals are released in the body, particularly growth hormone (GH). GH (chapter 3) is secreted by the pineal gland of the brain and stimulates bone and muscle growth in children; it is also responsible for tissue repair in adults. There should be no surprise, then, that teenagers spend most of their sleep time in deep sleep—something parents should think about before chastising their children for sleeping too much.

Recuperative functions are also carried out during deep sleep. For instance, ATP is replenished during this phase, giving us plenty of energy to use throughout the next day. Wound healing also increases during deep sleep. Damaged cells are replaced and new cells produced while old cells are killed off or "turned over" at this time.[123] Although the regenerative process occurs throughout the entire day—in every organ and tissue, keeping them healthy and functioning properly—it is during deep sleep when this process accelerates.

DNA repair is another form of regeneration that occurs during deep sleep. When we are awake, constant cellular metabolism leads to an increased formation of free radicals (chapter 2). Remember that free radicals can damage tissues and cause chronic diseases like cancer. During sleep, metabolism slows down, allowing the enzymes that neutralize free radicals to do their job. These vital enzymes are themselves regenerated in deep sleep.

Neurotransmitters like norepinephrine (controlling heart rate, blood pressure, and other vital functions) and serotonin (involved in mood regulation and sleep found in chapter 6) are replenished during non-REM sleep. These important molecules must be in ample supply to guarantee proper functioning of the nervous system. Sleep deprivation can cause depletion of our neurotransmitters, which can ultimately lead to varying forms of depression.[124] Studies have shown that people getting less than adequate amounts of sleep have a higher incidence of irritability and frustration and a decreased ability to modulate their moods.

The popular antidepressant medications Prozac, Paxil, and Zoloft are in a class of drugs known as the *selective serotonin reuptake inhibitors* (SSRIs found in chapter 6). This type of drug prevents the reuptake or replenishment of serotonin by the nerve cells, allowing neurotransmitters to be constantly present in the blood. Although serotonin is essential in regulating mood, these drugs may actually perpetuate the problem by taxing the supplies of the hormone as well as desensitizing its receptors. It is no wonder that people taking these medications often become reliant on them, eventually losing the wherewithal to cope without them.

Immune function also depends upon sleep.[125] Studies have shown that rats deprived of sleep develop sores on their paws and tails.[126] Researchers believe that this is a consequence of a depressed immune system (wound healing ability). Humans too are susceptible to a weakened immune system, as people who repeatedly deprive themselves of sleep are at a greater risk of developing colds and other infections.

Sleep may provide cosmetic benefits as well. During sleep, the body decreases the breakdown of proteins and, alternately, steps up their production. Proteins are the building blocks of all tissues including hair, skin, and nails; therefore, getting a sufficient amount of sleep is vital to the rejuvenation of our external appearance. Sleep gives people a healthy glow, but we often see the opposite in those continually deprived of sleep. Those who frequently rob the sandman tend to look old and haggard. They develop wrinkles, their eyes swell, and their skin gets dry and worn—the typical appearance of a regular methamphetamine user. Meth addicts typically sacrifice sleep for drugs. Loved ones stand by helplessly as the addict literally ages right before their eyes. This rapid aging process is as much a consequence of sleep deprivation as it is of the drug itself.

## Functions of REM Sleep

The benefits of deep sleep are numerous, yet REM sleep is equally important. During this stage, cognitive and memory functions are processed. Much of the information we gather or learn throughout the day is sorted out during this stage. Sleep deprivation, then, negatively affects our critical thinking process. People suffering from sleep deprivation find it harder to solve complex problems; and even routine tasks such as driving, using machinery, or handling tools can become impaired. Studies done on college students have shown that those who pull all-nighters consistently demonstrate poorer test scores than their well-rested counterparts.[127]

During REM sleep, signals travel in the brain from the pons to the thalamus to the cerebral cortex. The cerebral cortex is the area of the brain responsible for learning and memory. One study found that people who slept after learning and practicing a new task remembered more about it the next day than people who stayed up all night after learning the same thing.[128]

Another interesting event that happens during REM sleep is our propensity to dream. Some theorists believe that during REM sleep, the fragments of information we collect throughout the day are organized in the cortex. As pieces of fragmented material are put together for storage, the cortex tries to make sense of it by creating a "story" that we experience as a dream. Although some cultures believe that dreams have hidden messages and meanings, we are not yet certain of that theory's validity. Undoubtedly, this phenomenon will be better understood in the future. Sleep is not only restful for the body, but important for the many functions carried out during the process. Cell turnover, metabolism, immune function, and memory are all dependent on our sleep patterns—any disruption to these patterns and our capacity to function may be severely hampered.

## Sleep Disorders

The amount of sleep we get is not always our choice. There are several syndromes that can affect our sleep either by preventing it or by inducing it at inopportune times. According to the National Institute of Neurological Disorders and Stroke (NINDS), more than seventy sleep disorders have been discovered with sleep apnea, restless leg syndrome, and narcolepsy being some of the more common ones.[129] The most common sleep disorder, though, is one that we may actually have the most control over—and that is insomnia.

*Insomnia* is the inability to fall asleep. The National Institute of Health (NIH) reports that insomnia affects more than 70 million Americans, with 58 percent of adults experiencing symptoms a few nights a week or more.[130] People suffering from this disorder can go without sleep for up to a month or longer. This is a maddening situation that often leads to depression. Furthermore, chronic sleep deprivation has been shown to cause high blood pressure, heart attack, stroke, obesity, psychiatric problems, and mood disorders. Mental impairment, fetal and childhood growth retardation, injury from accidents, disruption of bed partner's sleep quality, and poor quality of life can all result from insomnia.[131]

Some of the many things that can cause insomnia are stress, jet lag, excessive caffeine before bedtime, nicotine, medications, dietary habits, and late-night exercise. It can also be due to an underlying medical disorder. Some people suffer from chronic insomnia, signifying a serious problem, yet many of us have experienced a minor bout at one time or another.

Unfortunately, many people try to combat insomnia with sedatives like pills or alcohol. Although sleeping pills may provide a quick fix, it is far too easy to become dependent on them. This can ultimately lead to an exacerbation of the sleep disorder, not to mention a whole host of other problems. Studies have shown that insomniacs taking prescription sleeping pills have been linked to many strange behaviors, like binge eating or having sex, while asleep; and worse yet, these people seem to remember none of their actions.[132] Alcohol, on the other hand, will depress the nervous system enough so that one can immediately fall asleep; however, once the effects of the drug wear off (about three to four hours), sleeplessness can return and is usually accompanied by a hangover.

A better way to combat insomnia is to practice good sleep habits. Start by waking up at the same time every morning. Because our circadian rhythms are sensitive to and can be set by light, waking up at dawn is the best option but certainly not a must. The rule is to keep a regular pattern by going to bed at the same time every night. This might be a difficult habit to acquire, particularly since many of us keep long and *odd* hours; but if you keep working at it, you should eventually be able to reset your sleep patterns. You will find that getting eight hours of sleep and waking up early in the morning far outweigh doing that extra report or catching that late-night television program.

Insomnia due to drugs, medications, or chronic illness cannot be overcome so easily. For instance, sleeplessness due to depression is often treated with tranquilizers. The use of tranquilizers to induce sleep can be counterproductive as drug dependence may ensue. These issues are serious and should be discussed with a qualified health practitioner.

Getting plenty of exercise also helps combat insomnia. Exercise not only gives you energy throughout the day, but also helps you sleep easier and more restfully at night. Be careful not to exercise too closely to your bedtime, though, since circulation and metabolism are increased during exercise. Doing so before bedtime might keep you energized and wide awake. It may take a few hours to slow these processes down, so if you must work out before bedtime, make sure you have a thick book to read as that will be more productive than tossing and turning the night away.

Insomnia can truly become more than just an annoyance. It can turn into a pattern that not only diminishes health, but can also keep one from realizing one's dreams in life. More and more people are staying up late so they can work more, play more, and watch more TV. This phenomenon is so prevalent that *Time* magazine aptly titled their December 20, 2004, piece about insomnia, "Sleep is for Sissies." According to the article, people are depriving themselves of sleep so they can have more time to do the things they consider necessary to live their lives to the fullest. Most of these people feel that they function just fine with minimal sleep and that they are the exception to the sleep rule. Unfortunately, they do not realize how much they are draining themselves, albeit slowly, just to squeeze a few more hours out of life.

One or two random days of sleep deprivation may not have a negative impact on one's health. However, the more one does it, the more it becomes a habit; and over time, the negative effects become cumulative. They can be so subtle at first that they may not even be noticed. Then, as time goes by, the lack of energy due to sleep deprivation may begin to affect one's work and maybe even one's *desire* to work. Many people at this stage are in denial; they may have difficulty noticing changes or an evolving pattern. As their sleep deprivation continues, they may actually finish their work, further reinforcing the notion that less sleep equals more production. As the weeks go by, though, their production diminishes.

Remember that REM sleep is necessary for memory; therefore, sleep-deprived people retain less information and forget things easier. They may get a little more tense (some mistakenly call this "intense" as it takes more concentration to complete each task) and irritable and may even start to lash out at others. They often get stressed out in situations beyond their control, like while sitting in traffic or waiting in line. As days turn into weeks, and weeks into months, they might start to feel overworked—desperately needing a vacation before they snap. At this point, their satisfaction with work may diminish, and they may begin to feel unfulfilled with their lives. They may try to counter this by taking a vacation; however, the same pattern of staying up late often continues. This vicious cycle can go on for years, eventually leading to ill health and depression—all rationalized by the false notion that "sleep becomes annoying once you realize how much [more] you can accomplish [without sleep]."[133]

Unhealthy sleep patterns usually begin in high school or college. Heavy workloads and full social schedules take up most of a student's time, especially for the "overachiever" type or "party girl or guy." Of course, their behavior is encouraged by society as there is always pressure to be productive. Sleep deprivation at the college level is so well known that at least one major American university has started to implement an individual wellness plan for all incoming first-year students, which educates them on the importance of sleep, exercise, and nutrition.[134]

What sleep deprivers fail to realize is that if they would just get a sufficient amount of sleep on a nightly basis, they would actually accomplish much more in less time. This is a secret shared by many successful people like Benjamin Franklin and Jimmy Carter.[135]

Those who work or play without proper rest *will* eventually fizzle and burn out. They run the risk of developing disorders like high blood pressure, heart disease, or mental illness. Plenty of people choose that path in life, but many of them end up being "too young to have a heart attack."

Let's face it—to maintain good health and increase overall productivity, sleep is as important as eating right or exercising. Without proper sleep, we lack energy;

and as a consequence, our life gets drained away from us like air from a tire with a slow leak. With less vigor, all of our efforts go toward performing tasks that we *have* to do instead of ones we'd *love* to do. No doubt, this pattern prevents many people from realizing their dreams. No matter who you are or what type of work you do, you will definitely do it better by getting plenty of sleep.

# Chapter 5 Summary

## Key Number 4: Sleep, Rest, and Recuperation

- Sleep at least eight hour per night.
- Keep a regular schedule. Early to bed, early to rise is best if possible.
- Take melatonin if you are having trouble keeping a regular schedule. Take the supplement on a regular schedule too.
- Any medications, which might keep you awake, should be taken earlier in the day (consult with your medical doctor before changing your schedule).
- Do not exercise too close to bedtime.
- Limit caffeine intake in the afternoon or evening. Drink caffeine during the morning hours, say before noon.
- Limit alcohol intake before bedtime.
- If you are tired, sleep. Don't burn the candle at both ends.
- Don't stay up to cram in that extra work. Get a good night's rest and continue in the morning.
- If you must miss some sleep, catch up the following night.

# CHAPTER 6

# Mind, Body, and Soul:
# The Triune of Human Existence

*There is no question that the things we think have a tremendous effect upon our bodies. If we can change our thinking, the body frequently heals itself.*
—C. Everett Koop, MD, former surgeon general of the United States

PHILOSOPHERS HAVE BEEN pondering the mind-body question for thousands of years. What makes up the entirety of man and his rightful place in the universe are riddles that have been mystifying great thinkers since the beginning of human existence. Today, we find ourselves asking many of these same questions: Are the mind and body separate and distinct, or are they connected in some concrete way? Is the mind the same as the soul, or is it merely part of a more complex neurobiochemical machine? Can our experiences transcend that which we perceive with our five senses, or must we be confined to the senses as our only means of evaluating reality? These are some of the many questions that we, like millions before us, continue to ask in order to better understand the connection between the mind and the body.

The idea of the mind as a major factor influencing health has not always been prevalent. In fact, it has only been until fairly recently that this theory has gained such wide acceptance. To be sure, there have been periods throughout history when people believed in a connection between the mind and body. Western civilization, however, has mostly viewed the mind as a distinct entity and, as such, has believed it to exert only a minor influence on health. Medical science operated from this ideology since the seventeenth century, and it was not until the middle of the twentieth century that a shift in thinking actually took place. To appreciate how much our understanding of mind-body dynamics has evolved, it will help to take a closer look at its long and intriguing history.

We will start in the fifteenth century BC with the Greeks who believed that health was not only a physical manifestation, but a spiritual one as well. When people became ill, they went to the temple to pray for health.[136] Clearly, the ancient Greeks respected the connection between the soul and the physical body.

Between the twelfth and fifth centuries BC, their belief system changed. It was the Greek physician Asclepius who started the practice of treating disease with medication and surgery, which then became the primary methods of patient care. Despite these new methods, some interest still remained in addressing *all* aspects of health, which included the body, the mind, and the spirit. Therapies like rest, music, massage, and dream interpretation were used regularly to heal the sick.[137]

In the fifth century BC, Hippocrates, the recognized Father of Modern Medicine, did away with any reliance on the supernatural in healing and, instead, encouraged a scientific approach to assess and treat patients. Doctors of that era commonly used social and psychological factors in addition to physical ones to evaluate those under their care. Health care, for the most part, remained a specialty of the physician; and as such, matters of mind, body, and spirit continued to be within the physician's realm—until the Middle Ages, that is.

During the Middle Ages, the mind-body question became a theological matter. The Catholic Church was at that time the sole authority on all issues pertaining to mind, body, and spirit. Academic scholars, though, began to study the anatomy and physiology of the human body; and their resultant findings helped to change the way the body was viewed. As a consequence of these new discoveries, the church, in an attempt to keep up with existing knowledge yet vying to maintain power, conceded to medical science the study of the body while maintaining control over the study of the mind, which it considered inseparable from the soul.[138] Despite this political and academic restructuring, most people still believed that the mind and soul were integral to the entire being and, therefore, were vital to the healing process.

It would take another two hundred years for contemporary thought to adopt the views held by the church that the mind and body were separate entities. The work of mathematician and philosopher René Descartes heavily influenced public opinion in the seventeenth century. His basic philosophy was that the universe could be described as "an impersonal machine strictly ordered by mathematical law."[139] He believed that all material phenomena, including the human body, were explainable by mathematical and physical principles. The mind was neither physical nor objective, in his opinion, but instead subjective and spiritual and, therefore, by definition, fundamentally different.

Descartes' philosophy was reductionist in nature, meaning that it started from the basic tenet that there exists a greater power called God (more on this method of logic later). The proof of our existence, then, could be derived from this basic belief. To keep in line with the teachings of the church—and especially out of his fear of persecution by the church—he taught that consciousness, or simply the mind, was a spiritual or religious matter. His influence on the collective philosophy over the next three hundred years created an even greater gap between the studies of mind and body.

The common belief at that time was that the body was a complex machine made up of many intricate and specialized parts. This type of philosophy is known as *mechanism* (chapter 1), and modern medical science has viewed and approached the human body in this way ever since. According to this paradigm, the body is seen as a conglomeration of separate parts and systems—the cardiovascular system, the pulmonary system, the digestive system, etc.—and most studies focus on each system separately. Of course, there have been benefits to approaching the study of the body this way—one of which has been the great strides made toward understanding the many intricacies of each separate organ system. However, what has been lost in the process is the understanding of the synergy that exists between all systems (chapter 8). In overlooking this, many important processes and functions of the human body remained hidden; this is especially true with regard to the mind.

The psychiatric profession tried to bridge the mind-body gap in the early part of the twentieth century, and to take on the task, they created the subspecialty of psychosomatic medicine. Their goal was to study the effects of the mind on the body and vice versa. Since they relied mostly on verbal analysis (speaking directly to subjects), they lacked any sort of objective measures; and their work was, therefore, never fully accepted by the nonpsychiatric medical community, as it was considered pseudoscience.[140] Furthermore, by relying solely on psychological protocol and ignoring physiological studies, they actually succeeded in creating an even wider gap between the studies of mind and body.

This failure to connect the mind and body mattered little to the overall picture of medical care at that time. Great advances were made in public health through vaccinations and antibiotics, and the desire to understand the mind-body connection soon faded. As surgical procedures became more sophisticated and medical technology blossomed, any further attempts to study mind-body healing fell by the wayside.

Just as in the time of Descartes, mind-body dualism was the prevalent philosophy in the beginning of the twentieth century. Medical science remained the authority on all things relating to the physical body while the psychology profession took hold of the study of the mind, basically liberating it from the confines of the church. Organized religion was not left out in the cold, though, as it continued to be the definitive authority on spiritual matters. What developed, then, was a triune of influence with regard to the three aspects of human existence—those relating to mind, body, and spirit—and it led to an even greater division of the many facets of man.

Medicine continued to experience great successes with the treatment of modern diseases. There were many medical breakthroughs achieved at that time, and the human lifespan began to increase dramatically. As a result, the concept of man as a complex machine persisted. It was not until chronic diseases like heart disease and cancer started to surge and old methods of treating people failed to produce consistent results that the old mechanistic model began to falter. Scientific evidence proved that chronic illnesses had many precipitating factors, with a great number pointing toward unhealthy lifestyle habits. Success continued in a fraction of cases, but the weakness of the one-treatment-fits-all approach was systematically exposed. Clearly, if chronic diseases were to be conquered, a new model would have to be constructed.

Renowned medical researcher George Engel apparently came to the same conclusion in his landmark article written for *Science* magazine.[141] In this piece, he outlined a new way of approaching health, one he called the *biopsychosocial model*. This model recognized health as a function of several factors including genetic, environmental, psychological, and social ones. This marked the beginning of mind-body medicine.

One of the earliest breakthroughs of this new discipline was the work carried out by Herbert Benson, MD, and his colleagues at the Harvard Medical School. In 1974, they studied a phenomenon called the *relaxation response*. At that time, it was evident that stress caused physiological changes to the body, many of which were harmful. These changes included increased blood pressure, heart rate, and respiratory rate—all of which played a part in the development of heart disease. If stress could cause illness, they reasoned, then perhaps relaxation would have a reversing effect.

Stress reduction is exactly what Benson and his colleagues studied. They observed people who practiced a form of meditation called *transcendental meditation* (TM), and they found that subjects who participated in this practice showed consistent decreases in blood pressure, heart rate, and respiratory rate, as well as positive effects on several other physiological functions. This was the first detailed study of its kind where a primarily Eastern practice was investigated by Western scientific methods. Science had finally validated what had already been understood by many cultures and civilizations throughout history that there were indeed physical benefits to the ancient practice of meditation.

Mind-body medicine (or behavioral medicine as it is sometimes called) now had a takeoff point. As a recognized subspecialty of the medical profession, studies on mind-body phenomena have been conducted regularly. Government-funded research followed, and today, many of the largest medical institutions offer mind-body-related treatment programs for patients.[142] In 1991, the National Institute of Health created the Office of Alternative Medicine, which eventually became the National Center for Complementary and Alternative Medicine (NCCAM) in 1998.[143]

Mind-body healing is at the forefront of alternative treatments regularly sought out by people. I think it is important, though, to make the distinction between mind-body *medicine* and mind-body *healing*. Mind-body medicine is a branch of the medical sciences that studies the use of the mind to affect healing. Using the mind as a tool for the healing process, though, can be done by anyone at any time. Being guided by a trained practitioner is helpful but not mandatory. There are many books and tapes available from which to learn different methods of mind-body healing; all it takes is a desire and the discipline to do so.

I will explain some very powerful mind-body techniques myself in the following pages. If you prefer to learn a technique under professional guidance, you have several options available. Choosing a medical professional is one option, but there are also effective techniques taught at yoga studios, meditation centers, and temples. Instructors at these venues can be as competent, patient, and effective as any medical professional and, in some cases, are even more so. For those seeking a more spiritual or philosophical path, these alternative sources may be a much better fit.

## Mental Illness: Biological or Psychological?

Although the study and practice of mind-body medicine have made great strides over the last few decades, the predominant method for dealing with "mental illness" is still traditional medical care. In other words, the mechanistic model, the basis for most modern medical interventions, has been the primary tool used to assess and treat mental health. To understand this further, it is important to investigate two schools of thought regarding mental illness: the biological and psychological models.

The *biological model* of mental illness views the mind from the same mechanistic perspective that modern medicine uses to view the physical body; that is, all mental processes can be explained by physical and biochemical laws. According to this line of thinking, all mental dysfunction is a consequence of chemical changes in the brain. These changes—due to either an overproduction or underproduction of hormones or neurotransmitters, or perhaps even to a flaw in the metabolic pathways of certain brain chemicals—can cause an afflicted person to behave differently than what society generally considers "normal." At least this is the rationale behind the biological model of mental illness. Proponents believe that the best way to treat these biochemical abnormalities are with drugs, surgeries, or other physical modalities like electroshock therapy.

The *psychological model*, on the other hand, believes that most mental disorders stem from the *mind*—that abstract component of human consciousness manifested in our thoughts, perceptions, emotions, will, memories, and imagination. Proponents of this model believe that the majority of mental disorders are due to psychological or social stressors, not chemical changes; and they point out that, as of yet, no modern instrument or technological devise has been discovered to effectively measure biochemical imbalances. In light of these facts, proponents emphasize that no convincing evidence exists that implicates genetics or biochemical imbalances as a cause of mental illness.[144]

I should point out here that there are some very distinct differences between the practices of psychiatry and psychology, both professionally and philosophically speaking. Psychiatrists are medical doctors; hence, they receive all the training necessary to become medical professionals. Not surprisingly, most psychiatrists subscribe to the mechanistic paradigm so predominant in the medical sciences—that is, the human body operates as a complex machine; and the brain, as its most complex organ, is no exception. The brain is comprised of an elaborate network of neurons and glial cells (support cells); and it carries out regular electrical, chemical, and hormonal actions. A psychiatrist, then, can be thought of as a specialist, one who focuses on an intricate neuroelectrobiochemical structure. Due to their philosophy, psychiatrists believe that mental disorders are brain disorders that can be treated effectively by electrical, chemical, and hormonal means; and their treatment methods generally reflect this point of view. The psychiatric profession is thus one of the strongest and most vocal advocates of the biological model of mental illness.

Psychologists, in contrast, are not medical doctors (MDs), but doctors of philosophy (PhD's). Their education is not bound by mechanistic ideology, but instead by the study of the mind. This discipline is best known for the work carried out by its forefathers: Sigmund Freud, Carl Jung, and William James. These pioneers focused on mental processes and human behavior, and the profession continues to use these principles as the foundation of its practice today. Most psychologists would not deny the physical and chemical nature of the brain; nevertheless, they consider the brain's chemical problems neurological, not mental. And they believe that neurological conditions should be treated neurologically, not biochemically. It is important to note that neurological disorders do, indeed, exist—Alzheimer's disease, Parkinson's disease, and Lou Gehrig's disease (ALS) are all very real. However, psychologists do not use the existence of these diseases as a rationale for attaching biochemical explanations to all mental disorders. Instead, they subscribe to the psychological model of mental illness.

Many people are unaware of the distinction between psychiatrists and psychologists. Most tend to think of these two professions as the same—not realizing that when they hire a therapist, they are generally hiring someone from the field of psychology. Psychologists are not qualified to prescribe medications; therefore, all psychotropic drugs are administered by psychiatrists. On the other hand, psychotherapists practice talk therapy, which up until very recently was the primary form of treatment for mental disorders. As you will see, times have drastically changed.

## Is There Really Such Thing as "Mental Illness"?

Depression is one of the most commonly diagnosed conditions in this country. Estimates report a staggering 21 million people suffer from depression at any given time, which is approximately seven percent of the general population of the United States.[145] With numbers so high, we have to wonder: Is the country really in such an endemic state of mental illness, or is depression simply becoming one of the most over—and *mis*—diagnosed conditions of our time? Or is it possible that our current definition of "depression" is perhaps a bit convoluted? Let's find out.

*Depression*, as defined by the World Health Organization (WHO), is "a *common* mental disorder that presents with depressed mood, loss of interest or pleasure, feelings of guilt or low self-worth, disturbed sleep or appetite, low energy, and poor concentration."[146]

Note that the above description classifies depression as a "common" disorder, something we all experience from time to time. If this experience is so common, should it really be qualified as an *illness*? According to the advocates of the biological model of mental illness, the answer is yes. In their opinion, depression is caused by biochemical imbalances in the brain and should therefore be treated by chemical means, despite the fact that a biochemical cause has yet to be proven.

During depression, the brain goes through physiological changes usually absent in a nondepressed state. We must ask the question, then: are these chemical and hormonal changes the actual cause of depression, or do they merely accompany the emotional state of the mind at that time? As we will investigate later, all emotional events have concurrent physiological responses, none of which can be truly implicated as the actual cause of those emotions.

To justify the claims of mental illness resulting from biochemical imbalances, proponents have formulated several tests to prove their hypothesis—none of which, so far, have been very successful. One method used in the past has been the Dexamethasone suppression test (DST) analysis. It is based on the theory that, during depression, a dysfunction occurs that increases the concentration of the hormone cortisol in the blood. Many hoped that this test would prove irrevocably that depression is a chemical event, yet it has failed miserably. According to several mental health experts, there were just too many cases of depression not showing a positive DST test. An article titled "Diagnosing Depression: How Good Is the 'DST'?" published in the *Harvard Medical School Health Letter* echoed this sentiment,

> For every three office patients with an abnormal DST, only one is likely to have true depression . . . . [And] a large fraction of people who are depressed by other criteria will still have normal results on the DST.[147]

But the DST was not the only test proponents were banking on; in fact, they still had a few other theories to cling to, most notably, the holy grail of chemical imbalance theories—the serotonin hypothesis. Based on the premise that depleted serotonin levels in the brain cause a state of major depression, this theory has been the foundation for the development of the megapopular antidepressants Prozac, Paxil, and Zoloft and has fueled their rampant use. Not all experts agree with this hypothesis, though. According to the U.S. Congressional Office of Technology Assessment,

> Currently, no clear evidence links abnormal serotonin receptor activity in the brain to depression . . . . the data currently available do not provide consistent evidence either for altered neurotransmitter levels or for disruption of normal receptor activity.[148]

In his book *The Anti-Depressant Fact Book*, medical doctor Peter R. Breggin states,

> Despite decades of research, thousands of research studies, and hundreds of millions of dollars in expense, no marker for depression has been found. To this day, the individual's personal feelings remain the basis for diagnosing depression.[149]

And regarding the serotonin theory, he says,

> Serotonin is one of hundreds of chemicals that affect brain function. Almost nothing is known about the relationships among the hundreds of millions

of neurons and these chemicals, and equally little is known about their relationship to the overall function of the mind or the brain (p. 31).

Clearly, the biochemical theory of depression is wrought with many holes; it simply does not stand up to the rigorous evaluation of the scientific process. Even so, it remains the basis of modern-day protocol for the diagnosis and treatment of depression. In effect, this unproven theory provides a ground for doctors to freely prescribe antidepressants to treat what they erroneously believe to be "chemical imbalances."

The question still remains, though: is depression actually an illness? A variety of experts think not; their opinion is that depression is not *necessarily* dysfunctional, especially since all of us experience feelings of sadness from time to time. What we would consider *clinical depression*—that is, a depression so severe, it disrupts a person's normal functioning—is characterized by feelings of sadness, loss, anger, or frustration for an extended period (two weeks according to some experts[150]). So the argument is, if we all experience sadness from time to time, then, to some degree, mustn't it be normal? And if the only thing differentiating "normal" from "abnormal" is the length of time we feel sad (two weeks?) or to the degree in which it affects our ability to function in our daily lives, then isn't the diagnosis of depression clearly subjective? The reality is that there is no definitive guideline with which to categorize this illness. Unlike diabetes, obesity, cirrhosis, or any other disease with specific parameters, depression is an arbitrary diagnosis. "I feel sad"; "I feel really sad"; "I feel really, really sad"—which of these should be considered depression, and which normal emotion? The time frame used to quantify depression is also completely random; nothing indicates two weeks to have any special significance. Furthermore, the ways in which our various emotional states affect us are as much a function of our perceptions, our tolerances, and our cultural upbringing, as they are of how strongly we experience any particular emotion. All these issues make categorizing depression as an illness very questionable.

Even if we do follow the reasoning behind the biological theory of depression, does it mean that psychological depression does not exist? Or are there two different types of depression: one biological, the other psychological? And what differentiates one from the other? What criteria are used to determine which form is present? Are intense feelings of sadness, anger, or frustration, that lead one to alcohol or drug abuse, psychological or biological? How about the feelings experienced following the loss of a job, the breakup of a relationship, or the loss of a loved one—which type of depression would these fall under?

By looking at these questions, it is not hard to see that we have overcomplicated the issue of depression, one which up until 1994 was still defined as an emotional or psychological state by every medical dictionary and psychology manual available. It was not until the advent of the selective serotonin reuptake inhibitor (SSRI) antidepressant medications that the definition of *depression* started to change. Suddenly, depression was no longer psychological, but instead a chemical dysfunction. Is it possible that our knowledge of human physiology was merely limited until that time? Or maybe the biochemical imbalances thought to cause depression are genetic and have somehow been favored during recent evolution? Perhaps, but there are still far too many inconsistencies and unanswered questions to make these assumptions. Either way, the number of depression cases diagnosed as chemical imbalances every year is highly suspect. Doctors and psychiatrists doling out these diagnoses really need to reevaluate their rationale and ask themselves if they are actually causing more harm than good.

To further call into question the biochemical theory of depression, it must be pointed out that cultural influences also come into play. The definition of *depression* heavily depends on the society that classifies it at any given time. Homosexuality was at one time considered a psychological disorder (as classified by the American Psychiatric Association up until 1972), but today, we would consider that belief completely ignorant. Suicide is still looked upon in our culture as a severe mental disturbance; but in Japan, it was traditionally considered to be an honorable act, especially in the face of military defeat. This illustrates how one culture's honor can be another's mental illness. Interesting when we put it into cultural perspective, isn't it? In light of the varying social definitions that exist, we can see that it is almost impossible to attach a one-cause-fits-all theory to depression.

## What Is Depression?

From the extensive research I have carried out on the subject, I believe that depression, at its core, stems from one of three things:

1. A perception that things should be different than they actually are.
2. Chemical intake (medications, recreational drugs, and alcohol).
3. Chronic disease (including chronic pain).

The first cause is a mental state, one of perception. It arises from the belief that one's life circumstances should be different from what they are now, or in other words, it stems from one's lack of gratitude for what actually is. I realize that this statement is going to make some of you very angry, but I ask you to really think about it. When you believe that circumstances should be different from what they are now—"I *should* be making more money," "my business *should* be doing better," "my family *should* treat me better," "I *should* be thinner"—then, naturally, you will feel depressed.

Desiring change is not in itself a bad thing; in fact, it can create purpose and fulfillment in our lives. However, a lack of gratitude for one's current life circumstances is not the same as desiring change. Ingratitude seems to be a ubiquitous human trait. As a result, every spiritual teaching has found the need to address it. In Buddhism, for example, ingratitude for "what is," or the want of different circumstances, is called the *attachment to desire*. One is said to find bliss when one can finally let go of this attachment. In Judaism, Catholicism, and Christianity, the tenth commandment discourages against the coveting of another person's property, spouse, or servants—which is just another way of addressing a person's desire for something outside of what they already have. Religious teachings were constructed precisely to answer questions regarding human behavior, and since our behaviors are heavily influenced by our minds, it makes sense that these teachings would evolve from our need to understand and direct our perceptions.

Some believe that depression actually results from life circumstances, traumas, or bad experiences. Although these situations definitely influence our state of mind, in and of themselves, they do not cause depression. I would argue, then, that the way in which we "see" the circumstances surrounding our experiences (our perceptions) ultimately determines how we end up feeling. In fact, two different people may see the same event in two totally different ways (our legal courts are a testament to this), so isn't it a generalization to assume that all traumatic events cause depression? On the contrary, some traumatic events actually lead to inspiration, others toward hope, and still others toward a state of gratitude. We simply cannot categorize all traumatic events as a cause of depression. Nor, for that matter, can we categorize all depression as the result of traumatic events since our perception of these events is purely subjective.

## Will the Real Chemical Cause of Depression Please Stand Up?

Although I have spent several pages disputing the notion that depression is caused by biochemical imbalances, the truth is that there are instances when chemical imbalances *can* lead to the development of depression. The chemicals in question are not what we normally produce in our bodies but, instead, the external or synthetic ones that many people ingest regularly. What I am referring to here are recreational and prescription drugs.

Some of the more common substances or "party" drugs people use that can actually lead to depression are alcohol, stimulants (cocaine and methamphetamines), and hallucinogenics (LSD and ecstasy). Alcohol, the most widely used recreational drug, is a central nervous system depressant; in small doses, it can lead to feelings of euphoria, talkativeness, and lowered inhibitions. But when consumed in greater than moderate quantities and over an extended period, alcohol increases the risk for both anxiety and depressive disorders.[151] We now even have evidence linking alcoholism to an increased risk of suicide.[152]

Other recreational drugs can also lead to depression. Cocaine, methamphetamine, and ecstasy, each causes depression rather quickly. If you routinely take these substances and also suffer from depression, then be warned—you are playing with fire. Incidents of suicide, homicide, and fatal accidents all rise when these drugs are mixed with depression. As an added risk, when people stop taking recreational drugs, they may go through withdrawals and, consequently, fall even deeper into depression.

Many frequently prescribed medications can also trigger depression. It is common knowledge among medical professionals that when evaluating depressed patients, it is important to find out which medications they are currently taking. To date, there are more than twenty-five classes of medications that can cause depression as a side effect.[153] They include antiviral drugs (acyclovir), antianxiety drugs (Valium, Xanax), beta-blockers (for high blood pressure and other heart disorders), corticosteroids (for inflammation, like prednisone, and allergies, like Flonase and Nasonex), estrogens (for female hormone-replacement therapy), heartburn medications (Pepsid, Tagamet), and cholesterol-lowering drugs (Lipitor, Zocor). There are many more medications that may lead to depression, so the first thing one should evaluate when suffering from a long-term bout of depression is the number and type of medications one is currently taking. As with any medical concern, it is imperative that you discuss all side effects with your medical doctor (depression or otherwise), especially before you decrease or discontinue the use of any medication.

## Chronic Disease as a Cause of Depression

The third thing that regularly causes depression is chronic disease. Along with the pain, discomfort, and loss of normal function that often accompany chronic disease, there are also psychological aspects that people must contend with. Feelings of helplessness, uselessness, guilt, fear, anger, and many other emotions are common with chronic disease. If the disease is lethal, like an aggressive form of cancer, then the psychological drain can be overwhelming. Obviously, there is no easy answer to this type of depression, but psychological and/or spiritual counseling may be helpful.

There are not many people who enjoy being in pain, particularly when it is constant or daily; but to further complicate the matter, chronic pain is often associated with disability. People suffering from chronic disease may not only hurt but may have a hard time functioning normally in their daily lives. Pain-relieving medications can be extremely useful in these circumstances; however, one must be careful—these drugs can be highly addictive. It is always better to find and resolve the actual causes of one's pain, but in difficult cases like cancer, medication is often necessary.

Not all pain is caused by chronic medical conditions, though. Many musculoskeletal dysfunctions cause pain too, and when they become long-standing or chronic, they can definitely lead to depression. These types of conditions can be effectively treated with regular bodywork like chiropractic care (chapter 4), so by taking the necessary steps to identify and resolve these physical ailments, you will be eliminating at least one major factor contributing to depressed feelings.

Whether a person's depression is caused by pain, drugs, or a psychological state of mind, solutions are available. I must again emphasize that no hard evidence shows depression to have biochemical origins. Physiological changes are a natural part of all mental and emotional events but are more likely the *result* of the psychological state than its actual cause.

The reality is that all people, regardless of national origin or cultural upbringing, suffer from some form of depression at one time or another. What becomes really useful, then, is the way in which we view the psychological state of depression and, consequently, how we choose to address it. By treating depression as a biochemical disorder, we may actually stifle a very vital function it plays in our lives—to help us grow and evolve as human beings.

## The Function of Depression

Since all people have feelings of sadness from time to time, some for an extended period, we must acknowledge that it is a ubiquitous human trait. Could depression possibly serve a useful function in our development and survival, then? If we really take the time to think about this, we can discover that depression actually fuels us and helps us evolve.

When people get depressed, it is often due to circumstances they are dissatisfied with, ones they ultimately wish to change. These circumstances might revolve around a job, a relationship, one's family, one's home life, or a number of other things people routinely become unhappy about. Whatever the situation, dissatisfaction often causes people to become frustrated; and when circumstances do not change on their own, they may eventually lead to feelings of sadness or depression.

Depression can be quite painful. Although it may make life seem unbearable during the time we are immersed in it, depression can create an intense desire for change—this can actually be a helpful tool. Depression acts as a catalyst to help push us forward to the next stage in our lives. A desire for change is often motivated by uncomfortable feelings like fear, guilt, boredom, or just plain dissatisfaction. These are generally considered negative emotions, but on the other hand, they can also serve to elevate us to the next level in our development. If we were never dissatisfied in our lives, we would never have an incentive to change, and this would make it very difficult to grow as human beings.

Not only is this true of people, but of cultures and societies as a whole. We have seen throughout history how societal dissatisfaction has led to enormous growth in human consciousness. Just look at the events leading to the abolition of slavery, the civil rights movement, and even the antiwar movement of today to get a good sense of this principle in action. Dissatisfaction and desire for change are necessary components for the evolution of humanity itself. As we will discuss later in this chapter, evolution is a universal law, and nothing can escape it.

The planet goes through its own process of change and evolution. An intriguing yet controversial premise called the *Gaia hypothesis* proposes that the planet itself is a living organism and, as such, maintains conditions necessary for its own survival. Although this hypothesis is presently unprovable, it does provide an intriguing model from which to view the earth as well as for our interactions with it. In any case, this example illustrates that all things need to change in order to survive.

Just as the earth has to maintain its environmental balance, so do people have to maintain their internal balance through the process of personal growth and change. The human experience is what acts as a catalyst for these necessary changes. By seeing things from this point of view, depression can actually be considered useful. All emotions, whether perceived by us as good or bad, are necessary for our personal growth and advancement. By pushing us to change our current situation, depression helps elevate us to the next level in our development. If we neglect to see the unpleasantries in life for what they really are—a catalyst for change and learning—and instead get stuck in our depression, then depression actually can become a "problem."

If we can, instead, appreciate that a real function exists to feelings of depression and use that knowledge to our advantage and create change, then there will be no need to *treat* depression as we do today, with dangerous psychoactive drugs and chemicals. In fact, people could seriously benefit from their therapists taking this approach when addressing depression. The therapist's role should be that of an evolutionary guide more than that of a professional trying to help solve a problem. This would certainly make a case for people to visit psychotherapists more regularly, even for those who wouldn't normally be classified as having a psychological problem. In fact, people could use psychotherapists for their mental health in much the same way they currently use medical doctors for their physical health—as a form of primary care. But they could do so in a preventative manner, not just when they are having trouble "coping." It would certainly make more sense this way, anyhow.

What is it that you are currently unhappy about? How are your perceptions unbalanced? And how can you work toward changing the perceptions that no longer serve you? These are the questions that need to be addressed when dealing with depression. Since we are all susceptible to depression at some time in our lives, let us take a closer look at how depression is approached and treated today so that we can better evaluate our options when having to deal with our own feelings of sadness.

## Antidepressants or Antievolution Medication?

Since current medical and psychiatric thinking leans toward a biochemical cause of psychological "disorders," mental conditions are routinely treated with chemical drugs. This practice has created one of the riskiest dilemmas of our times—the flat out overprescribing and abuse of dangerous antidepressant medications. Not only is the science behind the current antidepressant obsession unsubstantiated, but in many ways, it is also unsafe; and frankly, the results have not been exactly spectacular, either.

Antidepressant use is now so widespread that doctors often prescribed them for conditions other than depression. They are used freely to treat conditions like anxiety, panic and eating disorders, and general stress.[154] The question is, then: if antidepressants treat depression specifically, why would doctors need to prescribe them for other nonrelated conditions? The reason is twofold:

1.  There is a multibillion-dollar pharmaceutical industry aggressively marketing antidepressant drugs to doctors and psychiatrists, and many medical professionals rely specifically on the information provided by these companies when making decisions on whether to prescribe their drugs.
2.  It is the easiest thing to do.

The truth is that there is an enormous financial interest in perpetuating the biochemical theory of mental illness. Prozac, Zoloft, and Paxil—all antidepressants—are three of the most frequently prescribed drugs in the United

States. Zoloft alone accounts for approximately thirty thousand prescriptions *per month*![155] Combined, these three drugs account for approximately sixty-five thousand monthly prescriptions, making antidepressants the second largest-selling prescription drugs in this country.

When seeing these numbers, we become aware of how massive antidepressant use has become. It leaves one wondering: Are we the most depressed society mankind has ever seen, or are we merely being sold a myth that has tremendous marketability and great potential for profit? It is impossible to fathom that before the advent of antidepressant medications, human beings were essentially a mentally disturbed and emotionally confused lot, and not until the discovery of these miraculous drugs did mankind finally find what it had been missing.

But what else are we supposed to believe? How else are we to explain the astronomical numbers associated with antidepressant sales? One must wonder how we could have possibly made it this far in our evolution without these supposed miracle drugs. Unfortunately, most people do not ever stop and think about it in these terms. We have faith that the medical profession would never recommend anything unsafe or unproven to the public. However, bearing in mind the actual numbers of people currently taking antidepressant medications, we have to admit they are unusually high.

So what? What's the harm in taking antidepressants? We all know people who have been helped by them, right? Well, we just can't be too sure. A comparative analysis (meta-analysis) of thirty scientific studies has shown that the effectiveness of antidepressant medications is actually no better than that of a placebo (an inert substance like a sugar pill).[156] These same studies showed that only one-third of the subjects under investigation actually responded to the antidepressants, while one-third had the same response to both the medication and the placebo, and another third had no response at all.

In another recent study, the results were even more remarkable. A meta-analysis of the six most commonly prescribed antidepressants showed that, in nearly 80 percent of the cases, there was no difference between the medication and placebo.[157] The difference between the effects of the placebo and the drugs was so small that it led the authors of the study to conclude that "the pharmacological effects of antidepressants are clinically negligible."

Please, do not take this to mean that antidepressants have no effect on mental function whatsoever. On the contrary, physiological changes definitely take place in the brains of people who take these drugs. The aforementioned study merely analyzed the *clinical effects* of antidepressants or, in other words, the effects that are supposed to be beneficial. As you will see, there are many dangerous consequences of these drugs on the normal physiology of the brain.

Today's antidepressants form a class of drugs known as selective serotonin reuptake inhibitors, or SSRIs. True to their name, they prevent the reuptake of the hormone serotonin (or 5-HT as it is now preferably called) by the nerve cells of the brain. Serotonin is believed to play a role in mood regulation. The concentration of serotonin in the brains of depressed people has been found to be less than that found in nondepressed people, and this has led to the rash conclusion that serotonin levels must be the definitive factor involved in causing depression. Simply put, when serotonin levels are low, depression is believed to result. It therefore follows that in order to prevent depression, serotonin levels must be kept within "normal" limits. This is the basis of antidepressant therapy.

SSRIs were developed precisely to maintain serotonin levels at normal concentrations. They work by altering the serotonin transport molecule receptor. This receptor sits on the cell surface of neurons in the brain and allows the serotonin in the synapse (the space between adjacent nerve cells) to reenter the nerve cells where it can no longer pass its positive effects onto the brain (i.e., "good mood"). When SSRIs come into contact with these receptors, they alter the surface of the receptors and disrupt their ability to recognize serotonin; this, in effect, renders them useless. As a result, the receptors are unable to bring serotonin back into the nerve cells, and it causes serotonin concentrations outside the cell to remain high, leading to the maintenance of a "normal mood." In theory, then, the overall effect of this reaction should be to stop depression cold in its tracks and perhaps even reverse it. Sounds logical, right?

Well, unfortunately, some major chinks exist in this theory. For example, all we know is that concentrations of serotonin are low in the brain during depression. What we don't know is if this is the actual cause of depression, or if the change in serotonin concentration is a result of the depression itself. Mood might instead be regulated by a *change* in concentration of serotonin levels in the brain, not its absolute concentration, or it could be from something different altogether. We just don't know yet. It could also be a combination of things that we have not considered thus far. That's the most perplexing thing about the biochemical theory of depression: there is just so much about the brain we do not yet understand.

Even worse, we do not know entirely how antidepressants work on the brain. One of the long-term effects of antidepressant drugs that we do know, however, is that they can cause serotonin receptors (not the transport molecules we discussed above, but the ones that affect the brain to control moods) to become downregulated. Serotonin acts on these receptors, which then release other chemicals to affect brain function. The downregulation process occurs as a way for cells to maintain homeostasis (the process of maintaining balance or stability in an environment). Basically, the body stops producing receptors in response to the increased levels of serotonin in the synapse. Remember that SSRIs alter the function of the serotonin transport molecule, leading serotonin concentrations in the synapse to build. The body sees this as an unbalanced state since under normal conditions hormone levels must constantly change. As a result, the body reduces the amount of receptors in an attempt to regain balance.

Along with the downregulation of receptors, nerve cells may also stop their production of serotonin. This is another way the body decreases its levels of serotonin in the synapse. All of this occurs in response to the ever-increasing levels of serotonin brought about by SSRI use. Clearly, the body does not see "more serotonin" as beneficial. If it did, there would be no need to downregulate, or shut down, the production of this hormone. These changes occur as a response to an imbalance of the system. It stands to reason, then, that serotonin levels might not be the sole factor involved in the development of depression, although they may possibly be a marker for it—increasing and decreasing as our moods change.

The truth is that we have no way of knowing what the *actual* long-term effects of SSRIs are on the serotonin levels in living human brain tissue. Studies on the ground-up brains of animals have shown that antidepressants do not increase the overall serotonin levels in the brain at all.[158] This is most likely due to the strength of the brain in maintaining homeostasis. There is a constant battle between SSRIs and the brain to determine which will have the greater influence on the overall concentration of serotonin in the synapse. From these studies, it is clear that the human brain is much more powerful than the synthetic agents made by man to control brain function.

As we have said before, all emotional events have physiological consequences. When sad, we cry tears that are filled with serous fluid. This fluid contains different molecules like proteins, enzymes, and immunoglobulins. These constituents, in and of themselves, do not cause sadness. When angry or stressed, we release the hormone cortisol, which makes us tremble. Cortisol itself, however, does not cause anger. The molecules involved in sadness or anger are all by-products of an emotional event. In many ways, they can even become part of a conditioned response; that is, one can learn to control emotions in spite of one's feelings. Thus, one can experience a tearless form of sadness, or be calm, despite being angry. The point here is that we do not know what role serotonin actually plays in depression; and it is, therefore, presumptuous to implicate it as a causative agent without knowing all the facts.

Aside from the lack of evidence of serotonin's actual role in depression, there are also dangers involved with taking SSRI antidepressants. Many of these are not addressed adequately in the initial drug trials performed by manufacturers since it would not be in their best financial interests to do so. And the busy doctor does not usually have the time to scrutinize every drug in her arsenal; as a result, these dangers are rarely discussed with her patients. This fact has led the editors of eleven of the top medical journals—including the *Lancet*, the *British Medical Journal*, and the *New England Journal of Medicine*—to call for greater openness in the way pharmaceutical companies report their findings.[159] This, along with the numerous lawsuits filed and won against SSRI manufacturers by patients who have suffered complications from taking these drugs, has led to an increase in manufacturers' warnings being printed on their labels.

Some of the dangers inherent in taking SSRI antidepressants are possible brain damage, increased mania, sexual dysfunction, suicidal tendencies, and violent behaviors. This is especially daunting when we consider that children have in the past accounted for up to 8 percent of all prescriptions written in this country. Let's take a closer look at a few of the dangers posed by SSRI antidepressant drug use.

SSRIs have been shown to create changes at several different regions of the brain. For example, one study showed alterations in the frontal lobes following exposure to fluoxetine (Prozac).[160] These regions are responsible for our emotions and our personalities. They are also involved in motor function, problem solving, spontaneity, memory, language, initiation, judgment, impulse control, and social and sexual behavior. Changes in the frontal lobes could also cause problems with interpreting feedback from the environment. The frontal lobes, obviously, control many of our vital brain functions. In fact, all human behavior is controlled here; so wouldn't changes in this region create, well . . . changes? Even more ominous is the fact that antidepressants are routinely given to children, the group most susceptible to behavioral alterations since their brains are still developing. These changes not only occur in children, but also in adults, and we just do not know what the long-term implications are yet.

SSRI antidepressants (specifically Paxil) have also been shown to shrink brain tissue in the area of the thalamus.[161] The total functions of the thalamus are not completely understood; but some of them include sensory input to the cortex (sight, sound, and somatosensory function like position sense, vibration, pain, and temperature), motor input (movement), and cognitive function (arousal or responsiveness and memory). Can we really afford to chemically alter this region? Since it is the exact same area severed during the lobotomies of yesteryear, it doesn't take a brain surgeon to figure out that changes here can be disastrous.

Antidepressants can also affect other portions of the brain like the temporal lobes (organization of sensory input, memory, personality, language, and sexual behavior) and the basal ganglia (motor and learning functions). Because of the numerous regions influenced by SSRIs, it is no surprise that the side effects associated with their use are as varied as the regions themselves.

The most important issue with regard to changes in the brain is whether these changes are permanent. The truth is that we just do not know; however, evidence certainly points that way. Other than in the most extreme cases of depression, like those involving potential suicide, these drugs should in no way be used as readily as they are today. This is especially true for children. At a time when their brains are still developing, there is very little justification to add chemicals that may alter their behavior permanently. Thinking about it this way, doesn't it seem worthwhile to try to help children work out their issues psychologically? It certainly seems to me that this would be the healthiest option available, especially since the risk of dependence on antidepressants is high. It is also unfair to children to impede their learning in any way. By medicating them, their emotional responses are essentially numbed, and they'll never learn how to effectively handle mental challenges.

Unfortunately, many parents do not take the time to consider these consequences. Most just do not know the facts, and sadly, doctors rarely take the time to discuss them. The truth is that many doctors themselves are unaware of the dangers. They often rely on information provided by the pharmaceutical company's sales representatives who are unlikely to present facts that may ultimately hurt their sales. Furthermore, pharmaceutical manufacturers have yet to invest the time or money into studying the long-term effects of antidepressants on the brain or whether people can ever fully recover from changes that might occur.

Another side effect of antidepressant use is increased mania. The fourth edition of the Diagnostic and Statistical Manual of Mental Disorders (1994) verifies that *all* antidepressants cause mania. Mania is a form of intense overstimulation. It can lead to anxiety, agitation, insomnia, and nervousness. It is very similar to the effects of cocaine or methamphetamine. Feelings of elatedness, euphoria, and overconfidence are common in antidepressant users. The symptoms of mania are caused by the stimulant nature of having increased serotonin levels in the brain. Tragically, psychiatrists often misdiagnose these symptoms as a latent disorder; and as a result, larger doses of SSRIs are usually recommended.

SSRIs can also cause sexual dysfunction. Antidepressants cause hormonal changes that can directly impair the ability to experience and enjoy sex.[162] It can express itself as a loss of libido in men or women, ejaculatory problems in men, and the decreased ability to achieve orgasm in women.[163] Along with this, actual feelings of love can also be hampered by taking antidepressants. These drugs have the tendency to shut off emotions of empathy, caring, and sensitivity and therefore can seriously damage relationships. Through my own investigation on the matter, I have found that most people describe the feelings of being on SSRIs as "shut off," "even-keeled," or "not really being in any kind of mood whatsoever." These descriptions always sort of scare me since I liken this state to being an emotional zombie. Sadly, this is exactly what I have found most "heavily medicated" individuals to resemble.

Two other serious side effects of antidepressants are suicidal tendencies and violent behavior. SSRIs were shown to increase feelings of suicide in some people during the initial clinical trials of many antidepressants. Due to the brain's attempt to regulate serotonin levels, feelings of depression can actually *increase* in people using these drugs. Worsening symptoms often lead doctors to step up the dosage of these medications, which ultimately causes a more intense depression. It can get so bad that the depressed patient is pushed toward thoughts of suicide.

This fact was known by both the manufacturers of SSRIs and the FDA yet was largely ignored. Since we could spend massive amounts of time and ink on this, more than would be practical for this book, I would highly recommend reading *The Anti-Depressant Fact Book* by Peter R. Breggin, MD. Dr. Breggin has been the chief medical expert against Eli Lilly and Company (the makers of Prozac) and other manufacturers of antidepressants in legal cases contending that these drugs cause violence, suicide, and psychosis. This phenomenal book is an eye-opener and should be read if you are considering this type of treatment for yourself or a loved one—especially if that loved one happens to be your child.

SSRIs not only lead to increased feelings of suicide, but the manner in which it is carried out by people on these drugs is particularly violent. It often involves burning or stabbing oneself to death. For several years, American manufacturers of SSRI antidepressants withheld warnings of increased risk of suicide despite British and German warnings for their versions of the same types of drugs. In 2004, following a monumental report conclusively implicating SSRI antidepressants in increased risk of suicide in adolescents, U.S. manufacturers were forced to place the following black box warning on all product labels:

> Antidepressants increased the risk of suicidal thinking and behavior (suicidality) in short-term studies in children and adolescents with Major Depressive Disorder (MDD) and other psychiatric disorders. Anyone considering the use of [Drug Name] or any other antidepressant in a child or adolescent must balance this risk with the clinical need. Patients who are started on therapy should be observed closely for clinical worsening, suicidality, or unusual changes in behavior.

The black box warning is the most serious of all warning labels on prescription medications.[164] Once again, I must present the question: why would anyone want to give their children this stuff? And before you think that only children are at risk, think again. Recent studies show an increased risk of suicide in adults taking paroxetine (Paxil).[165] As it turns out, not only is the evidence for depression having biochemical origins severely lacking, but SSRIs as treatment are now known to be quite dangerous. Does anyone else find this disturbing? Does anyone else wonder why the prescriptions for these dangerous medications continue to soar?

To add insult to injury, antidepressants have been shown to increase violent behavior. We have already discussed the violent nature of the suicide attempts of people on SSRI therapy, but this violence can be turned outward as well. There are numerous cases pending against SSRI manufacturers alleging violent tendencies. Many of these cases involve the assaults and murders of the spouses of persons taking these drugs. Many involve the murders of family members by both adults and children.

Experts believe that violent tendencies in antidepressant users are a result of a combination of depression and anxiety. Remember that anxiety (mania) is a very strong side effect of SSRIs due to their stimulant nature. Many patients can become manic, psychotic, and paranoid—all which can lead to violent and bizarre behavior. The *Washington Post* reported that Columbine shooter Eric Harris was taking the SSRI antidepressant Luvox and had a "therapeutic amount" in his blood at the time of the shootings. He and another teen went on a shooting rampage, killing twelve fellow students and a teacher, and wounding twenty-four others before committing suicide. Since some reports have also suggested that Harris had a relatively good family life, it stands to reason that he was suffering from an antidepressant-induced mania.[166]

Proponents of the biological theory of depression point out that they see definite improvement in the patients who take them. It is my belief, however, that the improvements seen are due to a "shutting off" of emotional responses, a zombielike state that leaves the user unfeeling and devoid of any extreme emotions. For some, this may be enough to allow them to cope with difficult circumstances in their lives; but for many others, it renders them stuck in an emotional funk, unable to overcome their problems and evolve into the next phase of their lives.

So what can be done? you might ask. There are techniques that, when practiced regularly, can be used to gain a balance in one's perceptions. Only through mental and emotional balance can we hope to overcome emotional states like depression. One way to gain perspective is through psychotherapy. Remember that this is the treatment of choice by psychologists, but I will not spend any time on it here. If you feel that this is the road you wish to take, then I encourage you to do so; it is a superior alternative to antidepressant drug therapy. Balance, though, can be achieved on your own. It merely requires the understanding of a few universal principles and the diligent practice of a few powerful techniques. In the next few sections, I will present these principles and detail the methods of obtaining a healthy and well-balanced mental perspective.

## It's All in How You See It

The following section is quite possibly the most powerful in this book. The methods I present here are ancient yet timeless. They will help strengthen and condition your mind, just as we do the body. Although these techniques are the compilation of many different teachings, much of it is based on the brilliant work of Dr. John F. Demartini.[167]

The techniques I present here are not new; and they definitely take work, diligence, and patience. But if you can master them, you will experience great changes, both in your personal growth and in the way you respond to the world around you. These methods may not be the quickest and easiest ways to cope with depression, but they are powerful and have long-lasting results. The methods themselves will be difficult at first—unless, of course, you have been raised in cultures that actively practice them—but just know that they will get easier over time.

The beauty is that these techniques can be practiced over a lifetime, and they should—the more you do them, the more powerful you will become. There is no need to get discouraged if you drop off in your practice either. These techniques are timeless and can be restarted at any time. Your body and mind have memory, as does every one of your cells, and you'll easily pick up where you have left off. The most important thing is to first understand the theory behind the practices. From there, you can work on them slowly and steadily. If you use discipline and practice regularly, success will surely follow.

## Universal Laws

Before I disclose these powerful techniques that will sharpen your mind as well as help you develop a balanced perspective, it is important to first understand a few laws pertaining to the universe. Knowing these laws will make the techniques easier to apply. A universal law, as we discuss it here, is a philosophical construct, not a scientific proof. It is what we believe to be true based on thousands of years of deductive reasoning. A scientific law, on the other hand, is a generalization based upon empirical observation. That means we believe it to be true without exception since repeated testing shows it to be so and even strengthens it.[168]

Whereas philosophical laws are based on deductive reasoning, usually derived from a general premise, scientific laws are derived by inductive reasoning.

*Inductive reasoning* is the process of developing a conclusion by observing recurring phenomenal patterns. This can be done through experimentation or simply by seeing something occurring repeatedly—when an object falls after being dropped from a height, we know it will eventually hit the ground (law of gravity). With inductive reasoning, conclusions are often more generalized than the premise. In other words, we believe that because something has always been true in the past, it will continue to be so in the future. However, this way of thinking isn't always wise. For instance, just because drinking from a particular well has always been safe in the past doesn't mean that it won't be contaminated in the future.

There is nothing wrong with inductive reasoning. It is, in fact, a useful means for answering many questions. We need this type of logic to explain some of the common occurrences we observe on a daily basis. Most of what we know scientifically is due to inductive reasoning. We certainly would not have been able to realize the incredible advancements in the medical, computer, and aviation technologies were it not for inductive reasoning. However, it is not the only method of finding answers; in fact, it isn't even always the most effective one.

*Deductive reasoning*, by contrast, starts with a generalized premise and works its way downward toward a conclusion, one that is just as certain as the premise. A classic example is Aristotle's syllogism:

|  |  |
|---|---|
| All men are mortal | (major premise) |
| Socrates is a man | (minor premise) |
| Therefore, Socrates is mortal | (conclusion) |

In this example, the first line is the major premise; the second, the minor premise; and the third, the conclusion. We will use this type of reasoning to explain the universal principles. They are all major premises, and we will use them to formulate the mental techniques you can use to obtain a balanced perspective. These laws are taken from many different schools of thought, including modern science, yogic philosophy, and ancient spiritual and philosophical teachings. However, these laws are secular in nature and, therefore, easy to understand; they can be appreciated by anyone, regardless of religion or spiritual or philosophical belief.

## Law 1: The law of greater power

This law states that a greater power exists in the universe—one that organizes all matter, energy, events, and experiences. In fact, all things, both perceivable and unperceivable, are under the grand design of this organizing power. All major religious and philosophical teachings have understood this basic premise, the premise of a greater power. Whether we call it God, Allah, Buddha, or just Universal Intelligence matters not—only that we recognize that something greater than ourselves is directing the entire universe.

The only other option is for us to see the universe as a random series of events. In fact, there are a number of people who believe just that, yet is this way of thinking logical? Many of history's greatest thinkers—Einstein, Newton, Descartes—acknowledged the existence of a greater power. It is very difficult, if not impossible, to credit the wonders of the universe to random events. By seeing the universe as a random system, it completely removes our rationale for practicing free will. If things were merely random, then what would motivate us to carry out our lives? This would compromise the basis of our very existence.

Sure, there are some who believe our existence is merely tied to the pleasurable stimulation of our five senses: sight, smell, touch, sound, and taste. However, this way of thinking is one of the strongest precursors to depression that exists, as anyone who solely chases the feelings of pleasure eventually realizes how empty this pursuit is. Life doesn't always provide experiences to satisfy this principle.

The law of greater power is deeply philosophical, and we can spend a lifetime debating it. But for our intent and purpose here, we will use this as our most basic premise. If this is not your belief, don't worry, and definitely don't put the book down; this should not stop you from connecting to the other laws I present here, nor should it hamper your ability to get the most from the techniques I offer. If this law is something you connect to on a spiritual or philosophical basis, though, it will only serve to strengthen your confidence in what I present to you.

## Law 2: The law of mental correspondence

This law states that the universe is much greater than that which we can perceive with our five senses. It is vast and infinite, way beyond what we can comprehend, now or in the future. Since we are an integral part of the universe, there is a component of us that is deeply connected to it. Before you dismiss this as some unsubstantiated New Age rhetoric, understand that this is acknowledged by every branch of physics from the theoretical to the cosmological to the quantum physical.

So what is this profound connection we are talking about? The truth is we do not know exactly. The universe is so immense and incomprehensible to the human mind that we can only theorize about this connection. The only method we have to answer questions of this nature is through the process of deductive reasoning. Depending on the philosophy we draw upon, our connection to the universe is either through our mind or our spirit.

This law serves us by first acknowledging the vast and infinite realm the human mind encompasses. To explain it in practical terms, we have been able to use our minds to expand the human experience far beyond anything we have previously thought possible: We have constructed buildings that stand a quarter-mile high. We have technology that allows us to send pictures, sounds, and thoughts across the globe in seconds; and we can even travel in space! And we have accomplished all of this with the infinite power of our minds. The reality is that *everything* is possible, and we prove it every day.

Not only is this a mental law, but it is also a law of correspondence—it recognizes that we actually shape our experiences with our thoughts. By doing so, we affect the world around us, forming our own little portion of the universe. To what degree, of course, depends on the vastness or the extent of our thoughts. There is an axiom tied to this law that states "As above, so below," which in essence means that the thoughts we choose create the reality of our experiences on the material realm. This is not intended as a directive to simply practice "positive thinking," which, as you will see, would be an exercise in futility. It is instead a device for us to understand that we are constantly shaping what we experience through our mental faculties and which ultimately affects the collective human experience. This serves us by acknowledging that we are not merely insignificant beings in a vast random universe but are, instead, directly connected to everyone and everything around us. By understanding this law, we are in a position to act significantly as *creators* and not merely sit by as powerless *observers*.

## Law 3: The law of energy and vibration

In the early part of the twentieth century, a group of scientists discovered some pretty amazing things about matter that were not explainable by the reigning theories of the day. Essentially, their work uncovered the nature of subatomic particles, which they found were not solid matter at all but instead energy. This led to the development of the theories of special relativity and quantum mechanics.

Two very important principles act as the foundation of this third law. The first is that *all things in the universe are energy*. Albert Einstein formulated this with his famous equation $E=mc^2$ where E is *energy* and m is *mass* (c equals the *speed of light*, but it isn't really important for our discussions here). What this means is that all matter is made up entirely of energy. Therefore, human beings are basically energetic life-forms, and all their thoughts and actions are simply movements of that energy. Moreover, all nonliving things—rocks, trees, water, etc.—are energy forms too. The only thing differentiating living from nonliving matter (energetically speaking, that is) is the frequency at which each vibrates.

This brings us to the second important principle. All particles have the dual property of existing as a particle *and* a wave. Therefore, everything we experience as solid matter is really just a waveform, like light; and as such, it vibrates at a particular frequency. The reason we see things as solid is because we are only able to detect them as a concentrated image. If we had the ability to see very small particles, then we would see that all matter is mostly empty space with electric particles spinning around rapidly, forming a sort of energy cloud. However, we cannot see that small, so this concept is abstract and may be hard to grasp—but it is true, nonetheless.

We are only able to see that portion of energy detectable by our organs of sight—that is, our eyes. They have the ability to sense energy at wavelengths within the visible spectrum, but not at shorter or longer wavelengths, like ultraviolet light or infrared radiation. The same holds true for our hearing, smelling, touching, and tasting organs; they are also unable to detect energy frequencies outside a certain range.

The importance of this fact is twofold. One is that we can only experience those things that our sense organs allow us to. This means that we cannot be totally sure of what makes up the entire universe since we are not capable of sensing every form of energy present with the limitation of the machinery we possess. We cannot sense x-rays, microwaves, or gamma rays; yet we know each exists. The second important point is that we have an enormous power to move energy—through sound, movement, body language, and especially through thought and intention. We can use all these tools to our complete advantage, and we will discuss how later in the chapter.

Since all things are energy, each having its own distinct vibrational composition, we can surmise that human beings are also vibrational. Not only do our cells and tissues vibrate distinctly, but so do our voices and thoughts. The beauty is that we can change our vibratory patterns and draw different experiences and opportunities to us. We do this all the time, often without even being aware of it. The secret is to be fully conscious of our ability to change our vibration and then carry out this change by utilizing different methods, some of which we will touch on later in this chapter. In this way, we can truly enhance our life experiences.

It is important to point out here the scientific law known as the *first law of thermodynamics*. You probably remember its sibling, the second law of thermodynamics, which we discussed briefly in chapter 2. The first law states that the energy in a system can neither be created nor destroyed; it can only change forms. We see this law in action in many different instances, like when we convert the energy of food into the energy of action (movements, metabolism, etc.). But for our purposes here, suffice it to say that our primary energy is always present;

it merely changes into different forms around us. We will also learn how to use this principle to our advantage.

## Law 4: The law of polarity

This law states that all things in the universe exist along with their counterpart, an equal and opposite entity. This is most apparent with subatomic particles. *Electrons*, the particles that spin around atomic nuclei, have a negative charge as well as a direction to their spin. When two electrons are paired in a stable atom, they exhibit an equal yet opposite spin. We also know from atomic physics that there exists an exact opposite particle to an electron called a *positron*.

What this means on a practical basis is that nothing exists on its own or without its exact opposite. In other words, there can be no "up" without "down," no "happy" without "sad," no "black" without "white." Without its opposite to use as a reference point, we would not be able to identify anything since we would have nothing to compare it to.

This phenomenon has enormous implications, as it allows us to overcome our lopsided perceptions regarding the universe. This includes the one-sided views we have about people and ourselves. According to the twentieth-century Danish physicist Niels Bohr, one of the architects of quantum mechanics, "the same person can be good and evil, bold and timid, a lion and a lamb." This principle, as you shall soon see, is one of the most crucial in developing balance in our everyday perceptions and can also be very useful in overcoming depression.

## Law 5: The law of rhythm

We have already touched upon this law briefly in chapter 2 ("The Importance of a Healthy Diet") when we discussed keeping a rhythm to our eating schedules. However, this principle goes much deeper than that—all things in the universe follow their own rhythmic pattern. The rising and setting of the sun, the ebb and flow of the tides, and the change of the seasons all follow some form of rhythmic oscillation.

Although it may seem that human beings are the exceptions to this rule, we actually have rhythmic patterns to our many physiological processes. The beating of our heart, the inflow and outflow of our respiratory system, our hormonal secretions, and our peristaltic contractions all follow a pattern of rhythmic oscillation. And since we have determined that all matter is simply energy, then we can appreciate that every cell in our body also has a rhythmic oscillation that governs its birth, life, and death.

The law of rhythm will become important when we discuss the necessity of balancing our perceptions. This law works in conjunction with the law of polarity. By understanding that our perceptions may swing like a pendulum, from one pole to the other, we can use this law to understand the dichotomy of life—one which at times has us feeling up and at other times feeling down. This is the law that adds the spice to life. If there were not a shift in our mind from one experiential perception to the other, then we would not be able to appreciate all that life has to offer. Learn to understand this law, and it will help you find gratitude for all of your experiences.

## Law 6: The law of cause and effect

This law is pretty simple: it states that every action has a subsequent reaction. Whether we are talking about our physical actions, words, intentions, or even nonactions, it always results in a corresponding event, which ultimately unfolds to create yet another event. This law presumes that every choice we make—a result of our free will—not only has an effect on us personally, but on others as well. When we contemplate this on a larger scale, it becomes clear that our choices also impact the environment, the planet, and the universe as a whole.

This law recognizes an inherent order to the universe. Events may appear to happen randomly, but when we accept that every experience has a cause, we can then appreciate that a definite order guides the universe. This is not to say that our choices merely *create* an effect. In actuality, they *lead* to an effect. Therefore, we do not have to feel guilty when our choices lead to challenges. Instead, we can rest assured that the choices we make actually take us down a particular path, one that will lead us through our inevitable evolution.

This law is particularly profound since it teaches us that ramifications are inherent in every decision we make, each choice determining our next experience. Being in tune with this principle empowers us to make decisions more conscientiously and also leads us to a greater sense of certainty when making those decisions.

## Law 7: The law of evolution

This law states that all things in the universe evolve. People evolve, cultures and societies evolve, and human consciousness evolves too. Planets also evolve as do galaxies; in fact, the entire universe is constantly evolving. One could say that the sole purpose of existence is simply to evolve.

To what extent we evolve within our lifetime depends on the degree with which we choose to expand our minds. We have already discussed the infinite nature of the universe (law of correspondence), its dimensions containing no bounds. It stands to reason, then, that our own limits of expansion must be infinite as well.

We see this principle at play every day, in every facet of life. Whenever we think of that which we have already seen in our lifetime as unsurpassable, something else comes along to take our breath away. Michael Jordan, Oprah Winfrey, and Lance Armstrong are all testaments to this fact, as each has accomplished feats that in the past were considered unattainable. And who would have thought that we'd live in a world where cellular phones, high-definition television, and wireless Internet were the norm? Yet, we do. As impressive as these people and inventions are, we can be sure of one thing: something will eventually come along to exceed them. That is the process of evolution in full swing.

According to this law, every one of us changes and evolves constantly. By understanding this, we are better able to keep the current circumstances of our lives in perspective. We inhabit this material existence to grow and expand as human beings, to simply be all that we can be. Thinking of life in this way sure makes it inspiring, doesn't it? It gives us so much to be excited about. The possibilities are endless.

But our development does not just end with ourselves. We have the potential to affect the entire universe, becoming an integral part of *its* grand evolution. Everything we do or think has some effect on everything else around us (law of cause and effect), no matter how big or how small. We can choose to be a major player in this process or a modest one—there really is no right or wrong cither way. It is totally up to us. It just comes down to how far we want to expand our minds. Just know that whatever road you choose to take in life, change is inevitable; and as much as you might try to resist it, you can never stop the process of evolution.

## Powerful Tools to "Work Out" the Mind

We have already established that the mind and body share an inextricable link with each other. Although the extent of their interrelation has been the subject of much debate in the past, it would, in fact, be hard to find any health care expert who would deny this intimate connection between the two. So just as it is imperative to keep the body in shape by embarking on a regular exercise regimen, it is equally important to keep the mind conditioned through systematic mental exercise. In this section, we will discuss several methods that will not only assist you in keeping your mind sharp, but will also help you handle stressful situations more effectively, prevent prolonged and intense mental states like depression, and allow you to get the most out of your life by maintaining a balanced perspective—all while feeling complete gratitude for your life as it is today.

These powerful tools, if used properly and practiced diligently, can help you achieve the mental conditioning you need to develop optimal health and well-being. This section is by far the most powerful and exciting one of the program. Have fun with it because when you put these principles into practice, there is just no telling what you might accomplish.

## Keeping the Mind Sharp

As we age, one of our greatest fears is losing control of our precious mental acuity. Alzheimer's disease, a progressive brain disorder that gradually destroys a person's memory and ability to learn (as well as his ability to reason, make judgments, communicate, and carry out his daily activities), now affects one in every ten people over the age of sixty-five.[169] Alzheimer's disease is not a part of normal aging; on the contrary, people have the ability to keep their minds sharp and intact well into old age. Fortunately, there are measures one can take (both physical and mental) that may help prevent the development of this dreaded disorder.

Research has shown that the brain, like any other organ, needs continual stimulation to remain sharp. In one study, approximately seven hundred Catholic nuns were given examinations to test their mental acuity as they aged.[170] They were categorized according to information contained in their autobiographies, which they wrote when they first entered the convent about sixty years earlier. According to the results, the nuns that had the greatest linguistic ability—and consequently, the higher education levels—had the lowest risk for developing Alzheimer's later in life. And those nuns that had college degrees actually lived longer and led more independent lives than those who did not.

What was even more remarkable about this study was that when researchers looked inside the brains of the nuns who had died, they found plaques in a number of them. The plaques were the same as those generally found in the brains of people afflicted with Alzheimer's disease, yet these women did not actually have the disease. This extraordinary finding led researchers to the conclusion that the lifelong learning associated with a higher education actually prevented the onset of Alzheimer's. This was true even in the presence of physical factors that by all accounts should have caused the disease. Scientists believe that as we learn, nerve cells in the brain form numerous new dendrites. *Dendrites*—the extensions of a nerve cell's body—obtain information from and transmit it to other nerve cells. In other words, the process of learning forms a greater concentration of nerve pathways, which in turn increases one's ability to organize information. The result is sustained mental sharpness.

Continually challenging oneself with complex intellectual activities ensures a long life of exceptional mental acuity even into old age.[171] People who work in jobs requiring strenuous thinking, then, should be at a tremendous advantage. By having to constantly use their minds to solve complex problems, they create new neurological networks that not only strengthen their already existing ones, but also act as a reserve in case of a breakdown.

It is therefore important to engage in activities that use the mind, like reading, playing board games (like chess), learning a new language, or perhaps even learning to play an instrument. Each one can prolong your mental sharpness and prevent the deterioration of normal brain function. It is important to engage in mental stimulation regularly as this will give you maximum results. The activities should be mentally challenging too as it is the actual *process* of learning that stimulates dendrite growth in the brain. Just know that it's never too late to begin strengthening the mind—but the sooner you start, the better.

Some other ways in which you can affect the mind positively and keep it working in tip-top shape is by practicing the other five keys to optimal health. Nutritionally, you can supplement with a healthy regimen of antioxidants—vitamins A, C, E; the mineral selenium; and, of course, the superantioxidant alpha-lipoic acid. Experts believe that one of the major factors involved in the development of Alzheimer's disease is oxidative stress caused by free radicals. The body forms free radicals as it burns calories from food (while using oxygen) to generate energy. You may recall that oxidative stress damages cells and ultimately leads to their death (chapter 2). The brain happens to be more sensitive to free radical damage than any other organ in the body as it has the highest metabolic rate and also uses the greatest amount of oxygen. For this reason, it is imperative to supplement with both a good multivitamin and a strong antioxidant. By doing so, you will limit at least one factor thought to contribute to the onset of Alzheimer's disease.

Another nutritional measure you can take is to supplement daily with essential fatty acids (EFAs). About 70 percent of the brain is made up of fats and cholesterol. Fats are needed as a potent energy source for the high metabolic activity occurring in the brain. As we discussed in chapter 2, it is important to have a proper fatty acid balance in the body. This is especially true for the brain. Since the typical Western diet is high in the omega-6 fatty acids, supplementing with the omega-3s is crucial. You can find omega-3 fatty acids in fish or flax seed oil. Additionally, EFAs have strong anti-inflammatory properties and can therefore prevent any damage that might come about as a result of inflammation. Experts have found very solid evidence linking inflammation with the development of Alzheimer's disease. There is also a direct correlation between fatty acid imbalance and depression. Take no chances—supplement regularly with EFAs and you can help prevent the onset of this disorder.

Finally, leading memory loss researchers believe that overeating may play a role in the development of Alzheimer's disease. The theory is that free radical formation multiplies appreciably during the high metabolic process of turning excess food into energy. As free radical concentrations increase, so do the risks of developing Alzheimer's. To make matters worse, overeating may also increase inflammation in the brain, which, as we have said, has been linked to this neurological disorder. Studies done on rodents have shown a direct correlation between restricting caloric intake and slowing down degenerative changes seen with aging. Accordingly, caloric restriction without malnutrition (chapter 2) is a promising preventative measure toward halting Alzheimer's disease.

Another key that might be useful in preventing mental decline is regular physical activity. Exercise increases one's intake of oxygen, which we know is absolutely vital for proper brain function. Remember that the brain needs and uses more oxygen than any other organ in the body, so by exercising regularly, you are assured of importing plenty of oxygen to nourish the brain's delicate tissue. Not only does the current research show that exercise is a great preventative measure for warding off mental decline, but there is also evidence linking it to improved mental function in people already stricken with dementia.[172] As an added bonus, exercise has been shown to decrease feelings of depression by releasing endorphins during prolonged physical activity (chapter 3). So working out not only strengthens the body, but it strengthens the mind as well.

Exercise and nutrition are clearly powerful methods for keeping the mind sharp, yet there are a few other things you can do to improve your overall mental health. As we mentioned in chapter 4, regular chiropractic care can maintain the integrity of the entire nervous system, including the brain, by getting rid of physical barriers that stand in the way of its proper functioning. By removing subluxations, the brain, the spinal cord, and the nerves have a greater chance of functioning optimally. What's more, by correcting physical problems that may be causing pain, the brain has one less thing vying for its valuable attention and can therefore leave you with greater focus to tackle your daily tasks.

Sleep, as you saw in chapter 5, is vitally important for proper brain function. It allows our necessary repair processes to take place and is the time when information is stored into memory. No surprise then—getting a proper amount of rest is absolutely crucial in maintaining your mental health.

Finally, it is well known that heavy alcohol consumption can damage the sensitive brain tissue and can cause cell death. This can eventually lead to memory loss. While regeneration of brain tissue is, in fact, possible, it is not completely understood.[173] Hence, moderation of the drinking habit is the most sensible thing to do as it is better to preserve your brain than to hope for regeneration after damage has already set in.

Recreational drugs like methamphetamine and cocaine can also damage the brain and, as we have previously mentioned, so can the popular antidepressant medications, the SSRIs. Lastly, a recent study at the University of Michigan has found that long-term cigarette smoking can decrease mental acuity and lower IQ,[174] so kicking this habit will do wonders in keeping you mentally sharp.

## Gaining Perspective

Have you noticed that I have mentioned "perception" quite a bit in this chapter? Why is it that *balancing one's perceptions* is so important to one's overall health? The reasons are many as you will soon see. Every technique that I present in the following sections will attempt to bring you and your perceptions back into balance. Although you cannot always control every circumstance in your life, you can control how you perceive these circumstances, how you process or evaluate them, and how you respond to the challenges you encounter. These skills are the true secret to a healthy mind—no tricks, no gimmicks—just good old-fashioned balanced perspective.

But wait! Didn't I say earlier that you can *control* your life by simply using the power of your mind? No, not exactly. Trying to control the details of life, the little nuances that make up our experiences, is impossible. What I said is that you can *create* the life you would love to have, simply by using the power of your mind. I never said you could control it. In fact, it is precisely the desire to control the details of one's life that actually lead to depression. When we think life should be one way and it doesn't exactly comply, we end up suffering. We simply cannot control all the details of our lives; we can only manifest the final result we wish to achieve—be it a certain lifestyle, a certain type of relationship, or a certain level of professional or creative achievement.

Life works in a specific way whether we want it to or not. One could say it follows a certain set of laws and principles. If you understand and utilize these principles, you may have a much easier time keeping yourself together during times of stress. By learning to balance your perceptions, you will be able to make it through most of the rough patches in life and still remain grateful for all that is. And during those moments when life seems to be a breeze (i.e., when you seem to be operating "in the zone"), you can sit back and relish these moments even more since you will have already weathered the storm by keeping everything in perspective (law of polarity, law of rhythm).

Like everything else we have discussed in this book, I am only presenting the basics here. These concepts can be studied in much greater depth by checking out some of the titles I mention in the suggested reading list at the end of the book. I particularly encourage you to read the works by Dr. John F. Demartini, specifically *The Breakthrough Experience*. This book will give you a much deeper understanding of the principles I present here and more, so I cannot recommend it highly enough. If you read only one other book on personal and mental development, make it this one. Now let's move on to balanced perspective.

**Principle 1: Certainty**

The principle of certainty is possibly the most important concept we will discuss in this section. Without a doubt, it will also be the most difficult to master. In a nutshell, the principle of certainty states that in order to achieve anything in life—be it optimal health, enormous wealth, or deep personal and professional gratification—we must be certain of its presence in our lives *now*. In other words, we must be absolutely convinced that that which we want has already been accomplished. Whether you wish for physical attractiveness, happy relationships, or creative brilliance, it all starts with believing that our desires have already been fulfilled—the stronger our convictions, the greater the power of manifestation.

The principle of certainty is based on the first two laws we discussed earlier in the chapter: the law of greater power and the law of mental correspondence. First, to master the art of certainty, one must accept that there is a greater power at work organizing the universe and, consequently, organizing the grand design of your life. What this means is that you have a purpose to your life, one that you must determine on your own. Your life is yours alone, unique to you and your specific strengths, interests, and inspirations. Accepting the idea of a grand design does not mean there is an absence of free will. On the contrary, you have the choice to pick any path in life, just as it is your choice to change that path at any given time. Indeed, it is up to you to decide the direction of your life. Just remember the law of cause and effect: every choice you make leads down another road, bringing you closer to your ultimate purpose. There are no mistakes! When you look back on your life, now or in the future, you will see how true the law of cause and effect really is. Every decision you have made in the past has brought you to the place you are now, and every decision you make today will affect your life tomorrow. When you see things in this way, it is much easier to have a sense of certainty—at least when it comes to understanding your experiences. And certainty is exactly what you need in order to realize your dreams or at least make it through tough times.

So what does it mean to be certain? *Certainty* is having the complete conviction that whatever you wish to be true is true right now. Let us illustrate this principle as it relates to our health. Having certainty about health would mean seeing yourself as healthy—now, today—even if you do not feel so great at this very moment. Just knowing that you are a self-healing, self-regulating organism should help you develop your sense of certainty. Believe it because it's true. The biggest problem that many people face is that they actually believe the opposite to be true. They believe that a life of illness is inevitable and depending on the strength of their conviction might just make it so. This is really very unfortunate. Don't do that to yourself—be certain about your health.

Now comes the time for me to twist your mind a little. It is a fallacy to believe that you will never be sick again in your lifetime. This is not what I am talking about when I talk about certainty. On the contrary, according to the law of polarity, illness is inevitable—there is no such thing as health without illness. You cannot be totally healthy unless you are also occasionally sick (more on this in chapter 8). Neither is a life of illness alone possible. Everyone must experience health to some degree or another. The truth is that health and illness are always working together at the same time in every cell, breaking down and building up, and it is exactly what happens in the sum total of our bodies. Believing that life can exist solely in a state of illness or health is living a life of illusion.

What is important is how you view health and illness. One without the other is a delusion, but the presence of both in a proper balance is actually the true meaning of wellness. What you must develop, then, is a deep understanding of this principle, enough to create certainty. When you do, you will see your health flourish.

Certainty can be obtained by acknowledging all the laws we have discussed previously, including the law of energy and vibration. We are all energy forms, and illness is usually some blockage to the free movement of that energy. Nothing to get alarmed about—we merely need to find the means to undo that blockage. We also need to understand that the process of searching out and removing the blockage may actually have a function of its own—a spiritual significance, if you will. It may be to lead us into another level of our development or increase our consciousness of healing processes that we have not previously been aware of. Either way, be certain of your energetic essence; be certain that there is a function to all your illnesses and have an absolute conviction that the pendulum must swing back in the other direction, toward good health, since health is your birthright. And anyway, your return to health is inevitable because it's a law (law of rhythm).

The principle of certainty can be applied to weight loss, body shape, athletic performance, or anything else you wish to manifest. There is a caveat, though. To truly achieve certainty, you must be realistic in your expectations. If you are not a seven-foot behemoth now, you never will be. Likewise, if you are a naturally big-boned person, you'll never be a waif. Don't live those illusions. You may still be able to play a mean game of basketball, though, by constantly improving your skills. Or you can be in the best shape of your life, just know it will only be within your body's limits. Keep it real and don't try to achieve what is physically impossible. Just understand your parameters and work within them and, of course, be certain of the results. It will take work, but you have a lifetime to master it. Of that you can be certain.

## Principle 2: Presence

This principle is about being present in the moment, so we could just as easily call it a principle of consciousness. As an illustration, have you ever seen somebody drive their car right through a stop sign? I observe it all the time; you see, I live in Los Angeles. In this city, it is not only common for drivers to be speaking on their cell phones, but also to be veering into adjacent lanes, cutting off others, and simply ignoring important traffic signals. It is definitely not what we mean when we say being "present in the moment." Instead, it is moving through life in a distracted manner—unconscious, unaware, and unfocused—exactly what this principle is *not* about.

Being present means being completely focused on the task at hand. It means total consciousness. It means not thinking about your golf game while you are at work, not thinking about work while being intimate with your partner, and definitely not speaking on your cell phone while driving. It is also not about being caught up in the past or, likewise, not worrying about the future. It is about being present in the here and now since this is the only moment that really matters.

By being present, you will find yourself experiencing life to its absolute fullest. There is no other moment than the one you are experiencing now. Think about that for a minute. There is a real powerful implication in this notion. It means that no matter what you have done or have not done in the past, your experience at this moment is what counts; it determines the future, and more importantly, it determines the experiences you have today. Isn't that what life is all about, your consciousness of the present moment?

By following this principle, not only will you enrich your life, you will also master every activity you perform and enhance every one of your relationships. Your love relationships will flourish, your children will thrive, and your life will most certainly prosper. Only by practicing this principle can you ever hope to obtain optimal health. What is your health worth anyway if you can't enjoy it in *this moment*? There are many excellent literary sources on this subject, but the one I most highly recommend is *The Power of Now* by Eckhart Tolle. Read this fantastic book to get a deeper sense of how powerful this principle truly is. Start practicing complete focus and presence today. When you do, you will experience a much deeper enrichment of life.

## Principle 3: Affirmation

The principle of affirmation is the process of using a declaration, a firm statement, as a way to condition your subconscious mind. By saying this statement for a short but continuous period, it will lodge both into your short-term and long-term memory as well as into your subconscious mind. This principle is intimately connected to the one of certainty. You can effectively use affirmation to increase your current level of confidence.

Affirmations implant into your memory in exactly the same way that repeating a line over and over does. A repetitive thought converted into speech is one of the most effective ways we regularly use to memorize things. We do it to remember instructions, telephone numbers, and speeches. We do it any time we want to lodge something into our minds. How many times have you wanted so badly to remember the name of someone you just met, so you repeated it over and over while simultaneously picturing her face? You did this because it is the most efficient method for storing information into your short-term memory bank.

That is what we are doing when we say affirmations. We are repeating a statement that we believe to be true, like "I have perfect health," or "I am in great shape," or "I am my perfect weight and size." We say them over and over again until they become lodged into our long-term memory or they become a part of our very thought process. These statements actually become a part of us. When we say them continually, they become true in our minds.

Just think of how effectively this system works even when we do not want it to. How many of us have had the experience of that silly little song we heard yesterday playing over and over again in our heads? Advertisers know this, and it is why they have created those maddening yet completely effective jingles so that we will always remember their products. This process is powerful, and we can definitely use it to our advantage.

When an affirmation becomes successfully lodged into our memory, it has an astonishing effect upon the subconscious mind. The subconscious is the part of the mind that operates outside of the level of our conscious thought. One can think of it in much the same way as one does the autonomic nervous system, which we discussed in chapter 4. This branch of the nervous system does not need our conscious mind to carry out its operations—it works independently of our conscious thought. We need this system to control those functions of the body that must always be on, like heartbeat, respiration, and, of course, many of our mental processes. The subconscious mind is that portion of our mental operation that makes decisions as to what the conscious mind needs to perceive. It is almost like a distribution center where the functions that do not need conscious processing can be handled by the autonomic system. Processes that do require attentive decision making, of course, get shuttled to the conscious control regions of our brain.

A type of information that does not need to be constantly processed by the conscious mind is our belief system. Our beliefs become lodged into our memory banks and serve to influence our thoughts, words, and actions. They are bits of information that our brains use to process other forms of incoming data and are sometimes so firmly embedded that we have difficulty altering them. In fact, many times, our beliefs remain in place without us ever reevaluating them.

We can affect our subconscious mind directly—and thus, our belief system—through repeated affirmations. In reality, we all use this principle every day, sometimes without even knowing it. We all use affirmations in both a self-supportive and a self-effacing fashion. I am sure there are many of you reading this who can relate to your own use of affirmations to build yourselves up. We all have had moments when we have been pleased with our looks, our dress, our mannerisms, or anything else we have felt confident about. However, we also have the tendency to do the opposite; at times, we may affirm thoughts that can lower our self-esteem. The good news is we can choose the areas in which we wish to increase our self-confidence, and we can do it by saying affirmations.

The most effective way to do an affirmation is to keep it simple, say it in the present tense, and say it in a way that already assumes its reality. Short sentences spoken in the first person are the best. These would be things like "I am enjoying perfect health," "I am a perfect weight for my shape and size," and "I am a lean mean (add your own adjective here) machine." Also, saying an affirmation in the positive sense is more powerful than saying it in the negative. Therefore, affirming what you would love to be is preferred to affirming something that you do not want. "I am enjoying perfect health" has much more power than "I am no longer sick." It is a subtle yet important detail of this practice.

Furthermore, it is absolutely vital that you believe what you are affirming to be already true. This is sometimes hard, but by practicing the principle of certainty along with your affirmations, it will become much easier over time. Merely saying an affirmation without having complete conviction of its reality will unfortunately render it useless. Certainty adds congruency to the statement and allows both the conscious and subconscious minds to work creatively to bring about the experience. Remember the law of mental correspondence: we create our experiences in our minds first. This process is only strengthened by the use of regular positive affirmation.

A common criticism of this practice comes from a group that wishes to deny the power of affirmation in healing. They claim that it is dangerous to promote the idea that we can affect our physical experiences by conditioning our thought processes. They say it is foolish to practice this principle as a substitute for traditional medical care. I couldn't agree more. It *is* foolish to think that by simply saying affirmations, nothing else needs to be done. On the contrary, affirmations should serve only as a compliment to other treatments, protocols, or health practices you may be doing. Affirmations alone do not work—actions are also necessary. What the given action should be is a personal choice, but I assure you that by using positive affirmations, you stand a much greater chance of succeeding at your endeavors.

On a final note, affirmations are most effectively lodged into our memory and subconscious mind while we sleep. As you learned in chapter 5, sleep is when our short-term memories get moved into our long-term storage banks. Experts on the subject, then, recommend saying affirmations right before we fall asleep. Additionally, it is important to combine them with visualizations where you actually see yourself achieving your goals. That means you must *see* yourself in perfect health and at a perfect weight or shape or body size; and that will make both the affirmation and the visualization lodge into your subconscious mind more firmly and, eventually, bring them into actualization.

## Principle 4: Visualization

The principle of visualization is very similar to that of affirmation in that both work actively on the subconscious mind. Remember that all things, at their most basic, are simply different forms of energy. This is not only true with respect to our material bodies, but with regard to our words and thoughts too. When we use our minds to visualize a specific outcome, we create energetic and vibrational waves that are transmitted from our minds into the collective mental matrix.

Visualization is the process of seeing in your mind the outcome of something you wish to manifest. The law of mental correspondence states that whatever we experience on the physical plane always exists first as a thought. There is no exception to this rule. This is why purposeful visualization is so powerful. You are creating the experience in your mind first. With diligent and determined practice, it will be impossible for your visualizations not to manifest.

The same rules with which you use to perform your affirmations also apply to visualization. Seeing the outcome you desire in a positive light is a very powerful technique. Of course, you must believe it to be true for it to be congruent with your mind. By practicing visualization regularly and just before falling asleep, you will have the greatest effect possible on your subconscious mind. Where the practice of visualization differs from that of affirmation is that, when doing the former, you should use the greatest amount of detail possible. Simplicity is not the key here, but instead, it is the intricate details of your visual image that make this practice so powerful.

You can use this principle in every facet of your life—be it physical health, financial prosperity, or professional success. When practicing visualization, see what you would love to experience in your life in the greatest amount of detail possible and also believe it with absolute certainty; and you will see your dreams miraculously manifest, just as you have mentally envisioned them.

Unfortunately, this principle works in the opposite way as well. If you constantly imagine and visualize that which you do not want, you will ultimately create that experience. The power of your mind is that great—it brings about what you think about. Let us take weight loss for example. If you are trying to lose weight yet see yourself as fat, unsightly, or have any other image of yourself that is not exactly what you would like, then you are essentially sabotaging your own efforts. The reality is that no matter what physical techniques you use to lose weight, you will never be able to overcome a weight problem if your own mind is not in congruence with the thought of losing weight. This is why certainty is so crucial.

The way visualization, affirmation, and certainty work together is by actively conditioning your mind, which actually changes your vibrational energy. This, then, has the power to attract events or circumstance in your life that are congruent with your thoughts. Once again, remember, we are all energy. Energy can neither be created nor destroyed—it can only change forms. Since all energy exists as both particles and waves, and waves can change their frequency, then we can change our own cells' frequency by simply changing the way we think.

How does this work? To understand this incredible mechanism, we need to look at an interesting principle of physics. This principle is called *resonance*. The simplest way to understand resonance is by looking at a phenomenon that occurs with tuning forks. When a tuning fork is strummed so that it vibrates at its resonant frequency, it can be brought in the proximity of another tuning fork, which is not vibrating; and that tuning fork will start to vibrate at exactly the same frequency as the first one. This happens because sound waves from the first tuning fork actually travel through the air and strike the second nonvibrating tuning fork. The sound waves cause the second fork to vibrate, giving off its own sound waves at exactly the same frequency as the first fork.

So by changing our thoughts, we will be able to change the frequency of our cells—which, through the process of resonance, will begin to vibrate at the same frequency as our thoughts. This is a very important point: by simply choosing the nature of our thoughts to those that support the experiences we wish to create, every cell in our body begins to resonate at that frequency. Through this change in vibration, we have the ability to attract circumstances, events, and people into our lives that resonate at the frequency of our thoughts—it's simple physics!

Even more remarkable, though, is that modern science has shown that by simply visualizing an event or activity, it creates the same physiologic changes in the body as actually performing the activity itself. For instance, if you visualize yourself running a race, your brain waves will fire in the same way as if you were really physically running. Furthermore, as you improve your visualization skills, you may even increase your heart rate, respiratory rate, and begin sweating as you imagine yourself running. This is such a powerful point that I urge you to please take the time to digest it. If you can affect your physiology simply by visualizing an action, then what does it mean for your physical development, including weight loss? This is why visualization is so potent. When we see in our mind's eye that which we wish to create—perfect health, perfect weight, ripped abs, whatever—we vibrate at that specific frequency, and through the process of resonance, our bodies respond. It is truly a remarkable phenomenon.

Just as we saw with affirmations, we all use visualization to some degree already, sometimes without even knowing it. All successful people will admit to using this principle in some way. Sports stars, business people, and innovative thinkers in science, technology, and the arts all do it. There have even been studies showing the effectiveness of the visualization process. Numerous accounts abound of athletes who visualize themselves in their events, performing flawlessly and winning, all before it actually happens. Read the biographies of successful athletes, like Michael Jordan or Tiger Woods, to see this practice in action.[175]

## Principle 5: Meditation

This principle goes by several different names depending on the source of the information. It has also been referred to as the principle of silence, or the principle of prayer. I choose to speak of this principle as meditation because that is how I have learned it, but please understand that these terms are completely interchangeable.

*Meditation* is the practice of silencing the mind for a period that can range anywhere from five minutes to more than an hour to even days, depending on one's commitment level. Many methods exist including the use of mantras, visualizations, or counting the cycles of one's breath. The purpose of this act is to quiet the mind of the constant "chatter" that fills the empty space between our thoughts. The brain is an organ just like the heart, and as such, it performs its functions like most of our other organs without the need for our conscious mind to be involved. One function of the brain is to process information. This occurs whether we are conscious of it or not, and most times, we are not. Information being processed can present itself as mental chatter.

We are so used to this process occurring that we accept chatter as normal. And it is. However, chatter prevents us from connecting to our true essence, which is pure energy. When we can sit in silence and focus on nothing (an arduous task, indeed), we bring ourselves to a state where we will have the best ability to connect to our energetic source. This may be a difficult concept to understand intellectually. It would be very similar to describing how one feels when one is in love. One can describe it, but the only way another person can understand it is if she has had the experience herself. It is the same with meditation. I can describe it to you in complete detail, but you will actually have to experience it to ever understand what I am talking about.

Quieting the mind is more complicated than it may sound. It takes diligent practice to master, and many people give up in frustration as a result of its difficulty. However, I urge you to practice daily, even if it seems like you are not succeeding. I promise you, every time you do it, you will improve—each time bringing you closer to what you wish to achieve.

To quiet the mind, we can use one of a few popular techniques. The one most often used requires you to focus on and count the breath cycles. While sitting (which is better than lying down because it prevents you from falling asleep), you breathe in and out slowly. That counts as one breath cycle. Breathe again—that's two. And so on. Count to five cycles and begin again at one. This might sound easy to do but is most definitely not; it is actually maddeningly difficult to focus on one's breath for an extended period. When you try it, you may find that the first two cycles give you no problem at all. However, I assure you that if you have never practiced this before, your mind will wander; and it will start the mental conversations that generally fill the space in your mind, or in other words, the chatter. It will bring up every other thing that currently occupies your mind—your work, your grocery list, your golf game, or whatever you might have wished you had said to your boss. However, don't let this discourage you.

Over time, you will master this practice. Be easy on yourself, though. I have been practicing for years, and I have only been able to extend my practice recently to thirty minutes. Some days are better than others, but quite a few are still really tough. I accept it, I try to do my best, and I move on. Tomorrow is another day.

Another method is to close your eyes and visualize a light and just focus on it; yet another is clearing your mind by saying a mantra. A *mantra* is a sacred invocation repeated during prayer or meditation. The most common mantra is the word "om." It has spiritual and energetic properties, but to explain it here would be outside the scope of this book. If you are interested, there are many books on the subject of mantras. You should not have any problems finding a great source to this ancient practice.

Whichever way you choose to clear your mind, the end result is the same. What you will accomplish when you are actually able to experience this state is a dimension between your thoughts. The best description I have heard is that it is similar to the brain state you enter just before falling asleep. As we have discussed in chapter 5, your brain waves change during this process—from the fast beta waves that are present during conscious activity, to the slower alpha variety, and eventually on to the even slower theta waves.[176] The theta waves are associated with deep meditation. This state has been accurately described as *conscious unconscious*, not quite awake yet neither asleep.

Aside from allowing us to connect to our true essence, meditation provides many other physiological effects that are beneficial. Studies have shown that meditation actually lowers blood pressure, heart rate, and serum concentration levels of several substances like cortisol (stress hormone) and cholesterol.[177] This makes sense to those already practicing meditation as many report decreased levels of stress and anxiety with regular training. The evidence to support this comes from studies showing meditation to lower muscle tension as seen on *electromyogram* (EMG, a tool used to measure muscle activity).[178] Many other studies are available that show meditation to be beneficial with the following:[179]

- Reduction of symptoms associated with PMS
- Reduction of blood sugar levels in diabetics
- The treatment of asthma
- Reduction of psoriasis
- Reduction of symptoms associated with fibromyalgia
- Alleviation of pain
- Improved memory and problem solving
- Reduction in reaction time and reflex motor response
- Increased alertness
- Improved concentration
- Increased empathy and emotional sensitivity

- Increased creativity
- Increased self-actualization (potentials for personal growth)

Some medical experts have even established, through case studies, the effectiveness of meditation to decrease the discomforts associated with cancer. Further studies in this area would be enormously beneficial, but even with what we know now about meditation, the benefits can greatly assist those suffering from this disease.

The most important benefit practitioners derive from meditation, though, is the connection and awareness they develop to their own bodies. I believe that this is the highest level of optimal health we can achieve, being in touch with our own bodies. This concept is something we have discussed before in nearly every chapter. The ability to recognize and understand the subtle messages given off by your body is absolutely vital to your health and well-being, and the benefits of this intuitive skill are incalculable. By practicing meditation regularly, you will hone your ability to intuitively understand your body. Nothing will serve you better than this skill. Start practicing now and be consistent. Evidence is plentiful showing the effects of meditation to be cumulative. That means the beneficial effects of meditation multiply exponentially over time. But remember, be patient—this is a practice that will only get stronger as you do it.

## Principle 6: Gratitude

The sixth and final principle, and perhaps the most important one I will present, is the principle of gratitude. Gratitude is a state of being; it is the state of thankfulness and appreciation for our life exactly as it is right now. This means accepting all of our life's circumstances as a necessary stage that we must experience to help us move toward our life's purpose.

When we can look at our life in this way, it is easier to appreciate the details of our lives, even the seemingly "bad stuff," since it gives us the insight that each one of our experiences is necessary. Every experience has the function of bringing us into balance. Remember the law of polarity: it states that something does not exist without its opposite. Therefore, we cannot have "good" or supportive experiences without having an equal amount of "bad" or challenging ones. This is only part of the equation, though. In reality, there is no such thing as good or bad. All events are neutral until we analyze and label them. These labels are just mental constructs that man has developed to give reference to things; in this way, he can make better decisions. These constructs, in turn, are governed by the emotions. That is why we develop such intense emotional charges to things that do not resonate with our value system. Isn't it interesting that the things which charge us seem to differ in degree and content from person to person? For instance, you may get charged about the current presidential administration. I, in turn, may also get charged but not as much as you do. And we may have a mutual friend who doesn't get charged at all. This shows just how important the emotional reference system really is—it guides us toward making decisions and leads us down our own individual paths. We certainly have to be grateful for that!

It would seem, then, that our goal should be to develop a perpetual state of gratitude; however, this is not realistic. The truth is that we can only *approximate* a constant state of gratitude. Despite our desires to reach even the slightest state of appreciation, actually doing so takes work and diligence. Like all the other principles we have discussed, mastering gratitude is a process that will only get better the more you practice it. The degree to which you are able to master this principle, though, will have great implications for your health as well as for every other facet of your life.

So how do we do it? How do we enter a state of gratitude? The following comes from the teachings of Dr. John F. Demartini. The first step is to acknowledge that our perception of a situation is purely that—a perception. No experience is either all good or all bad. We can, therefore, start to look for both the benefits and the disadvantages to any situation, even with regard to our health. This might be hard at first as it is our natural tendency to deny one side of an experience or the other; however, if you can see both sides to a situation, then you will be better able to balance the perception of that situation. You will also be able to remove or neutralize any charge that you have associated with this particular situation. Please note that a charge does not have to be anger or hurt; it could just as easily be an infatuation or elation. When you balance your emotional charges, and consequently your perceptions, you will experience a deeper sense of gratitude. And more importantly, you will experience unconditional love. If you are able to walk away from a situation that appeared bad to you at first and still feel gratitude for it, or for the lesson it has taught you, then you have opened the door to unconditional love.

When you enter a state of unconditional gratitude, you will appreciate all aspects of your experiences, and those experiences will become more meaningful to you. You will also become more powerful because in this state, you will transcend any obstacles that may prevent you from growing. As a result, you will be able to move on to the next stage of your development. Just understand that we are talking about one experience and not all of them; every situation that charges us in some way or another stands alone. Therefore, each experience will need to be balanced separately. And when we grow, we do so in relation to the particular experience we have just balanced. So this type of skill lasts a lifetime. We will subsequently need a lifetime to master it as there will always be the next experience for us to balance. No problem, that's life. We will never reach the top of the mountain since its height is infinite. Life is merely the journey we take up the mountain—how far you wish to climb is up to you.

Now please forgive me for making all of this sound so simple; it is not. In fact, as I have said before, we develop many mental blocks that can make it difficult for us to achieve a state of gratitude; and sadly, some people never reach this state at all. Fortunately, there is a technique that you can learn that will greatly enhance your ability to enter this state of gratitude at will. It is called the *Quantum Collapse Process*, and it is one of the most useful techniques I have ever learned. This tool is based upon physics, neurophysiology, and human dynamics; and it was developed by Dr. John F. Demartini. You can learn more about it through his book *The Breakthrough Experience* (see Suggested Reading).

The human mind is one of the most fascinating and wondrous entities we know of. It has the capacity to create and shape all our experiences. Quantum physics teaches us that we are continually creating our universe, and we do it primarily with our minds. I am in deep gratitude for the gift of this magnificent power. When it comes to influencing your health, really, the sky's the limit. You are capable of achieving great heights with the power of your mind—you merely have to believe it. I personally practice all of the mental principles I have discussed, and I am completely certain that they are the wave of the future with regard to human health. These principles are on the cutting-edge of mind-body dynamics. Start practicing them today, and you will understand exactly why this is so. Knowing what we know about the human mind—and also knowing what we *don't* know—really makes me wonder why anybody would want to take the chance of harming it by taking powerful and dangerous psychotropic drugs. Let the power of your mind work for you, in health and in life, and watch your experiences soar.

# Chapter 6 Summary

# Key Number 5: Mental Health

- Identify the areas in your life that you are dissatisfied with, those causing you to be depressed. If you don't know exactly, list everything you are unhappy about. Find out where you desire change, and either work toward changing it or accept it.
- Get help with eliciting change: hire a therapist, join a support group, and become proactive.
- Identify any medications you take that may cause depression and speak to your medical doctor about alternatives.
- Take essential fatty acid (EFA) supplements daily.
- Take a daily multivitamin.
- Limit alcohol intake; reduce recreational drug intake.
- Have your pain evaluated by a doctor (MD, chiropractor, etc.).
- Put your depression into perspective. Its presence is to stimulate change or growth.
- Discuss an alternative to antidepressant drugs with your medical doctor.
- Exercise at least three times per week.
- Engage in mental activities like crossword puzzles, playing chess, reading, or learning a new skill (language, instrument).
- Get at least eight hours of sleep every night.
- Be certain but keep it real.
- Be mentally present in everything you do.
- Do daily affirmations for at least five minutes per day. Be certain in your affirmation.
- Meditate at least one time per day. Buy a book on meditation (see Suggested Reading).
- Visualize what you wish to manifest. Be detailed and specific.
- Practice gratitude. Read *Count Your Blessings* and *The Breakthrough Experience* by John F. Demartini (see Suggested Reading).

# America: The Great Toxic Society

*The economic and technological triumphs of the past few years have not solved as many problems as we thought they would, and, in fact, have brought us new problems we did not foresee.*

—Henry Ford

I N 1978, THE front page of the *New York Times* reported,

NIAGARA FALLS, N.Y.—Twenty five years after the Hooker Chemical Company stopped using the Love Canal here as an industrial dump, 82 different compounds, 11 of them suspected carcinogens, have been percolating upward through the soil, their drum containers rotting and leaching their contents into the backyards and basements of 100 homes and a public school built on the banks of the canal.

The city of Niagara Falls purchased a small area of land in 1953 that was once owned by the Hooker Chemical Company—the cost, one dollar. What the inhabitants did not know was that this site, at one time planned to become a dream community, was in fact a chemical dumpsite. The chemicals leaching up through the soil killed off the plant life, formed toxic puddles in yards, basements, and school yards; and they caused burns on the hands and faces of the children out at play. Even more tragically, they caused a number of illnesses and birth defects that plagued this small community.[180]

A toxin is a poisonous substance. We are exposed to hundreds of toxins every day—in the air, in our water, and in our food. Their presence is a consequence of a highly productive industrialized society where consumerism is a way of life. Loads of chemical substances have leaked into the environment in the form of by-products and wastes that result from a constant produce-and-consume cycle. Sadly, when we place more importance on technological advancement than on environmental safety, we end up paying the price with our health.

Whether talking about smog, household cleaners or pesticides, toxins are everywhere; and it is almost impossible to be in a totally toxin-free environment. It reminds me of a movie I saw when I was a child called *The Boy in the Plastic*

*Bubble.* It was about a kid with a critical immune disorder who could not survive outside a sterile environment. He had to live in an airtight room, or "bubble"; and if he ever ventured past the walls of his sanitary confines, he would die. In this scenario, the main character had to go to extremes to reduce his exposure to infectious agents and toxins. Obviously, we do not have to undertake such measures yet; nevertheless, when we become conscious of the vast array of toxins we come into contact with every day, the thought of a plastic bubble does not seem so crazy after all.

Over sixty thousand chemicals have been used commercially in the United States since 1984, and the numbers have been growing at a rate of approximately one thousand new ones per year.[181] But this is only the half of it. Over seven hundred organic chemicals have found their way into our drinking water, forty of them carcinogenic (cancer-causing materials), and every year four billion pounds of toxic chemicals are released into the air by twenty thousand industrial facilities.[182,183,184]

How does this affect our health? From 1976 to 1991, a study was conducted measuring the amount of toxic substances accumulated in human fat tissue. Samples were taken from all over the United States with startling results. High concentrations of five toxic substances were found in 100 percent of the samples, nine others were found in 91 to 98 percent of the samples including DDE (a by-product of the neurotoxin DDT—baby boomers will remember this one), and an astonishing twenty toxic compounds were found in 76 percent or more of all samples.[185]

So what can we do to minimize the risk of toxic exposure? First, we must understand the problem at hand. A *toxin* is described as any poisonous substance that can cause disease or illness. Many classes of toxins exist, including venom (from a snake or spider), neurotoxins (botulism toxin), and carcinogens. During the first half of the twentieth century, most toxins that jeopardized human health came from bacteria, microorganisms, and other pests. Man-made chemical agents, like pesticides and antibacterial agents, were eventually designed to combat these invaders. Unfortunately, many of these agents were also toxic to fish, plants, and animals—including man.

Toxic chemicals contaminating the air, water, and soil are a consequence of urbanization and industrialization. Beyond industrial pollutants, there are other toxins that exist as a result of our modern-day lifestyles—ionizing radiation from x-rays, carbon monoxide from auto exhaust and cigarette smoke, and synthetic hormones that come from cattle ranch runoff and infiltrate our drinking water. Repeated and long-term exposure to these and other toxins increases our chances of becoming ill dramatically.

With so many toxic substances in our environment, it is no wonder that cancer is the second leading cause of death in the United States.[186] The American Cancer Society estimates that over half a million Americans will die from cancer this year. That equates to over 1,500 people every day. Over the last fifteen years, cancer has been diagnosed in over 18 million people, and 1.4 million new cases will be diagnosed this year. As with heart disease, many cases of cancer are a consequence of lifestyle choices—the foods we eat, the water we drink, the substances we use.

The best thing we can do to reduce our risk is to try to minimize the amount of toxins we are exposed to on a daily basis. Like anything else, consistency is the key—what we do over and over again is what really makes the difference. Smoking a cigarette occasionally will probably do very little to damage your health, yet one pack a day for thirty years can be a disaster. A little mercury here, a little carbon monoxide there, not a big deal, but consume these toxins over a lifetime in your food and water and you might find yourself in serious trouble.

Over the following pages, I will discuss several of the more serious threats to our health and environment. These issues are some of the most controversial political topics in the world today. I will attempt to present these facts the best I can, but you will see that I definitely have my biases. In addition to the facts, I will also attempt to provide you with some viable options to the practices in question. The most important thing will be to gather all the information you can on these subjects. Do not solely take my word for it: do some research on your own; learn every side to the story. By doing so, you will get the information you need to make intelligent decisions. When you minimize the amount of toxins you are exposed to on a daily basis, you will reduce the possibility of developing one of the many diseases that plague our modern society.

## How Do You Like Your Poisons Served?

One area in which we are exposed to toxins on a regular basis is in our food. How is it possible for foods sold under the guise of "safe and natural" to contain toxic material? Well, most people would be shocked to learn how tainted some of the foods found on supermarket shelves can actually be. Many are laden with pesticides, hormones, antibiotics, and other chemicals; and they are sold to us as sound, wholesome products.

Various conventionally grown produce items, those not grown organically and representing the majority of crops sold in the United States, have been found to contain high levels of pesticide residues.[187] In 1996, the U.S. Department of Agriculture (USDA) discovered the residues of thirty-eight different pesticides on apples alone.

What are pesticides used for? They are intended to prevent the destruction of crops by any insect, plant, or fungal species that use these crops as food or compete for the soil and resources needed by the crops to grow. The Environmental Protection Agency (EPA) defines *pests* as "any living organisms that occur where they are not wanted or that cause damage to crops or humans or other animals."[188] This classification also includes insects, mice and other animals, weeds, fungi, and microorganisms (bacteria, viruses, and *prions* [organisms that cause mad cow disease]).

Pesticides are not only toxic to pests, but to animals and humans too. A variety of pesticides are used today—some chemical, some biological, and some antimicrobial. Since listing every type of pesticide here would be outside of the scope of this book, we will discuss only the most common one, organophosphates.

*Organophosphates* act by disrupting the nervous system in both insects and mammals. These chemicals were developed in the nineteenth century and were later used as nerve agents in World War II. Organophosphates disrupt the regulation of an important neurotransmitter called *acetylcholine*, which is essential for communication between nerve cells. Exposure to an organophosphate neurotoxin can lead to severe muscle weakness, spastic paralysis, headaches, fatigue, shortness of breath, memory and concentration problems, anxiety, and depression.[189] Although generally requiring a single high-dose exposure to cause such drastic complications, long-term, low-dose exposure has not yet been studied fully; so we do not know how the pesticide residues found on crops might affect our health. The EPA is currently undergoing studies to test the dosage levels that actually pose a risk to the population.[190]

A major concern regarding organophosphates is that their use as a pesticide is so widespread. Numerous crops in this country are sprayed with organophosphates mainly because they are considered broad-spectrum; that is, they kill a large variety of pests. According to the EPA, 60 million pounds of organophosphates are used on 60 million acres of agricultural land annually. Approximately 17 million pounds are also used nonagriculturally for ornamental plants and lawns found in many homes and commercial properties. At 77 million pounds per year, it is by far the most commonly used pesticide in the country.[191]

Another problem with organophosphates is that their residues may remain on treated fruits, vegetables, and grains for a long period. When we consume these foods, we are also ingesting the pesticide residues. For that reason, it is important to thoroughly wash produce before eating it. This is especially true for thin-skinned fruits and vegetables like apples, peaches, potatoes, and carrots in which we eat the skin (that has been sprayed directly with pesticide) along with the fruit. Since organophosphates are used on such a wide array of crops (including corn and wheat), washing produce may not completely decrease our exposure. Even processed foods like applesauce, tomato sauce, and baby food are at risk from contamination since they also come from crops sprayed with organophosphates.

Contamination resulting from residue runoff, or seepage of the chemical into groundwater (our drinking water), is yet another way we might be exposed to organophosphates. Fortunately, these compounds are broken down in the environment faster than any other chemicals previously used as pesticides; however, this does not mean that we are not exposed to low levels of the neurotoxin. What remains unknown is whether long-term, low-level doses have chronic and dangerous consequences to our health. With idiopathic (cause unknown) disorders like Parkinson's and Alzheimer's on the rise, it would seem prudent to minimize our exposure to organophosphates as much as possible.

## The Benefits of Buying Organic

An excellent way to minimize exposure to pesticides is by consuming organically grown produce. Organically grown food is farmed using renewable resources and, through its practices, conserves both soil and water. Its purpose is to produce high-quality food with minimal pesticides and "to enhance environmental quality for future generations."[192] Organic farmers use almost no pesticides, no synthetic fertilizers, and no sewage sludge to grow their foods. Organic meats, poultry, eggs, and dairy are produced without hormones or antibiotics. And organic food is never subjected to ionizing radiation or genetic engineering (another method commonly used in the United States to render produce unappetizing to pests).

Not just any farm can claim to be organic. To be certified, a farm must first be inspected by a U.S. government agent to make sure the farm actually complies with United States Department of Agriculture (USDA) standards. Additionally, companies that distribute or process organic foods must also pass federal inspection before their product reaches the supermarket.

There is some public confusion regarding the labeling of organic foods. With the popularity of these foods rising, many companies would like to jump on the bandwagon by labeling their products Organic; but since only a portion of their contents (in cereals or other prepared foods like soup) may actually be organic, stringent labeling is now in place. To be labeled 100 Percent Organic, a food must contain 100 percent organic material. If the food's organic content is between 95 to 100 percent, then it must be labeled simply Organic. If a product has between 70 to 95 percent organic content, then it may be labeled Made with Organic Ingredients. Anything containing less than 70 percent organic material must not use the label Organic at all on the front panel of its packaging but may list its organic ingredients on the side information panel. Stiff fines are levied against any company caught mislabeling its product.

When we become aware of the potential hazards in eating foods treated with chemical pesticides, it starts to make sense to buy organic. Remember the study that we mentioned earlier in which high levels of five different toxic substances were found in every sample of human fat tissue taken and twenty additional toxins were found in 75 percent of the samples? By buying organic, you avoid taking in many of the toxins people ingest on a daily basis. True, organic foods can be more expensive, but it is certainly worth the investment. When we consider all the benefits organic foods provide for our health, why wouldn't we spend the extra cash to minimize toxic exposure? Today, almost every supermarket carries some type of organic products on their shelves, and their volume seems to be increasing yearly. Most cities have grocery stores that specialize in organic "health" foods. And farmers' markets, which sell produce coming directly from the grower, are increasing in popularity. Clearly, not all food is the same. Naturally grown, pesticide-free foods are better for you than those treated with chemicals. For a few extra bucks, you can rest assured that you and your family will enjoy the most nutritious and wholesome foods available.

## GM Food: The Controversy Over Mutant Edibles

One of the most heated issues in the world today is the development and distribution of *genetically modified* (GM) *foods*. GM foods are also said to be *genetically engineered* or *transgenic*. They are produced by using advanced molecular biology techniques that genetically alter their natural composition. By introducing the genes of another organism, new plant species may manufacture substances like preservatives, pesticides, medicines, or vaccines—which ultimately become a constituent of the plant itself. This process is used extensively throughout the United States and is also practiced in countries like Argentina, Canada, and China. An estimated 60 to 70 percent of packaged foods contain GM ingredients, with corn and soy being the most often modified. [193,194]

Genetically modified foods are developed with the promise that they will virtually wipe out world hunger. Proponents claim that by developing new plant varieties—particularly those that can produce their own pesticides and herbicides—crops will be less susceptible to pests and, as a result, will produce greater yields. They also point out that fruits and vegetables can be manipulated to grow larger and more flavorful by introducing genes that produce growth, flavoring, or hormones that accelerate ripening, which should make the produce more attractive to consumers.

But not everyone is singing the praises of GM foods. According to some prominent scientists, many dangers lurk within these mutant edibles. To fully appreciate the risks, one must first understand the details involved in genetically altering foods. A *gene* is a unit of heredity, composed of a length of DNA, which occupies a specific location on a chromosome. It codes for a particular characteristic of an organism (perhaps hair color in humans or flavor in strawberries). Whatever the characteristic, the genes that code for those traits have been present in the species for a long stretch of time (e.g., gills on a fish, feathers on a bird, or seeds in a grape).

When a DNA sequence changes, even if by only one single unit, then the gene is said to have mutated; it will no longer code for the exact same characteristic. Instead, the gene may be rendered useless (turned off or unable to influence the characteristic), become overly expressive (constantly turned on like the genes in cancer cells), or may code for something entirely different (like a toxin). Mutations may result from exposure to radiation, toxins, or even from certain microorganisms. Mutations can also result from the genetic engineering process itself.

In natural breeding methods, organisms of the same species combine genetic material through sexual reproduction. Usually, each parent contributes half the chromosomes to their offspring and, consequently, half the genes. These genes are then paired-up in the offspring in an orderly fashion, and the sequence of genetic material remains fixed. On the other hand, in genetically modified organisms, biotechnicians take the genes from one organism and splice it forcibly into the DNA of another, quite often into one of a totally different species. For example, engineers may combine the genes of a bacterium with that of a plant or animal. In this way, new hybrid species are created with the hopes of solving some of today's most difficult medical problems or, at the very least, increasing the efficiency of the world's agricultural production.

Although control of gene expression is maintained through a highly sophisticated regulatory system present in all cells, GM organisms are unable to fully utilize this system on their own. An additional stretch of DNA called a *promoter sequence* is needed to recognize and turn on the newly introduced gene. While necessary for proper gene expression, adding promoter sequences to the hosts DNA has several potential drawbacks, some of which we will discuss later.

Nevertheless, the arguments supporting the practice of genetically modifying foods are many. Proponents such as the Food and Drug Administration (FDA) contend that the inheritance of traits due to gene splicing in the lab is equivalent to that which takes place during natural sexual reproduction. They believe that introducing genes artificially is not only in tune with nature, but scientifically sound and virtually risk free. They say that as long as a product of an introduced gene is generally recognized as safe, then it should be safe whether it is produced in its natural environment or inside a foreign host.

Another argument in favor of genetically engineered foods is that we can produce newer, heartier, and more pest-resistant crops. Supposedly, these crops can now withstand drought, insects, and weeds—which in the past might have destroyed the crops or at least have competed for valuable resources. In theory, then, this "improvement" in agriculture should increase overall yields and finally put an end to world hunger. Proponents also believe that GM crops will be larger and more flavorful, adding yet another advantage to this practice. Additionally, genes for preservatives can be spliced into fruits and vegetables increasing the shelf life of the produce. Ultimately, this will lead to bigger profits for farmers and grocers—and this is good—but it will also lead to larger profits for the big biotech manufacturers who hold the patent rights to this technology. This, as we shall see, can result in a serious conflict of interests.

Proponents also believe that GM organisms are better for the environment. They claim that with decreased maturation time, fewer resources like water, soil, or energy will be needed to grow GM foods. Since crops can also be engineered with fertilizers, waste management will be more efficient as it should decrease the need for animal manure. "Better for the environment, better for the world" is how genetic engineering is sold to the public.

So with all the benefits that GM foods supposedly provide, why would there be any arguments against them? Well, some inherent problems exist, including issues of human safety, environmental concerns, and freedom of choice; it also brings up ethical questions regarding corporate control over the world's food supply. The opponents to GM foods include prominent scientists who believe that genetic modification has neither been rigorously tested nor demonstrated as safe. As of this writing, several American and British scientists have filed suit against the U.S. FDA precisely on these grounds.

By far, the biggest scare regarding GM foods is that they may pose serious risks to our health. When one gene is spliced into another, the location of its insertion can only be estimated to a certain degree—being exact is simply impossible. Some genes may therefore insert haphazardly into another already existing gene, changing the latter gene's sequence. A disruption in a gene's sequence, or its genetic code, is known as *genetic recombination*. If the recombined sequence disrupts an already existing gene, that gene is rendered useless and the organism loses a trait—quite possibly a necessary nutrient, enzyme, or cofactor. It could also disrupt the host gene in such a way that it might produce an undesired substance like a toxin or an allergen. This is what happened in 1989 when a GM batch of the supplement L-tryptophan was contaminated by several toxins that were a metabolic by-product of the genetic engineering process. The product was neither tested nor analyzed for contaminants before going on the market and was unfortunately sold to an unsuspecting public. As a result, thirty-seven Americans died, fifteen hundred were permanently disabled, and five thousand more made ill from the toxic GM product.[195]

The potential health risks involved in using biotechnology to alter our food supply should be reason enough to be cautious, but environmental concerns stand out too. Cross-pollination of GM plants with wild plant species can create new "superweeds," which develop resistance to pesticides. Recombination that occurs between *transporter viruses* (carries the new gene into the host organism) and *wild viruses* (already existing inside the host) can likewise cause "superviruses." These, in turn, can create potentially new and dangerous diseases.[196] Some of these concerns may seem alarmist in nature, but they do point out hazards that should be studied further.

Cross-contamination becomes even more frightening when one considers the notion of *pharmfoods,* future crops designed to produce medicines such as vaccines, blood clotting agents, and antibiotics. Although this may sound like a great idea in theory, there is a real risk of pharmfoods contaminating our food supply. Outdoor crops are continuously exposed to winds, which may blow pollen from pharmfood crops to adjacent nongenetically engineered crops. This is a frightening thought for anyone wishing to keep their foods and medicines separate. Imagine the horror of accidentally eating someone else's blood-thinning tangerine—definitely not the way to start your day.

Opponents of GM foods have not merely conjured up this scenario to promote a state of panic. On the contrary, cross-contamination of our food supply is actually happening right now. Researchers have found evidence of genetically modified DNA in human gut bacteria originating from GM crops, even though biotech officials have repeatedly said it could never happen.[197] If we can just keep in mind that government officials and corporate businesses have their own agendas, we can avoid basing our own decisions on their steadfast assurances.

As one can see, the bioengineering of foods poses numerous questions with regard to our health, yet equally disturbing are the issues surrounding its effects on the environment. Completely containing GM crops is impossible—their seeds may be carried by wind, birds, or insects that can eventually contaminate other crops. So there is a real risk of introducing genes haphazardly into the environment.

Unfortunately, buying organic will mean very little in this case since organic crops are also at risk from cross-pollination by their GM counterparts. A recent British study uncovered this fact: 40 percent of the organic foods tested contained some transgenic material with soy being the most commonly contaminated. Would anybody care to guess which "healthy food" ranks as one of the top sellers in the world today?[198]

Experts predict that it is only a matter of time before GM material contaminates the entire world's food supply; this could eventually change many of the earth's species and may even impact the earth itself. In 1999, researchers found that GM corn is endangering the Monarch butterfly. Plants growing in or around cornfields have been dusted with enough GM pollen to kill significant numbers of Monarch caterpillars feeding on these plants—and it may eventually lead to their extinction.[199] The implications for our own species are, as of yet, unknown. But surely, by tampering with the earth's natural balance, there will be consequences to every life-form on the planet, including man.

Obviously, health and the ecology are at the center of the genetically modified foods debate, but questions involving freedom of choice are also at hand. The biggest problem has been that the public has had very little say in the matter. The FDA and federal government approve genetically engineered foods, yet many Americans are unaware of the practice, let alone the facts surrounding the issue. We are sold foods containing GM ingredients that have no labeling whatsoever. The FDA and corporations manufacturing GM foods provide limited information that is often one-sided and deficient in many of the necessary details. Their assertion that GM foods are no different from naturally produced foods is far too simple and happens to be unproven at this time. Even so, we are fed GM ingredients indiscriminately without having a choice for an alternative. No other commodity outside of fluoridated water is forced upon us without a choice in the way GM foods are.

We may have no choice in the United States whether to consume GM foods or not; but they do in Europe, and they refuse to have genetically engineered foods forced upon them. Many countries of the European Union have rejected American food products that contain GM materials; they scrupulously refuse to consume untested and unnatural products. The United States taking exception to this refusal has filed suit with the World Trade Organization (WTO) citing restriction of free trade. The Europeans have since allowed American-manufactured GM foods into their countries but require them to be labeled as such. That seems fair enough. Why not let those not objecting to GM foods have them, but give those of us who prefer natural foods the option to choose? This can only be accomplished through proper labeling practices.

Yet another fear looms in the minds of opponents: they believe that the world's food supply could be controlled by the corporations that produce GM foods. The reality is that biotechnology is big business with major corporations owning the technological patents of GM products. By advocating genetic engineering in food production, countries that are major producers of GM foods will have a strong economic advantage in the world as well as direct control over global agricultural commerce. It is no surprise, then, that the United States adamantly opposes labeling GM foods, seeing that they are one of the largest producers. Understandably, the fear is that consumers will reject these foods if given the choice. Others besides Europeans have turned away from GM foods: several African countries have refused seeds coming from the United States for fear that they have been genetically modified. In 2000, despite being ravaged by famine, Zambia declined U.S. relief, citing fears of contamination by GM organisms as well as the risk of dependence on American agribusiness.[200] For these countries, accepting U.S. food relief must seem like entering into a pact with the devil—damned if they do, damned if they don't. But for the time being, they have decided on other options.

According to the United Nations' World Food Programme, "Enough food is being produced to provide everyone in the world with a nutritious and adequate diet—in fact 1.5 times the amount required,"[201] yet over 800 million people are still chronically hungry.[202] GM foods will not solve the world's hunger problem because economic interests control the world's food supply. By turning food into a patented product, it will only increase the existing problem and succeed in shifting this economic power from agriculture to biotechnology.

The bottom line with GM foods is not that we shouldn't have them. On the contrary, if that is what *some* people want, then, by all means, make it available. But wouldn't it be prudent for us to have stringent testing policies and controls as well as natural alternatives for those of us who do not want modified foodstuffs on our plates? We have no evidence yet of the safety of GM foods, so why take the word of policy makers who might be wrong (or have their own interests in mind)? These same officials argue that we can never expect to be guaranteed "total safety" and instead should be relieved that no evidence shows GM foods to be unsafe. Incredibly enough, this is the same argument used by the tobacco industry for years, and we know how that story turned out. We should definitely not impede scientific progress but we should have the option to feed our families 100 percent safe and natural foods until a *proven* alternative is available. Only then should we accept man-made food as superior to Mother Nature's.

## Pumped-up and Ready for Dinner

If worrying about GM foods is not enough, there is yet another concern surrounding our food supply that has to do with the cultivation and processing of meat products, particularly beef. Crowded and sometimes filthy feedlots, as well as the liberal use of hormones and antibiotics, are some of the dangerous practices connected to beef products.

The birth of the U.S. cattle industry dates as far back as the Civil War. Starting as a small-scale industry in the 1850s, cattle drives grew along with the migration of people to the West. With the advent of refrigeration and railroads, it became easier to transport beef to eastern cities, further expanding the beef trade.

It did not take long for beef to become the primary protein consumed in the United States. The cattle industry today accounts for almost half of the total sales of all farm products in this country, totaling approximately $98.3 billion in 2003.[203] Traditionally, it has been a family-run business with only five major players controlling 80 percent of all beef production. Although these five companies control production and distribution, they use over fifty thousand ranchers to raise their cattle.

As the demand for beef has increased, so has the need for larger and more efficient production capacities. As a result, cattle-raising practices have switched from open-ranged grazing to fenced-in farms and crowded feedlots. Today, cattle graze on wild grasses for a short period lasting only a few months and are then transported to feedlots where they finish out the remainder of their days before going on to slaughter.

Many experts believe that a decrease in grass feeding has disrupted the normal nutritional and hormonal balance of most cattle. Feedlots generally provide a grain diet for the animals, which many consider nutritionally inadequate for healthy growth and maturation. As a result, many farmers are forced to provide hormones to the cattle to fatten them up as well as to increase their tenderness.[204] These hormones are usually androgenic (primarily testosterone), which means they are similar to the steroids used by bodybuilders and other athletes.

The practice of injecting hormones into cattle has both its defenders and opponents. Proponents contend that these hormones are the same as those already produced by the animals, so they merely supplement the cattle's own natural substances. In their opinion, no safety concerns are present with this practice whatsoever. They defend their position by pointing out that the added hormones affect the tenderness of the meat, making it more palatable for consumers.

On the other hand, opponents to hormone supplementation believe that an increase in hormone exposure may have the same health ramifications for cattle as it does for humans. All of us are aware of the severe health consequences suffered by athletes who have used steroids like former NFL star Lyle Alzado. Steroids are banned substances in all professional sports—not only because they enhance performance, but because they can also damage one's health. Hormone use, however, is the norm in the cattle-raising industry. If we declare the use of hormones dangerous for human health, then why would we want to eat beef that has been pumped up with it?

There is currently no proof showing a causal relationship between beef raised with growth hormone and the development of chronic diseases like cancer. Despite the lack of concrete proof, wouldn't most health-conscious people prefer naturally produced beef over beef raised on crowded feedlots or with supplemented hormones? Why would anyone risk potential harm, even if that risk is minimal? It seems to me that any cattle needing hormone supplementation to make it more palatable for human consumption is by all accounts a defective animal. The question must be asked, then: why would anyone want to eat the meat of a deficient animal in need of artificial enhancement?

The argument to this question is usually that today's cattle-raising practices keep beef prices down. In my opinion, it makes very little sense to choose savings over safety. Just as with organic produce, which is grown without pesticides or genetic engineering, naturally produced beef is well worth the investment. Eating healthy foods is prevention in the truest sense of the word, and prevention is the most cost-effective insurance policy money can buy.

Aside from the possible health risks inherent in hormone supplementation, an even greater threat exists from hormonal runoff from cattle waste products, like feces, into our water supply. Hormone residues can find their way into water sources, exposing other wildlife and even humans to high concentrations of steroids. Studies have shown that fish living downstream from conventionally raised cattle farms have higher incidences of physiological mutations than those living either upstream or downstream from natural farms.[205] The effects on human health, however, are at this time unknown.

To further darken the picture, farmers in the past have mixed bits of sheep's neural tissue into the cattle's grain feed in an attempt to minimize costs. This unnatural and dangerous practice has led to the development of *mad cow disease*, an always-fatal illness (to cows) caused by the development of malformed proteins called *prions*. When ingested by humans in beef, prions cause a disorder called *spongiform encephalopathy*, or new variant Creutzfeldt-Jakob disease (nvCJD).

Spongiform encephalopathy, or spongy brain, is exactly as it sounds: portions of the brain are eaten away by the prions, forming holes or craters.

Several years back, millions of infected cows turned up in Europe while the United States discovered its first documented case in 2003. Unfortunately, the practice of feeding sheep tissue—and sometimes even other cows—to cattle was not outlawed in the United States until 1997. As a result, a large number of cattle may be infected today; however, it is impossible to know exactly how many. Cattle are generally slaughtered before they turn two years old, which is far too early to detect the presence of mad cow disease. Beef raised on conventional farms may therefore be infected and may even end up on our dinner table. [206]

Under these circumstances, it seems the wisest practice would be to buy and consume beef raised naturally on open-ranged farms. Cattle raised on these farms are allowed to feed on grass for their entire growth period; no hormones are used, and distributors won't purchase beef that comes from animals failing to live up to growth standards. This ensures that only the most fit and healthy cattle are sold for consumption. There is no danger of developing mad cow disease as the cattle are only fed grass diets. Since conditions on these farms are not crowded, other diseases and infections are minimal, reducing the need for antibiotics so prevalent in conventional cattle-raising practices.

Consumers are becoming more aware of how cattle are raised in this country, and many have started buying their beef from alternative sources. The increase in natural beef, pork, and chicken farms in the United States is on the rise; and many health-conscious grocers carry their products. With all this information at hand, wouldn't it make sense to buy natural whenever you have a choice? After all, what price can you put on your health and that of your children?

Colorado State University professor of animal science Tom Field has said it best, "If an organic product better suits your needs, desires and value systems, go for it. The reality is in the marketplace. Some people want food produced with minimal technology and minimal scientific protocols. Others want their food produced as safely and as cheaply as possible."[207] As consumers, we can only hope that safety is always the main consideration and that quality is never sacrificed for cost.

## Cage Free: What's All the Hype Anyway?

Raising animals for mass consumption is a tricky business. Farmers must be able to balance production with cost, and to be profitable, they must sometimes use cost-effective measures. There is certainly nothing wrong with minimizing costs, yet when savings compromise the safety of the end product, especially when that product is food, health watchdogs go on alert. For exactly this reason, the poultry industry is now under scrutiny. Poultry farmers have been accused of treating their chickens inhumanely as well as raising their fowl under filthy conditions. On "conventional farms," the standard practice is for up to ten thousand chickens to live in the same shed from chicks to slaughter. They are subjected to 23.5 hours of continuous light, which denies them sleep. This is done so that the chickens remain active, leading to increased muscle growth and maximum plumpness. Chickens that are "quick growers" are generally favored over slower ones; they are usually injected with growth hormones to help speed up the process. In fact, broiler chickens—those we buy for meat—can grow so rapidly that they often outgrow their legs, leading to hip fractures and dislocations.

On many farms, sheds are not cleaned during a chicken's lifetime; it is only done between each new "crop" so that the birds spend most of their lives trudging through their own urine and feces. The ammonia levels resulting from the stagnant urine can get so high that it can cause blindness in the chickens (it is not very safe for the humans that work the sheds either). The crowded conditions and filth can also lead to infections like *Salmonella* and *Campylobacter*, which are well-known causes of food poisoning. To prevent infections, antibiotics and vaccines are routinely given.

Knowing the details of mass poultry production does not exactly leave one with hunger pangs. Yet there is an alternative—one that promises cleaner, more humane breeding practices as well as greater health benefits. It may also offer better taste. That alternative is pasture-raised or grass-fed meats.

Pasture-raised animals (poultry, beef, and pork) live on open-ranged farms and graze on grasses and other vegetables. They eat plenty of legumes, insects, and worms too. Studies have shown that animals raised predominantly on grass-fed diets have higher levels of omega-3 fatty acids (chapter 2).[208] They also have greater concentrations of CLA (conjugated linoleic acid), a fatty acid known to reduce the risks of cancer, obesity, diabetes, and various immune disorders.[209]

Grass-fed meats are generally hormone and antibiotic free. The term *organic* is used only if the animal feed is grown under organic guidelines. The use of organic feed is less important than whether the animal is grass fed or pasture raised since the type of food (in this case: grass, clover, alfalfa, and other leafy greens) is what leads to the high concentration of omega-3s and CLA.

There are a few obstacles to purchasing grass-fed products, though. One is availability. Pasture farms are mostly small and independent, and they cannot produce enough to satisfy the demand of the larger chain grocery stores. For this reason, most producers sell their goods out of local farmers' markets. As more people learn about the benefits of eating grass-fed meats, demand will surely rise, and it will lead to more grocery chains carrying this option.

Unfortunately, many food manufacturers have tried to jump on the "natural" bandwagon in an attempt to exploit a marketing label that actually has very lax regulations. This is especially true in the poultry industry, where the term *cage free* is used quite freely. *Cage free* may conjure up visions of birds roaming without restraint in wide-open pastures, scratching dirt and grazing on insects; but the term can be used in any case where chickens have access to an open space, no matter how small the space is. Many farmers, in fact, simply attach a ten-foot outdoor pen to the sheds with a swinging door leading in and out. They do this so that they may sell chickens under the cage-free guise, regardless of the fact that the majority of chickens never actually make it outdoors. What we end up getting is a highly overused and misleading label. This is maddening since the chickens are not any different than what you would get from a conventional farm. But you end up paying more for it just because it carries the deceptive classification.

It would be helpful for the FDA to adopt guidelines and standards to regulate the Cage Free label in the same way they do for organic produce. Standards would ensure that cage-free chickens were truly pasture raised and grass fed and that you could pretty much bank on getting a higher concentration of omega-3s and CLA than with conventionally grown chickens. Most health-conscious people would pay extra to know they are getting the added benefits of grass-fed meats, but charging more for essentially the same quality product is practically begging for stricter regulation.

In France, regulation is mandatory; and it seems to be working well, particularly with their premium Label Rouge chicken. This "red label" is used to mark the highest quality poultry available and is produced under strict guidelines: small number of birds per shed, genuine free-range access, and high food safety standards.[210] The chicken feed they use cannot contain any animal products, hormones, antibiotics, or other additives.

In her doctoral thesis on the marketability of free-range chickens in the state of Illinois, Liz Neufeld explains that people are willing to purchase free-range chickens, especially if the poultry promises increased health benefits. In a survey conducted to study the public's poultry-buying habits, the researchers found that cost was not a factor in determining whether one would purchase free-range products. Most respondents said they would be willing to pay substantially higher prices for the more healthful birds. By far, the most important consideration given for buying any chicken, whether free range or conventional, was taste: respondents said that if the product did not taste good, they simply would not buy.

Another interesting result of the survey was that the most common reason people cited for not purchasing free range in the past was that respondents had never heard of this label. They also found that people who tended to buy free range, and organic for that matter, had a higher education level. One could deduce, then, that people who are sufficiently informed of the latest health information (i.e., more educated) will make food purchases based on health considerations rather than on price alone.

Once again, the main obstacle to buying free-range or grass-fed meats is the lack of availability to consumers. This is especially true for people living in major cities who are often dependent on the products purchased by their grocers and do not have access to local farmers' markets. There is an option, though, even for city dwellers. One can find nearby farmers specializing in grass-fed, pasture raised meats anywhere in the United States and Canada just by visiting http://www.eatwild.com where they are listed by state. But remember, beware of the most overused and overhyped label in the poultry industry, Cage Free. Even the most reputable natural grocery stores will sell meat, poultry, and eggs shamelessly under this label. Until there is FDA regulation of the poultry industry, you will be better off buying your free-range products from small local farmers who specialize in them. If your health is a priority and you want to enjoy the benefits that come from eating grass-fed meats, do not hesitate—find a grass-fed farm near you.

## Whatever You Do, Don't Drink the Water

Water is essential to all life—without it, no living thing could survive. Water is known as the universal solvent because it can dissolve more substances than any other liquid, and this property makes water the quintessential medium for all biological and chemical processes in the body. It is no surprise, then, that human beings are comprised of approximately 60 percent water. Without this composition, nutrients would not be absorbed, enzymatic processes would not be carried out to completion, and macromolecules would not be transported between cells. When we take in an insufficient amount of water, we experience dehydration, which can harm every system in the body including our heart, our lungs, and our brain (see chapter 2). Because of its importance to life, 71 percent of the earth's surface is covered with water, making it one of the most vital resources we have. As the world's population continues to rise, the value of this already precious commodity will surely increase as well.

For years, Americans have taken the safety of their water supply for granted. They trust that the water pumped into their homes is relatively safe for drinking.

But is it? To answer this question, we have to take a look at where our drinking water comes from, its source, and its method of transportation into our homes.

The source of our water supply depends largely on where we live. Big cities receive their water from surface sources like lakes, rivers, and reservoirs while rural areas generally receive groundwater pumped from wells. Anybody can check the source of their tap water at the following Web sites:

Environmental Protection Agency: *http://cfpub.epa.gov/surf/locate/index.cfm*
U.S. Geological Survey: *http://water.usgs.gov/data.html*

All the water that reaches your home via a community water system (CWS), a public water system that supplies most people in the United States, should be treated for various contaminants like microorganisms (viruses, bacteria, and parasites), heavy metals, fertilizers, pesticides, and other chemicals.[211] However, despite the stringent regulations on water safety, our drinking water is far from pure; in fact, in many cities, it can be downright appalling.

The National Resources Defense Counsel (NRDC) conducted a study in June 2003 of nineteen U.S. cities and found a wide disparity in water quality among them.[212] In its report titled *What's On Tap?*, the council concluded that many of the cities had one or more of the following problems: polluted source water, outdated treatment processes, or poor maintenance of the water treatment and storage systems.[213] The report states that tap water may contain a "vast array of contaminants" with a number of particularly harmful ones like lead, pathogens (like Cryptosporidium), by-products of the chlorination process (which can cause cancer), and toxins like pesticides and arsenic.

The NRDC made four major recommendations to the government in their report. The first was to upgrade the deteriorating water systems in place in many cities, including replacing many of the old pipes currently in use. The second recommendation was to upgrade treatment technology. Most cities use outdated techniques that have been in place since World War I and which are unable to remove many of the man-made chemicals released by modern industries. The third recommendation was for the government to increase source-water protection—water suppliers, Congress, and the EPA should identify sources of pollution of our surface and groundwater. Some of the many sources of pollution today include animal feedlots, farms, urban and suburban storm water runoff, sewage leakage and overflow, industrial facilities, and other toxic waste sites (like those releasing perchlorate, a.k.a. rocket fuel).

With so many substances contaminating our water supply, it is mind boggling that the United States continues to use a dangerous practice that has been in place since 1945—the fluoridation of its nation's drinking water.[214] Fluoridation of the public drinking water is a highly controversial practice, yet the average citizen knows very little about it. Even though many people accept that fluoride prevents cavities, there is much debate among experts about fluoride's effectiveness or safety in our drinking water.[215]

According to the American Dental Association (ADA), water fluoridation is both safe and effective in preventing tooth decay. They correctly point out that all U.S. groundwater contains some fluoride. This fact led scientists at the turn of the twentieth century to discover a decreased rate of dental caries (cavities) in populations drinking naturally fluoridated water. Today, fluoride is simply added to water sources that are considered *deficient* in this chemical with the rationale that fluoridated water helps prevent cavities. The ADA reports on their Web site that "145 million people in the United States are consuming fluoridated water today." They also proclaim that "fluoridation is the single most effective public health measure to prevent tooth decay and to improve oral health over a lifetime."[216] But is it?

As the largest and most powerful dental organization in the world, it is really no wonder that the general public accepts the ADA's opinions on water fluoridation as dogma. After all, where else would we get dental health information from other than our trusted national dental association? Unfortunately, they may not be providing us with all the information we need to formulate an educated opinion. Many other organizations and health professionals oppose water fluoridation based on facts that show it to be a highly toxic substance.

The first and most remarkable fact I would like to present is that the positive effects of fluoridation are achieved through its topical application, *not* through oral ingestion as we had once believed.[217] Fluoridated drinking water predates fluoride toothpaste, so at one time, it stood to reason that oral ingestion was the most effective way to receive the benefits of fluoride. But now that we have other options—toothpaste, mouthwash, dentist-administered fluoride—do we still need to increase our exposure by adding it to our drinking water?

It has been shown that populations receiving fluoridated water have the same rate of tooth decay as those receiving nonfluoridated water. A 1986-87 national survey conducted by the National Institute of Dental and Craniofacial Research (NIDCR) showed "no difference in tooth decay [between populations drinking fluoridated water and those not] when measured in terms of DMFT (Decayed, Missing, and Filled Teeth)."[218] Additionally, 98 percent of Western Europe does not fluoridate its drinking water, and the rates of tooth decay in these countries have declined at the same rate as those fluoridating their drinking water.[219] Many foreign officials speak out against the practice of water fluoridation. You can see what they have to say by visiting *http://www.fluoridealert.org/govt-statements. htm*. In light of these facts, one can surmise that the fluoridation of our water supply is neither necessary nor good for our health.

What makes fluoride so dangerous to human health is its chemical composition. Unlike sodium fluoride (NaF), which is the fluoride used in toothpaste, the sources of fluoride in drinking water—silicofluorides ($Na_2SiF_6$ or $H_2SiF_6$)—are known to be highly toxic. Sodium fluoride, on the other hand, is the only source of fluoride that has been tested as safe. According to Myron J. Coplan, a chemical engineer and outspoken proponent of testing silicofluorides,

> Silicofluorides are highly toxic compounds whose addition to water supplies has never been tested for safety. The assumption on which their use was originally authorized (virtually complete dissociation after addition to water) has been contradicted by subsequent laboratory experiments. Epidemiological studies have associated communities using silicofluorides with increased uptake of lead from environmental sources (such as lead paint in old housing). And finally, controlling for other risk factors, there are higher rates of violent crime, substance abuse, and learning disabilities in communities where silicofluorides are added to water. Because all of these behaviors have been associated with lead neurotoxicity, silicofluoride enhanced lead uptake could be a factor in this association. In addition, however, silicofluoride-treated water has also been found to be a cholinesterase inhibitor and exposure to fluorinated silicic acid may contribute to protein-misfolding (either or both of which could contribute to adverse health or behavioral effects). On each of these four points, evidence is persuasive.[220]

Mr. Coplan bases his opinions on forty-five years of experience as a practicing scientist who has performed or supervised research under contract with dozens of U.S. government agencies and hundreds of commercial corporations. In the course of his consulting activities, he has had firsthand experience with silicofluoride, the agent used to fluoridate 91 percent of all fluoridated water in the United States.[221]

In his position paper titled "Toxicity of Silicofluoride Treated Water, Health, and Behavior," cowritten with Roger Masters, a research professor of government at Dartmouth College, Mr. Coplan points out that:

> Because sodium fluoride or naturally fluoridated water do not have the same effects as silicofluorides, fifty years of debates about "fluoridation" have been flawed. To a large degree, neither critics nor supporters have addressed

the chemical and biological characteristics of the specific compounds in use. Without prejudicing decisions on fluoridation with other chemicals, the facts summarized more than justify an immediate moratorium on the use of silicofluorides pending studies of their toxicity and effects on health and behavior.[222]

Silicofluorides are known to act as very strong competitive inhibitors for the enzyme *acetylcholinesterase*, which breaks down the neurotransmitter acetylcholine (ACh). ACh is necessary for muscle contraction; therefore, when breakdown of the neurotransmitter is prevented through the inhibition process, muscle spasms result.[223]

In 1977, the National Toxicology Program (NTP) was ordered by Congress to determine whether fluoride causes cancer. They found that rats given fluoridated water had a higher risk of *osteosarcoma*, a rare malignant bone cancer.[224]

According to the National Research Council's Subcommittee on Health Effects of Ingested Fluoride, 50 percent of the fluoride humans ingest accumulates in the body, primarily in the bone but also in the soft tissues.[225] High levels of accumulated fluoride cause a crippling skeletal disease known as *skeletal fluorosis*. This disease starts out mimicking symptoms of osteoarthritis, such as painful joints and bones; sensations of burning, pricking, and tingling in the limbs; muscle weakness; chronic fatigue; and gastrointestinal disorders. It can lead to calcification of ligaments and eventually osteoporosis of long bones.[226] The end stage of skeletal fluorosis is fusion of the skeletal bones.

This disease has reached epidemic proportions in China and India. The Chinese government now considers any water supply containing 1 ppm fluoride a risk for skeletal fluorosis. Here in the United States, the ADA considers a safe dose of fluoride in the drinking water as 0.7 to 1.2 ppm. Especially scary is that the National Institute of Arthritis and Musculoskeletal and Skin Diseases (NIAMS) reports that 21 million Americans suffer from osteoarthritis.[227] What we do not know is how many of these cases are misdiagnosed cases of skeletal fluorosis.

In 1995, a study published in the scientific journal *Neurotoxicology and Teratology* showed that fluoride accumulated in the brains of rats led to behavioral deficits typical of most neurotoxic agents.[228] The primary author of the study, Dr. Phyllis Mullenix, stated that "the rat study flagged potential for motor dysfunction, IQ deficits and/or learning disabilities in humans."[229] Studies in China have demonstrated decreased IQs in children exposed to high levels of fluoride.[230]

Finally, a British study published in the scientific journal *Caries Research* found high fluoride accumulation in human pineal glands.[231] This finding is significant since the pineal gland regulates many processes, including the production of serotonin and melatonin (chapter 5). The author of the study expressed concerns over the effects of accumulated fluorine on the regulation of puberty. This is especially alarming since the groups primarily targeted for fluoride supplementation through drinking water are children and adolescents.[232]

A final complication of fluoride on human health is its effects on the thyroid gland. Up until the 1950s, European doctors used fluoride to decrease thyroid activity in patients with a hyperactive gland.[233] The dose used to depress the thyroid (2.3 to 4.5 mg/day) is exceeded by the amount people routinely ingest on a daily basis from fluoridated water supplies (1.6 to 6.6 mg/day). This is a frightening thought as Synthroid, the drug used to treat hypothyroidism, was the third leading drug prescribed as late as 2003.[234] Many experts are concerned that fluoridated water may have a hand in the elevated numbers of Americans suffering from hypothyroidism.

With all the potential dangers inherent in water fluoridation, the only possible reason this practice persists today is that not enough people are aware of the facts. Couple this with the government's refusal to consider the current available research on the dangers of fluoridation and the ADA's support of the practice, and we can see why silicofluorides continue to be added to our drinking water.

In spite of all this, many experts publicly denounce the practice. In 2000, the National Treasury Employees Union at EPA Headquarters had voted to oppose fluoridation and called upon Congress to issue a "national moratorium" on the fifty-year-old policy.[235] In 2001, the Sierra Club also voiced its concerns:

> There are now valid concerns regarding the potential adverse impact of fluoridation on the environment, wildlife, and human health. The Sierra Club therefore supports giving communities the option of rejecting mandatory fluoridation of their water supplies. To protect sensitive populations, and because safer strategies and methods for preventing tooth decay are now available, we recommend that these safer alternatives be made available and promoted.[236]

At this time, more and more European countries are rejecting fluoridation of their drinking water.[237] In the United States, many voters are also rejecting fluoridation proposals. The Fluoride Action Network reports that since 1999, "51 communities in the U.S. have voted against fluoridation, while recent attempts to pass mandatory statewide fluoridation bills have failed in Hawaii, Oregon, Pennsylvania and Washington."[238] For a complete list of these communities and links to the news articles reporting on this phenomenon, please visit *www.fluoridealert.org/communities.htm*.

## How Can We Get Clean Drinking Water Anyway?

When we consider all the contaminants that infuse our drinking water today, is it any surprise that the bottled water industry has exploded, enjoying thirty-five billion dollars in sales worldwide? More than half of all Americans (54 percent) consume bottled water regularly, with 36 percent drinking it more than one time per week.[239] Sales in the United States have now topped nine billion dollars and are rising rapidly.[240] According to the Beverage Marketing Corporation, bottled water sales have been increasing at a rate of 9.1 percent per year.[241] That makes it the fastest growing beverage segment in the United States, second only to sodas as the most consumed beverage by volume.[242]

The quest for health has led Americans to consume bottled water at astonishing rates. Although most people poled in 2003 replied that health was the major reason for drinking bottled water, taste and convenience were also cited.[243] Is bottled water really safer than tap, though? The answer to that question may actually startle you.

The EPA regulates public tap water. Bottled water, on the other hand, is a packaged product and is therefore considered a food item: that means it is regulated by the Food and Drug Administration (FDA). The FDA has standards for bottled water that are as stringent as those set by the EPA's for tap water. However, as reported by National Resources Defense Counsel (NRDC) Senior Attorney Eric Olson in his 1999 report, the FDA has a "weak regulatory framework," which unfortunately "may allow careless or unscrupulous bottlers to market substandard products."[244]

What this means is that you do not always know how pure bottled water is. No law prohibits bottled water manufacturers from using a label with a picture of mountains or springs, regardless of the actual source of the water. Companies are therefore free to bottle tap water and market it with a label depicting some scene from nature. Seems misleading, right? Well, unfortunately, it's completely legal. There are rules, though, which require bottled water labels to disclose the origin of the water (spring or mineral), the manufacturer, and the volume. If the water is from a municipal source and not treated any further, the label must say From a Municipal Source or From a Community Water System.[245] Where this whole process starts to become convoluted is when a company takes regular tap water and treats it further; this can be something as minor as chlorinating the water, which is usually a pretty good sign that it is municipal tap water. Treated municipal water is not required to be labeled as such; therefore, companies can call their water "purified."

According to government and industry estimates, about 25 to 40 percent of all bottled water is actually bottled tap water.[246] Some cities have announced that they too will get into the bottled water business by selling their tap water without further treatment. And if those were not enough, the two largest beverage companies in the world, PepsiCo and Coca-Cola, have also entered the bottled water race with their brands Aquafina and Dasani respectively. "Aquafina reportedly is treated tap water taken from 11 different city and town water supplies across the nation," says the NRDC.[247] PepsiCo executives explain that anybody can find out the true source of Aquafina by calling the 800 number on the bottle top. Sure, just let me call the number on this bottle top while I take a break from reading the inserts my utility company has sent me—give me a break! With mountains pictured on the label, I should assume that it means I am drinking pure mountain spring water, right? But there you have it—bottled tap water from the makers of liquid sugar. Today, Aquafina is the number 1 branded noncarbonated bottled water in the country.[248]

So if 40 percent of bottled water is just tap water, how come it is so expensive? Industry experts disclose that 90 percent or more of the cost paid by consumers for bottled water go to things other than the actual water like bottling, packaging, shipping, marketing, retailing, and profit.[249]. And being tap water, bottled water from municipal sources may be contaminated with agents like fecal matter, bacteria, arsenic, and other carcinogenic chemicals. The NRDC did a four-year study to test bottled water safety and found 22 percent of brands tested chemicals at levels above strict state health limits. They concluded that "if consumed over a long period, some of these contaminants could cause cancer or other health problems."[250]

To be fair to many of the nation's largest bottled water companies, most bottled water did pass the safety standards set by the NRDC in their study. Consumers can find out the source of their bottled water by visiting the International Bottled Water Association (IBWA) at *http://www.bottledwater.org*. The IBWA is a trade organization that helps the FDA set safety standards on bottled water. Members of this organization must submit to an annual, unannounced inspection administered by an independent, internationally recognized third-party organization.[251] This inspection ensures that its members are bottling and selling safe water. Please visit their Web site to check on your local bottler, supplier, or distributor.

Making a decision about whether to buy bottled water comes down to a couple of key points. First, are we getting something more than just tap water, which we know often has unsafe levels of contaminants? The only way to know for sure is by checking the IBWA Web site for the participation of your local water companies. Also, checking the label to determine if the water has come from a municipal source is helpful; but as we have pointed out, the labels do not always tell the whole story. Even treated municipal tap water, like Aquafina, is better than tap water alone since it passes through additional filtration.

Second, how much are we paying for this water relative to what it is worth? If the average cost of tap water in California costs about one-tenth of one cent per gallon, then can paying ten thousand times more for bottled water at about $1.50 per half liter be justified? In my opinion, it can—provided I am getting more than just tap water. I have no problem paying more for spring or mineral water because these classes generally promise less contamination than your standard tap water with its old piping and outdated treatment systems. However, if the choice is between bottled municipal source water and water from the tap, why spend the extra money for the packaging? I would even buy treated tap water if I was in a pinch, but for that price, I would just as soon use a home filtration system and treat the tap water myself.

When reflecting on the options regarding drinking water in this country, I am of the opinion that the best, most cost-effective way to enjoy relatively clean water is by using a home filtration system. These systems come in many varieties; and finding the right one for you can, undoubtedly, be overwhelming. To help ease in this search, the National Science Foundation (NSF) International program is a third-party testing organization for home water-treatment systems. To be certified with NSF, a filtration system must pass rigorous testing. A complete listing of systems can be found on their Web site at *http://www.nsf.org.*

By having your own filtration system, you can receive relatively clean municipal water and treat it further, ensuring an even cleaner product. For approximately four hundred dollars, you can enjoy cleaner, safer water that won't cost you a fortune. On the other hand, if purchasing such a system is out of the question, then the bottled water option is fine, provided the company is listed with the IBWA.

When it comes to clean and safe drinking water, the real answer lies in keeping our sources free from contamination and pollution. By following the recommendations laid out by the NRDC, lawmakers and regulatory agencies can nip the problem in the bud right from its source. Until these recommendations become policy, though, we will all have to continue to play Russian roulette with our water. In the meantime, write your members of Congress, the FDA, the EPA, and your governor. Insist that they adopt strict requirements for bottled water safety and laws to prohibit and deter the pollution of our water sources. And please, stay informed—by staying abreast of the current legislation, particularly as it applies to water fluoridation, you will have a greater chance of having a say on these very important issues. If you feel that we are entitled to a choice in the matter, keep on top of things and leave these issues neither to government nor to chance—our health depends on it.

## Mercy, Mercy Me

"Oh, mercy, mercy me. Things ain't what they used to be. No, no." Marvin Gaye was not being prophetic when he sang these words in 1971. In fact, he was merely reflecting what was already happening to the ecology at that time. One unfortunate consequence of the industrialization of our modern world is that its waters and fish are showing the effects of pollution. Mercury from processing plants, mining operations, and garbage incinerators has been seeping into the waters of lakes, streams, and oceans for years.

Aquatic mercury in its most prevalent form is methylmercury. This organic form of mercury binds tightly to the proteins in fish tissue. Because it tends to accumulate, large predatory fish have higher concentrations of methylmercury since their diets are rich in fish that have also been exposed to mercury. The species with the highest concentrations of mercury are shark, swordfish, king mackerel, and tilefish.[252]

Mercury poisoning was first experienced en masse in Minamata, Japan, in the early 1950s.[253] The Chisso Corporation, a major plastics manufacturer, fueled the local economy at that time. In the process of producing acetylaldehyde for plastics, mercury was spilled into the bay and, over a twenty-year period, accumulated in the fish inhabiting it.

First, cats in the village were observed "dancing" and even collapsing and dying. Shortly thereafter, the people of the village started exhibiting strange behaviors. Stumbling, loss of motor control (inability to write or button their buttons), loss of hearing, and tremors were just some of the disorders they developed. Over one hundred of the inhabitants became ill, and twenty died. It took six years for investigators to discover the symptoms were due to heavy metal poisoning.

The Minamata tragedy was the first major episode of methylmercury poisoning of our times, and since then, we have learned much of its devastating effects. Mercury poisoning leads to neurological damage to both nursing mothers and children. Additionally, because of its tendency to accumulate, it can build up in women before they become pregnant and can later be passed across the placenta to the fetus. It is estimated that 630,000 children are born each year "at risk for lowered intelligence and learning problems caused by exposure to high levels of mercury in the womb" states the Environmental Protection Agency (EPA).[254]

Although most experts would agree that fish is an excellent dietary source of nutrients like essential fatty acids (EFAs), limiting one's intake of certain types of fish is a wise health practice due to possible contamination. Along with large predatory fish, tuna steaks and albacore also have suspect levels of methylmercury. The EPA and FDA both recommend no more than one serving (six ounces) of tuna or other large fish species per week for women of reproductive age or children. Because light canned tuna is made from a smaller fish, it is generally considered acceptable, but it should probably be consumed in moderate amounts as well. Most other fish species also have some degree of methylmercury contamination, but the concentrations are low enough for one to eat them up to two times per week (twelve ounces). Either way, it is prudent to be moderate in one's weekly fish consumption while enjoying fish regularly enough to reap its benefits.

Unfortunately, the latest EPA warnings regarding fish consumption have not been met with open arms, particularly by the U.S. Tuna Foundation (USTF). Understandably, government warnings have decreased tuna sales leading the foundation to accuse the government of unfair finger-pointing. The USTF has waged a campaign to raise the allowable mercury levels to be safe for consumption. It points to studies showing women and children in Japan whose diets are high in fish but have no more neurological disorders than those who eat no fish at all.[255] The tuna industry's concern over diminished sales are understandable, but instead of focusing on raising the allowable levels of mercury, it might behoove them to lobby for more stringent controls on air and water pollution instead as this seems to be the root cause of contamination.

Whatever the economic and political climate surrounding the issue, eating high-risk fish species in moderation will decrease health risks for women and children. This advice is especially important for people living in urban centers or suburbs where eating sushi has become very popular. Fish is enjoyable and one of the best sources of essential fatty acids available, but the risk of methylmercury poisoning is great enough to adhere to EPA and FDA recommendations.

## Air Pollution and Exercise

We all know that smog and air pollution is bad for our health; but do we know it on more than just an intellectual level, and are we actually taking precautions to minimize our risk? My friends and family used to chuckle at my idiosyncratic habit of closing the car window any time I would find myself pulled up alongside a garbage truck or bus. Although I was not aware of why I did this every time, something was intuitively telling me that the mushroom cloud of truck exhaust spewing from the big rig next to me—and which was about to come wafting into my car—was probably not very good for my health.

Air pollution is classified as two types: primary and secondary. Primary pollutants are formed directly from industrial sources, like factories and automobiles. These include carbon monoxide (CO), sulfur oxide, hydrocarbons, and ash. Secondary pollutants are formed when primary pollutants react with other natural substances, like air, to create toxins like ozone ($O_3$), aldehydes, and sulfates. Smog is a combination of both primary and secondary pollutants.

To get a better idea of how pollution acts as a toxin in the body, one must first understand the basics of respiratory physiology or how our respiratory system works. The lungs are the organs responsible for taking in oxygen ($O_2$) from the air and removing carbon dioxide ($CO_2$) from our bodies. This occurs through the breathing process (chapter 3). Inhalation is initiated by contraction of the diaphragm muscle. The process is directed by the autonomic nervous system (ANS) and is done outside our conscious control. As the diaphragm contracts, the thoracic cage expands and the lungs are allowed to fill with air through the process of negative pressure. Air enters the alveoli (little sacs) of the lungs and comes into contact with a vast supply of blood. Here, oxygen binds to hemoglobin, which is attached to our red blood cells. The oxygenated red blood cells then move to all the other tissues in the body including the brain, heart, and muscles. Oxygen is essential for the large energy production occurring in the tissues by using a process called *aerobic respiration*. While oxygen is deposited, $CO_2$ is picked up by the red blood cells and brought back to the lungs. $CO_2$ is moved from the deoxygenated blood in the lungs to the remaining air; the exchange of $O_2$ and $CO_2$ in the lungs happens simultaneously. Following this exchange, the diaphragm relaxes and allows the thoracic cage to contract, pushing the $CO_2$-rich air out; this is known as *exhalation*.

Respiration, then, like most physiological processes, is essential for life. Without oxygen, the brain and heart would not function nor would we produce energy or remove $CO_2$ from our tissues. $CO_2$ in high concentrations in the blood can lead to asphyxiation or suffocation and, eventually, death.

The ability of red blood cells to uptake oxygen is dependent on several factors, one being high $O_2$ concentrations in the alveoli of the lungs. The higher the $O_2$ concentration in the air, the higher its concentration will be in the lungs and thus the greater the amount, which will eventually be taken up by the red blood cells. Pollutants like CO and $CO_2$ compete with $O_2$ for binding sites on hemoglobin, leading to respiratory toxicity. It is therefore essential for the air we breathe to be as clean as possible, ensuring a high oxygen concentration as well as lowering toxic exposure.

What are the physiological consequences of breathing polluted air? Smog contains ozone, which can damage the lung tissue directly by causing inflammation and swelling. People with existing heart and/or lung dysfunction (asthma, emphysema, etc.) are especially at risk, although "healthy" people can be affected too. Other physiological effects are chest pain, cough, and shortness of breath. Air pollution is also believed to be a possible cause of cancer of the lungs.[256] A study done at Brigham Young University found that air pollution could decrease life expectancy by one to three years in some of the most polluted cities.[257]

Athletes who exercise outdoors may be at the highest risk of all. According to Dr. Henry Gong of University of California-Los Angeles (UCLA), outdoor exercisers may begin to suffer at an ozone level of 0.12 ppm, which is the federal health standard. To put this in perspective, health advisories are generally issued at 0.15 ppm and first stage smog alerts at 0.20 ppm. Outdoor exercise should therefore be avoided when the ozone levels begin to reach the federal health standard. Exercising outdoors during smoggy conditions poses a greater risk. As oxygen need increases during aerobic respiration, mouth breathing is initiated; and it brings an even greater volume of air into the lungs as well as anything else residing in it, including pollutants. During mouth breathing, the nasal passages are bypassed, and air cannot move through the natural filters present in the nasopharynx; the air can therefore not be cleaned before it is passed on to the blood via the lungs. As a result, a greater amount of pollutants are inhaled into the body.

Carbon monoxide (CO) is a pollutant formed primarily from car exhaust. It is also what is inhaled when smoking cigarettes. CO competes with $O_2$ for the binding sites on hemoglobin. Because CO is a much stronger binder to hemoglobin than $O_2$, it will prevent proper $O_2$ uptake and utilization by the body's tissues. This is one of the reasons why smokers may become hypoxic or oxygen deficient. It is also another reason to close the windows while sitting in heavy traffic.

With so many ill consequences to our health, what can one do to minimize the risk of air pollution? There are several solutions. First, minimize exposure to the outdoors, especially on days of health advisories or flat-out alerts. One can obtain the current air quality readings at the EPA Web site (http://airnow.gov). Exercise indoors, especially in air-conditioned environments as air conditioners generally filter out some pollutants. If one must exercise outdoors, one should do it early in the morning or later in the evening when pollution is generally at a lower level, and one should avoid exercising near congested roads and highways. Another precaution is to purchase a high-efficiency particulate air (HEPA) filtration unit. These units are reported to have a minimum particle-removal efficiency of 99.97 percent and remove particles as small as 0.3 microns in diameter (that's small!).[258] The American Lung Association recommends using HEPA filters to reduce indoor pollution while the federal government requires these filters to be available in government buildings in the event of an act of *bioterrorism* (release of microorganism like anthrax or tuberculosis). I personally prefer HEPA filters to ionizers as ionizing units can cause a buildup of ozone, which is itself a pollutant.[259] HEPA filters can be small and mobile, cleaning one room at a time; or they can be part of a central unit, cleaning an entire home or building. A final precaution is to keep the car windows closed, especially when sitting in traffic. And of course, quitting smoking will be a great way for you to reduce the effects of air pollution, both directly and indirectly.

## Cigars? Cigarettes?

So since we're on the subject of smoking, I think I should take the time to say a few words on this habit. I am not going to bore you with another why-smoking-is-bad-for-you lecture—we have all heard it before. There probably isn't an adult or teenager around who doesn't know the dreadful health consequences associated with smoking. Instead of going through all the dangers, then, I would like to take this time to add a bit of perspective on the smoking habit.

Why should you want to listen to what I have to say about smoking? Well, I happen to be a former pack-a-day smoker who finally kicked the habit after twenty years. That's right—twenty years! How did I do it? Why did I do it? I will explain, but first, let me tell you how I personally feel about smoking. I love it! Yes, you heard me right—I said I love it. Smoking was one of the most pleasurable activities I had ever engaged in. It was social. It tasted good. It went well with coffee, liquor, and soda. It was a good breakfast substitute. It made me drive better. It made me speak on the phone better. Heck, it even made me go to the bathroom better. You smokers and former smokers know exactly what I'm talking about. Smoking was fun, and it was my favorite pastime. Not a day goes by that I do not wish I could have a smoke. That is the positive stuff.

Even though I had all those positive experiences surrounding my smoking habit, I still chose to quit. I did so because I was able to attach enough negative aspects around smoking to *balance out* the positives. This is a very important process that one needs to undergo in order to succeed in quitting. Smoking is a habit, and one must attach as many negative consequences as positive ones to any habit if one wishes to break it. All habits are hard to break, but very few are as difficult as kicking the smoking habit. Nicotine is one of the most, if not the most, addictive substances known to man. Regular nicotine use causes physical addiction; that is, changes occur physiologically that the body gets used to. When the drug is removed—yes, nicotine is a drug—the body goes through physical stress. This stress alone makes quitting very difficult, but unfortunately, there is more.

Smoking, like most drug addictions, has a psychological component—mental dependence develops. I would even go so far as to say that there is a deep emotional dependence involved. Think about it: anyone who smokes regularly will tell you that his or her use increases under times of intense mental and/or emotional stress. Stressed out? Have a smoke. Sad? Have a smoke. Angry? Have a smoke. Happy? Have a smoke. Good sex? Have a smoke. And the appropriate occasions go on and on and on.

Smoking acts in the same way any addiction does—as a way to comfort, to forget, and to deal. Smoking becomes that best friend, the one that is there for us at all times. We develop an extreme attachment to our cigarettes. This is an unconditional love. Cigarettes do not care what we look like. They do not care what we smell like. They do not care if we have an attitude problem. Cigarettes are always there for us, 24/7. They are there whenever we want them, and we *always* want them. As a smoker, I could generally go up to an hour without a cigarette. However, if I was down to my last smoke, I had to have another one—*immediately*. If that is not an emotional dependence, then I do not know what is.

Quitting smoking will be one of the hardest things you ever do, and I do not profess to have any easy answers to this problem. There are a few things, though, that may help. First and foremost, if you do not smoke now, don't ever start. That is the absolute best way to avoid the pain and suffering associated with smoking and quitting. Here is a stark reality: if you have children and you smoke, be prepared for your children to smoke too. That's right—you are teaching them to do so. Do not even fool yourself into thinking that if you only tell them not to smoke, they will listen. Children learn by watching. True . . . Some children may listen, but do not bet on it. I smoked, my parents smoked, and my grandparents smoked. Let's just say it was a family tradition. As reported on CNN's Web site, children of smokers are two to three times more likely to smoke as teenagers than those raised by nonsmokers.[260] That alone should encourage you to quit.

But of course, the question remains: how does one quit such a highly addictive habit? The first step is to truly want to. I know that I'm oversimplifying this, but not really wanting to quit smoking is the absolute greatest obstacle to doing so. I have seen more people fail than I can remember because they were not in touch with this reality. Quitting for any other reason than absolutely wanting to quit is hopeless. One might succeed for a week, a month, or even a year; but one will start again—guaranteed. I speak from experience on this one. I quit for a year once because the girl I was dating hated it. I quit for her, not me! And as it happens so often, we broke up, and I got back together with my cigarettes. Good ol' nicotine, there for me through thick and thin. That's more than I could say for ol' what's her name.

How, then, does one convince oneself to quit? As I mentioned before, it is absolutely imperative to attach as many negatives to the habit as positives, at least as it relates to you (this is true of breaking any habit).[261] First, you have to write down all the positive aspects of smoking. I have mentioned several above, but we all have our own reasons why we *love* to smoke. Write them down. Then write down all the negative aspects. You might have to do some research here. You might need to read again all of the many ways in which regular smoking can destroy your health. You might want to look at some pictures of black lungs and cancers that are caused by smoking. Write these down. Write down how it endangers the health of your family through secondhand smoke and how it also might teach your children to smoke. Write those down. Write down how it not only decreases the length of life, but also how it eventually destroys the quality of life too. Write that down.

At this point, not only do you want to write down the negative aspects of smoking, but you should also write down the positive and negative aspects of *quitting*. This is very important. Don't think that there are no negative aspects to quitting—there are. For instance, you'll probably miss it. You might also lose that best friend—you know, the one that's been there for you through thick and thin. Of course, there will be negatives—write them down. Withdrawal is painful, and it surely isn't fun. Write that down too.

Then write down all the positive aspects associated with quitting. Let me tell you, there are many. You will smell better. You will have more energy. Your teeth will not be stained yellow. Your lung tissue will regenerate. Your circulation will improve. Your ability to breathe deeper and more fully will improve. Athletic performance and endurance will improve. Not an athlete? Try this one: your sex life will improve! That's right—increased circulation equals increased stimulation and, consequently, increased erection for both men and women. Essentially that is how compounds like sildenafil citrate (Viagra) work: they merely improve circulation. Quit smoking and your Viagra bill will go way down. What a plus!

After you have written down all the positives and negatives to smoking and to quitting, read them over and over again every day. I promise you, if you can attach as many negatives to smoking as positives and as many positives to the idea of quitting as negatives, then you will soon be very ready to quit. If after all this you still cannot find the reasons to quit, then you probably won't. It's as simple as that.

The next step is actually quitting. There are many organizations and programs dedicated to helping you. I strongly suggest you visit their Web sites and, at the very least, get their free literature. One site you can start with is the Centers for Disease Control and Prevention's Tobacco Information and Prevention Source (TIPS) at *http://www.cdc.gov/tobacco/how2quit.htm*. This type of research helped me enormously. You will find tips on behavior modification—things I found valuable, especially later on when I was a nonsmoker but still had strong cravings.

The first month is the hardest due to the physical dependence and the withdrawal symptoms, but it is merely a hump. Once you get over that hump, it becomes much easier. There are many products on the market that help make this stage a bit easier such as gums, patches, and medications meant to ease the physical symptoms associated with withdrawal. Products that continue to give you a form of nicotine and aid in weaning you off the drug generally increase the length of withdrawal, but some people prefer these methods. Cold turkey, on the other hand, is a tough road; the mountain is steep, but the trip is shorter. In other words, it is the most uncomfortable way to quit initially; but in my opinion, you get over the withdrawals the fastest.

There is another aid available that may assist you in quitting. It is an antidepressant drug called bupropion HCL (Wellbutrin and Zyban are the brand names) that has been used successfully by many, including myself, to overcome the physical discomforts associated with withdrawals. Obviously, not everyone will be able to use this drug since there are side effects that might be contraindicated for some. However, with the availability of these types of drugs, the physical discomforts of quitting smoking can be minimized, leaving you to deal only with the psychological component of your addiction. Therefore, not to sound like a broken record, but it is absolutely imperative to establish a complete and passionate desire to quit. Without that much, your efforts will likely go up in smoke.

## Party All the Time

Everybody loves a party, right? Bright lights, big city, fast women, hard liquor, coke, speed, ecstasy, and every other drug that may lend itself to a good time. These types of drugs are called *recreational drugs*. Some are legal, some are not.

There is nothing wrong with having a good time; in fact, our mental well-being depends on it. Some people like to have a good time with booze, others with substances classified as hard drugs. Is there really anything wrong with ingesting substances that help us feel good? On the surface, I would argue no. What is the occasional drink or smoke? Will it really harm one's health if one uses recreational substances once in a while? Well, let us investigate.

There are different classifications of drugs in the United States based on their medical use, level of abuse, level of dependency, and harmfulness.[262] Schedule 1 drugs have no recognized medical uses, have a high level of abuse, and have a high dependency rate. They are also known to be harmful to the user's safety.

They include drugs like heroin; lysergic acid diethylamide (LSD); methylenedioxy methamphetamine (MDMA), or ecstasy; marijuana; and methedrine (an early form of methamphetamine). By law, a citizen must not be in possession of these drugs at any time.

Schedule 2 drugs have some medical uses, a high potential for abuse, and a high rate of dependency. They also have a high rate of harmfulness to the user. These substances include opium, morphine, cocaine, methadone, and methamphetamine. A citizen may be under the influence of these drugs only if administered by a licensed physician. Ritalin, a drug used to treat ADHD in both children and adults, is classified as a Schedule 2 drug because of its high potential for abuse and dependency; and unlike other Schedule 2s, it can be obtained through a prescription.

Schedule 3 drugs have a definite medical use, a lower but still definite potential for abuse, and a moderate risk of dependency. These substances also have a high risk of harm to the user. They include amphetamines (especially diet pills), barbiturates, Valium, Xanax, codeine, and anabolic steroids. These drugs can only be obtained through a medical prescription.

Schedule 4 drugs have a high medical utility, a limited potential for abuse, and a limited risk of dependency. These drugs include sedatives (like chloral hydrate, a la Anna Nicole Smith), antianxiety pills (like meprobamate, which is similar to but less potent than barbiturates), depressants (like paraldehyde), and phenobarbital (a barbiturate). These drugs can also be obtained only by prescription.

Schedule 5 drugs are a mix of prescription and over-the-counter (OTC) medications and are typically preparations of the above drugs in limited amounts. Although medical and pharmaceutical representatives would never admit it, there is little doubt that these are some of the most abused drugs in our society.

Drugs that are used recreationally are generally Schedules 1 to 3. The more a drug is used recreationally, the higher up in class it goes. For instance, MDMA (ecstasy) was eventually classified as a Schedule 1 drug after its recreational use spread throughout college campuses, bars, and nightclubs. It received this classification in 1985 despite being also used by psychiatrists to successfully treat many of their patients.[263]

Like any drug, recreational ones have effects and side effects. Many of the direct effects can be harmful to the body. For example, cocaine can increase the heart rate so high that it can cause heart failure and death. Studies have shown that during the first hour after using cocaine, the risk of heart attack increases twenty-four times, even in subjects who never had any symptom of heart disease.[264] Heroin, a very powerful central nervous system depressant, can essentially cause the respiratory center of the brain stem to shut down the breathing process and cause death.[265] We have all heard of musicians and celebrities who have overdosed on both of these drugs while rock legend Jimi Hendrix overdosed on a combination of barbiturates and alcohol.

Most everybody knows the effects and dangers of recreational drugs, but there is a drug that is used widely in many societies and is equally as dangerous although the destruction and devastation it causes is slower and more insidious. The dangers lie in its social acceptance, which allows its negative effects to often be ignored. The drug we are talking about is alcohol.

Alcohol, liquor, or booze has strong roots in our country and culture. According to the National Institute on Alcohol Abuse and Alcoholism, 17.6 million Americans—nearly one in every ten adults—abuses alcohol or is an alcoholic.[266] Millions more engage in binge drinking, an activity that can easily lead to alcoholism. But what are the consequences of alcohol abuse to human health?

The physiological effects of alcohol are the most extensive of all the recreational drugs. It affects every system of the body, every tissue, and every organ; and ultimately, it affects every cell. It is a slow form of poisoning that breaks down the strength and resilience that is usually inherent in all of us. Some of the damages it causes are

- increased risk of cancer of the liver, esophagus, throat, and larynx;
- cirrhosis of the liver;
- peptic ulcers;
- hypertension;
- decreased immune function;
- peripheral neuropathies; and
- brain damage.

In men, it can also cause hormonal dysfunction leading to testicular atrophy, gynecomastia (development of breasts), and impotence. Because it is a depressant, it can also lead to depression and anxiety disorders.[267] This substance is so toxic that it can cross the placenta during pregnancy and harm the fetus. These are the direct physical consequences of alcohol abuse, and they do not even include the indirect dangers to health such as automobile accidents and violence, which so often accompany heavy drinking.

It is not the goal of this book to make a plea for social change with regard to the use of drugs and alcohol. I merely wish to point out that these substances directly impact one's health. If the use of drugs and alcohol becomes a consistent habit, then one should expect one's health to decline accordingly. For the most part, drug and alcohol abuse are a way to render its users numb to the emotional pains that we all must feel and overcome at some point in our lives (chapter 6). When we anesthetize ourselves with substances, we prevent our emotional growth—replaying the same dysfunctional experiences over and over, leading to an even greater need to sedate ourselves. It becomes a vicious cycle of depression and dependence with seemingly no way out. The reality is that there is a way out. Many people have successfully overcome their addictions, and most would admit that not only have their lives improved in every sense, but so has their health.

Recreational drugs take a heavy toll on the body and the health. They prematurely age their user visibly, causing bags and wrinkles, as well as invisibly damaging the internal organs like the brain. Studies show that alcoholics lose a greater amount of brain tissue than nonalcoholics do.[268] The damage to the heart and blood vessels caused by cocaine is also well documented. Interestingly, heroin in its pure form is not toxic to the body, and it does not appear to damage the tissues and organs.[269] On the other hand, street heroin is usually mixed with various impurities (called being "stepped on"), which are often so highly toxic that they lead to heart damage, hepatitis, abscesses, tetanus, pneumonia, and bronchial infections. Most ominous, though, is that heroin is highly addictive. It consumes the addict's every thought and action, making it very difficult to stop using. When a user does stop, withdrawal symptoms are severe; and include diarrhea, convulsions, cramps, and depression.

The bottom line is this: drugs and booze can kill. They can either kill you quickly through an overdose or slowly by poisoning your tissues and organs. Either way, it ain't pretty.

## Our Real Drug Problem

As damaging as regular recreational drug use can be, there is an even greater drug problem in our society that has yet to be adequately addressed: the overuse and abuse of prescription and over-the-counter (OTC) medications. In 1997, research showed that 49 percent of American adults were taking some form of prescription drugs while 30 percent were regularly taking OTC medications.[270] Spending for prescription drugs is now one of the fastest-growing components of the national health expenditure.[271] These numbers are even more alarming when we consider the fact that drug spending has increased by a shocking 17 percent per year.[272] What is the current obsession with prescription and OTC drugs, and why do Americans seem so hooked on them? The answers may surprise you.

The use of medicine during the nineteenth century was neither scientific nor effective, let alone safe. During that period, medicines were a blend of tinctures, soups, and teas made up of herbal extracts and animal products such as bone and fat as well as various minerals, mercury being the most popular.[273] Most medicines were highly toxic and often killed those they were meant to help. In other words, things were not that much different than they are today.

During the nineteenth century, the microbial theory of disease was the most prevalent of the day. Practicing good hygiene had not yet taken hold; and many people were thus exposed to an inordinate amount of dangerous pathogens, including those that caused typhoid fever, botulism, and small pox. Needless to say, many people died as a result of being infected by germs. As Western science developed a more thorough understanding of microbes, chemical and pharmaceutical technology flourished. By the end of the nineteenth century, the first two "legitimate" medications were synthesized—antipyrine and aspirin. The creation of these drugs led us into what is now known as the Pharmaceutical Century.

There is no doubt that the development of medicines, especially antibiotics and antitoxins (antibodies isolated from treated animals against microorganisms and their toxins), saved many lives during the early years of the Pharmaceutical Century. As the success of pharmaceuticals continued to grow, so did society's confidence in their effectiveness. With the advent of vaccines in 1885, the public had further reason to hail pharmaceuticals as miracles.

During the twentieth century, further advances were made toward understanding the human body and its various systems (cardiac, pulmonary, digestive, etc.). This new comprehension led to a greater opportunity to develop drugs that could intervene in what were considered abnormal physiological processes, including blood clotting, vascular and bronchial constriction, and even erectile dysfunction. Prosthetic manufacturing became so advanced that prosthetics were almost as good as, if not better than, the actual body parts they replaced. With all these new discoveries, it certainly started to appear as if all physiological processes could be manipulated by man to his advantage.

Modern medicine's early successes made it easy for society to develop a false sense of security in taking prescription and OTC medications. Pharmaceuticals, so far, had shown great promise in curing man of all his health woes; and it further promised to return him to his rightful state of well-being. It appeared as if man could eat, drink, or smoke anything he wished because he took for granted that a magic bullet would be waiting for him, which could alleviate all his ensuing health problems.[274] And wasn't health at that time seen only as an absence of symptoms, anyway?

Unfortunately, no one counted on the fact that synthetic drugs could also act as poisons when taken in large quantities or when taken consistently over an extended period. Prescription drug dependence has become a very real calamity in this country, and it has taken its toll on human health in the form of addictions, organ toxicity, and overdoses. A 1998 report featured in the Journal of the American Medical Association (JAMA) showed that during a twenty-year stretch, adverse drug reactions were between the fourth and sixth leading causes of death in the United States.[275] That puts prescription drugs just behind heart disease, cancer, and stroke as the leading killers of Americans every year. The reasons for this tragic reality are many, including overprescribing, heavy marketing by the pharmaceutical industry (Big Pharma), and the public's misperception of prescription drugs—their uses, side effects, and dangers.

More than 50 million unnecessary antibiotic prescriptions are written for patients outside of a hospital setting each year in the U.S. alone.[276] Additionally, the Centers of Disease Control and Prevention (CDC) estimates that 40 percent of all antibiotics that doctors prescribe are for viral infections, despite the fact that these drugs are only effective against bacterial infections. Since antibiotics are useless against viruses, why do doctors continue to prescribe them so readily? One reason, doctors say, is that patients demand them. Presumably, patients do so in order to feel that *something* is actually being done for them. Another reason for overprescribing has to do with time pressures on physicians. It is no secret that medical doctors are overworked, and it is much quicker—and easier—to prescribe a medication first and then see how a patient responds to it than to spend an inordinate amount of time searching for a specific diagnosis. In medical circles, this practice is known as *diagnosis by treatment*. A final reason for overprescribing is simply diagnostic uncertainty. This is when a doctor is unsure of the cause of illness and prescribes a medication in the hopes that it will help the patient. This is also a form of diagnosis by treatment.

The overprescribing of medications not only perpetuates society's dependence on drugs but also creates another and even more harrowing problem—antibiotic-resistant bacteria. Bacteria that are exposed to antibiotics, but not completely killed off, can mutate and develop resistance. Antibiotic resistance is not a new phenomenon—it was recognized as early as 1947 when penicillin was first introduced to the public.[277] Overprescribing of antibiotics, then, is helping to create new strains of "superbacteria," which have developed resistance to many antibiotic drugs designed to kill them. Particularly alarming is the fact that many strains of drug-resistant *Staphylococcus aureus* are now contaminating hospital settings. Some have become resistant to all useful antibiotics, including vancomycin, which is the major weapon used against resistant bacteria. It isn't hard to see what the outcome will be if one is infected by a vancomycin-resistant strain of *S. aureus* (VRSA). Fortunately, only eight cases have been reported in the United States at this time; but at the current rate of development, even this strain may find its way out of containment. To illustrate how very real the threat of resistant bacteria is to public health, a recent outbreak of methicillin-resistant *S. aureus* (MRSA) has found its way into the training facilities of several teams of the National Football League (NFL). It has also been found in many private health clubs, infecting thousands of people and bringing this once-contained danger into the public sector.[278]

The overuse of prescription drugs in the United States is also attributable to the massive marketing conducted by Big Pharma. Marketing directly to consumers (DTC advertising) was virtually nonexistent up until the early 1990's but has since become big business netting over two billion in advertising dollars.[279] DTC advertising is illegal in almost every country in the world except the United States where consumers of prescription drugs spent $162 billion in 2002—and that number is growing at a rate of 14.5 percent annually.[280] Today, we are flooded with television, radio, and print advertisements touting the benefits of the latest drugs. DTC advertising has worked so well that the National Institute for Health Care Management (NIHCM) has reported that the top twenty-five selling medications have led the majority of the increase (40.7 percent) in retail sales for pharmaceuticals.[281]

Several problems are inherent in DTC advertising. To begin with, some critics point out that this type of marketing leads to patients demanding prescriptions even if they do not need them. Meredith Rosenthal, PhD, of the Harvard School of Public Health wrote in the *New England Journal of Medicine* that "71 percent of family physicians believe that direct-to-consumer advertising pressures physicians into prescribing drugs that they would not ordinarily prescribe."[282] Case in point: health officials in San Francisco report that young gay men are taking Viagra in combination with illegal drugs to enhance their sexual experiences.[283] These young men, who by all accounts probably do not *need* Viagra, are getting their prescriptions from somewhere. This is the power of DTC advertising. Prescription drug abuse, however, is not solely relegated to the gay community; in college campuses across the country, students partake in an activity called "pharming," whereby they swallow pharmaceuticals down with ice-cold beer or a cocktail chaser.[284] Whether these drugs are obtained directly from a doctor or illegally on the Internet, it is the effectiveness of DTC advertising that has placed them into the public's consciousness.

Another problem with DTC advertising is that it promulgates medication as the primary, if not the sole, answer to all of man's health woes. Why this is so dangerous is that people, as a result of this intensive advertising, turn to medications even when a nondrug solution may actually be more appropriate, like adopting better lifestyle habits. When one has trouble sleeping, for example, is it really because one needs medication, or is it better to investigate one's lifestyle instead? By advertising sleep aids so excessively, it merely encourages people to look for the quick fix and not the real solution.

DTC advertising is used so heavily in the United States for one simple reason: it works! Prescription drug advertising has definite effects—it creates a positive public perception of pharmaceuticals. As a result of this hype, there comes a greater reliance on drugs as a panacea, or magic bullet, even to the point of believing that we need drugs to improve our otherwise normal functions like sleep, digestion, or sex. And even if there is nothing wrong with us, we may be convinced there is just because it was suggested in a commercial. Medical physician, biologist, and author Lewis Thomas addresses this eloquently in his book *The Medusa and the Snail*,

> We are, in real life, a reasonably healthy people. Far from being ineptly put together, we are amazingly tough, durable organisms, full of health, ready for most contingencies. The new danger to our well-being, if we continue to listen to all the talk, is in becoming a nation of healthy hypochondriacs, living gingerly, worrying ourselves half to death.[285]

Yet another problem with DTC advertising is that it can often lead to misleading information. DTC advertising just does not allow objectivity as manufacturers have a vested interest in showing their product in the best overall light without regard to impartiality.

Although one can see how overprescribing by physicians and DTC marketing has increased pharmaceutical drug use to epidemic proportions, we can hardly blame these two sources alone. The bigger problem lies in our own perceptions regarding prescription drugs. Due to our obsession with magic bullets, as well as our glorification of pharmaceutical's past successes, we have simply placed pharmaceutical drugs on a pedestal. It is no surprise, then, that pharmaceuticals are now the fastest-growing class of abused drugs in the country. More than 8.2 million people, or 4 percent of the U.S. population, have used prescription drugs for nonmedical purposes in the past year.[286] The most popular drugs seem to be narcotics (Vicodin, Percocet, OxyContin), tranquilizers (Xanax, Valium), stimulants (Alderral, Ritalin), and sedatives (Soma).

For some of these drugs, like Ritalin, abuse has reached epidemic proportions. The Drug Enforcement Agency (DEA) lists Ritalin as one of the top ten most stolen drugs in the country.[287] The frightening thing is that it isn't just adults who are abusing these meds, children as young as twelve years old are becoming regular users. As much as 2.5 percent of eighth graders abuse Ritalin while 3.4

percent of tenth graders and 5.1 percent of twelfth graders do too.[288] Students are turning to Ritalin more and more to help them stay awake and study. Research shows that Ritalin use doubles the chance a child will turn to future substance abuse like smoking, cocaine, or other stimulants.[289]

Until people recognize the multitude of dangers involved in the indiscriminate use of prescription medications, overuse (and abuse) will likely continue. Unfortunately, many people mistakenly believe that because a physician prescribes these drugs, they must be safe. However, nothing could be further from the truth. All medications have side effects, and they can even be toxic at very high doses or when taken for extended periods of time. As sixteenth-century alchemist Paracelsus once said, "All things are poison and not without poison—only the *dose* makes a thing not a poison."

In other words, all medicines are toxins to some degree; the only thing separating the two is the amount one takes. To get a better idea of the toxic nature of pharmaceuticals, please see Appendix at the end of the book for a list of side effects accompanying some of the more popular pharmaceuticals on the market.

# Chapter 7 Summary

## Key Number 6: Toxin Avoidance

- Eat organically grown fruits and vegetables.
- Eat hormone-free meats, fish, and dairy as much as possible.
- Limit processed food intake.
- Wash all fruits and vegetables thoroughly.
- Check the quality of your source water (check EPA or U.S. geological Web sites).
- Check to see if your favorite bottled water brand is truly spring water (check IBWA Web site).
- Buy a water purifier for your home (check quality at http://www.nsf.org).
- Keep up with the latest information on water fluoridation. Write your Congress representative. Vote on fluoridation measures.
- Limit fish intake to two servings per week.
- If pregnant, limit fish intake to one serving per week.
- Exercise indoors on smoggy days.
- Wash your hands thoroughly after working out at the gym.
- Buy an air purifier and run it regularly (HEPA is best).
- If you are thinking about quitting smoking, quit.
- Moderate your alcohol consumption.
- Limit recreational drug use or quit altogether.
- Discuss alternatives to prescription medications with your doctor.
- Question the rationale behind every medication recommended to you.

# CHAPTER 8

# Integration: Creating Synergy with the Six Keys

*A person who has a cat by the tail knows a whole lot more about cats than someone who has just read about them.*

—Mark Twain

*Knowing is not enough, we must apply. Willing is not enough, we must do.*

—Johann Wolfgang von Goethe

## Why Choose Health?

W E HAVE JUST spent a great deal of time discussing the six key areas that, if focused on regularly, can dramatically increase our health and well-being. Having so much to attend to in our daily lives, why should health consume such a significant portion of our time and energy? The truth is that for many people, it just doesn't. Many of us, especially if relatively young and healthy, simply take our health for granted. In this final chapter, we will discuss why striving for optimal health is such a worthwhile endeavor; we will show you how to maximize your results by integrating each key one by one and how by doing so, every aspect of your life will improve as well.

So why should we focus on health, anyway? What difference will it make in the long run? The truth is that without our health, we have very little. Think about it for a moment: how can we enjoy any of our material possessions, our professional accomplishments, or our creative endeavors without one of our greatest assets, our health and well-being? Ask anyone who suffers from illness or injury what he desires most, and with very few exceptions, he will respond that he wishes a return to good health. Baseball legend Mickey Mantle expressed this sentiment exactly while lying on his deathbed. Racked by cirrhosis of the liver and hepatitis C following years of chronic alcohol abuse, he was asked whether he wished he had done things differently in his life. Expressing regret for some of his lifestyle choices, he said he would indeed do things differently if he could do it all over again. Why? Because a life of neglected health is essentially a life of unrealized potential.

The reasons to strive for health seem fairly obvious since it gives us many of the personal advantages that we have discussed throughout this book; yet there are many other, albeit less apparent, reasons for doing so. To begin with, our health affects not only ourselves, but everyone and everything around us. We are not isolated beings. Remember that all things in the universe are energy (chapter 6). When we operate at our highest potential, our vibrational patterns change, and this has an effect on the way we interact with all the other energetic forms around us.

This fact is most evident in our daily experiences as well as in our personal relationships. When we do not feel well, it is much harder to handle stressful situations, to express tolerance, or to even express love toward other people. And when one is ill for an extended period, it often takes all of one's energy just to make it through the day. Physiologically speaking, this is because our bodies have to work overtime to maintain balance. Balance in the body is called *homeostasis*, and as a living organism, the body does everything it can to maintain this balance. The property of homeostasis is the greatest mechanism a complex living system has to ensure its survival. When we are ill and all of our faculties are working overtime to regain balance, we have much less energy to carry out our daily functions, let alone be conscious of our actions or express tolerance toward other people. We have all experienced illness at one time or another, and we can therefore appreciate how hard it is to maintain awareness of our responsibilities or to have peaceful, courteous interactions with the world around us when we are not feeling well.

Most people feel that there are conditions in the world that need changing. Whether we are consciously aware of it or not, we all have a sense that everything in the universe must evolve (law of evolution found in chapter 6). People, however, often desire change in the world without realizing that changes must occur within themselves first, the only area over which they truly have power. Only by focusing on those areas over which we have power can we ever hope to create change in a world where so many things fall outside of our immediate control.

Within our personal life, then, are numerous areas where we can exert our control—in our financial practices, in our social life, in our spirituality, in our acquisition of knowledge (learning), in our professional and creative pursuits, and in our family life. But none is more basic or more encompassing than our physical health. True, each one of these areas has profound and direct effects on all the others, but none more so than our health and well-being. Failing to care for one's physical body will lead to its inevitable breakdown and will ultimately hinder all of one's other endeavors. Worse yet, when debilitation results, it usually requires a majority of one's time and energy just to function in any capacity whatsoever. In my opinion, it is just too high a price to pay for neglect, especially when this consequence can be completely avoided by practicing the six keys to optimal health.

When we focus on our physical health, the changes we create as a result have the possibility of improving our lives so immensely that it will be impossible for these changes not to extend well beyond our immediate circle. President John F. Kennedy understood and reflected this sentiment when he said, "Physical fitness is the basis for all other forms of excellence." We cannot hope to be productive, conscientious, or even ecologically aware if we cannot take care of ourselves first. This is a fundamental principle, yet so many people have lost touch with it. Don't get me wrong, it is extremely important and, indeed, highly admirable to work toward creating change in the world—whether it be of a political, ecological, or humanitarian nature. However, how can we affect change in the outside world if we can't even change ourselves?

We can control our immediate environment—our bodies, our homes, our families, and our communities—and there is not a more powerful way to do so than through healthy living. In fact, we cannot ever wish to have an impact on our surroundings if we do not first seek health. If, through our pursuits, we act as a living example for our loved ones, then they too will benefit directly and be encouraged to emulate us. The Buddhist monk Thich Nhat Hanh, in his famous letter to his colleagues during the Vietnam War, so eloquently expressed this concept of living to affect our immediate surroundings,

> We talk about social service, service to the people, service to humanity, service for others who are far away, helping to bring peace to the world—but often we forget that it is the very people around us that we must live for first of all. If you cannot serve your wife or your husband or child or parent—how are you going to serve society?[290]

Because our experiences reflect our perceptions (chapter 6), when we improve our internal environment, we cannot help but have an improved outlook on the world. We have discussed that a healthy mind is essential to a healthy body, but it works the other way as well—healthy body, healthy mind! When the frequency of our vibration changes as a result of our attention to wellness, then through the principle of resonance, our experiences will change too.

This is such a powerful phenomenon that we must remember to embrace it. When we see the world through the eyes of great health, we develop a greater appreciation for every thing around us. All things exist interdependently: the planet provides us with the air we breathe, the food we eat, and the water that nourishes every cell of our body. Equally important is that every human being provides a function to maintain life on this planet. Farmers, lawyers, doctors, and civil servants all have a vital function in society as well as in the continuation of life itself. This includes you! Your contribution to the world is absolutely essential. Regardless of what you do for a living, you provide an important service to humanity. For this reason, it is important that we all care for ourselves to the best of our abilities. When we do, our contributions to the world will be that much greater than if we simply allow ourselves to deteriorate physically.

The most significant legacy we can leave to the world is to adopt values that enhance optimal health and well-being and pass them on to future generations. What we teach our children today will have such wide-reaching consequences tomorrow that we must not minimize the importance of these vital concepts. Our generation can leave its greatest mark on the future by instilling in our children the desire to achieve optimal health as well as to provide them with the necessary tools to do so. Do not take this responsibility lightly. It is up to us, today's free-thinking society, to pass on the principles of health to future generations. In this way, we can truly make our mark on posterity.

## Health and Evolution: Who Will Survive?

In chapter 6, we discussed the law of evolution at length. According to this law, all things change in order to develop and expand. In biology, the theory of evolution explains that

> Groups of organisms change with the passage of time, mainly as a result of natural selection, so that descendants differ morphologically and physiologically from their ancestors.[291]

In layman's terms, *morphologically* means "in appearance" and *physiologically* means "with regard to function." Natural selection is the concept that

> only the organisms best adapted to their environment tend to survive and transmit their genetic characters in increasing numbers to succeeding generations while those less adapted tend to be eliminated.[292]

Even in the most basic definition of the term, then, *evolution* means that some type of change must take place. With regard to the scientific theory, it explains this change in purely genetic terms; and indeed, with regard to simpler organisms (bacteria, fruit flies, or algae), this is the only change necessary for evolution to occur. However, in more complex systems (human beings, societies, nations, or the planet), changes can be genetic, behavioral, or, conceivably, can even relate to human consciousness.

How does this concern our discussion here? Since this is a book on health, it will be valuable to investigate the evolutionary process as it relates to health. From this analysis, we may attempt to evaluate how our future might then be affected.

But first, it will be useful for us to discuss a few important facts. Throughout history, man has had to contend with famine, war, natural disasters, and, of course, disease. Each one of these has served to act as a natural form of population control and, therefore, as a catalyst to the evolutionary process itself. For each new and successive challenge, man has been forced to use his ingenuity to overcome any and all obstacles before him. If unable to manipulate his external environment, then he would have to adapt physiologically. In this way, man has been able to withstand the pressures of living on this planet and, as a result, to continue his existence. This is how the amazing process of natural selection works in its most apparent and practical application.

Just as man has had to adapt to his environment to ensure his survival, so has the multitude of other organisms inhabiting the planet along with him. Animals, plants, and insects have all gone through their own evolutionary processes as have microorganisms like bacteria and viruses. Even these organisms, which are typically associated with human disease and death, must change and adapt in order to survive.

But we must ask ourselves: are the organisms that cause human illness actually a threat to our existence, or are they simply different life-forms with which we must learn to coexist? Obviously, we can be as much a nuisance to bacterial and viral microorganisms as they can be to us. Since they usually do not possess the machinery to exist and multiply on their own, microorganisms need a host organism (human, animal, insect, or plant) in which to dwell. When that host actually ends up attacking the microorganisms, these life-forms must also adapt to their environment or risk being killed off. Both bacteria and viruses adapt by mutating, which makes them better able to evade detection. This is vital as their surroundings may suddenly become saturated with a poisonous antibiotic or perhaps even get invaded by dangerous (to them) white blood cells. Very often, these organisms are placed under the most extreme and stressful conditions. At these times, they will respond by multiplying rapidly in a final attempt to survive and often kill off their host in the process.

So on an evolutionary level, viral and bacterial organisms have actually been paramount to human existence. Without them, the human immune system would have had very little stimulus to elicit its own development, perhaps even weakening the human species as a whole. We simply cannot disregard these life-forms when contemplating our own evolution. They have been vital in helping us develop into the living beings we are today (as well as being our oldest ancestors, but that is another story entirely).

Interestingly, humans have been playing a game of cat and mouse with microorganism for decades, all in a futile attempt to eradicate them from the planet. Our efforts, however, have not only failed to remove them completely from our lives, but have even led to the creation of superspecies that have successfully adapted to our weaponry (chapter 7). Even as we have succeeded in ridding ourselves of diseases like polio and smallpox, new forms of microorganisms have surfaced to take their place. The SARS-associated coronavirus (SARS) and the avian influenza (bird flu) viruses are two current examples; they are some of the newest microorganisms to threaten human health. Human influenza virus is yet another—this virus is itself a rapidly mutating pathogen, and as such, we have been unable to effectively control it. As a result, a new flu vaccine must be developed and administered every year to fight new strains.

The importance of these examples is to illustrate a very fundamental principle of human health. The virulence (strength) of an organism is not the only factor involved in our response to infection—that is, whether or not we'll get sick or what our chance of survival are if we do. In fact, virulence may not even be the primary factor involved in illness at all. It is becoming more and more evident that the environment in which the organism lives is what plays the greatest role in determining the outcome. Healthy individuals (those with strong and well-functioning immune systems) have the greatest ability to ward off illness and, in the process, become even stronger with each successive exposure as coming into contact with virulent microorganisms serves to strengthen their immunity.

We can see examples of this with every infection known to man. Take HIV for instance; when homosexual men first started showing signs of infection in the latter part of the 1970s, the initial prognosis was of a sure and swift death. We now know, however, that it is possible to live for many years, and even thrive, despite being infected with the HIV virus. Yes, it's true that people still die from AIDS; nonetheless, we can all glean a glimmer of hope from people like Ervin "Magic" Johnson who conducts his life in a healthy and productive manner even in the face of being HIV positive. Magic Johnson and others like him not only serve as inspirations to anyone diagnosed with HIV, but also remind us that our current views on health may no longer be adequate—in other words, we may be in need of a new model.

Essentially, the message I would like to get across here is that as long as human beings inhabit the earth, there will be organisms that we must contend with; organisms that may compromise our health and even cause death in epidemic proportions. It would probably be wiser to strengthen our immune system or the environment in which these microorganisms must dwell than to solely rely on outside interventions to combat what are otherwise worthy life-forms. By adopting the practices outlined in this book, you will do more to ensure your survival and, subsequently, to pass forth your genes than by doing nothing at all and leaving your health to chance.

We would be better served to appreciate all life-forms inhabiting our earth as not only worthy of their existence, but also as vital contributors to the evolution of this planet and, indeed, of life itself. The energetic configurations that form microorganisms clearly serve many vital functions. They act as decomposers of other energy forms (for example, organic materials found in nature as well as food in our digestive tracts), producers of vital gasses and other biologically active substances, transporters of genes among different species, and, yes, even as a form of population control. Why, then, should we attempt to eliminate organisms that have such a high degree of functionality?

It does not make sense for us to attempt to eradicate any other life-form as we cannot be sure with our limited knowledge what their functions might be. It seems logical, then, to accept all living forms as our cohabitants on this earth. Of course, we must always remain on guard as it would be foolish to allow an overgrowth of microorganisms to compromise our resources or our health. However, despite a certain amount of individual risk, our species can certainly exist symbiotically with all other life-forms. In fact, it appears that we even need them to continue our own physical evolution. It would seem much more practical to focus our attentions on health-enhancing behaviors, those that enhance and revitalize our own energy, than to focus on eradicating microorganisms.

The stark reality is that we have to learn to live with many different species, some that have yet to be discovered and perhaps even some that have not yet evolved. Some new species will likely be created by our own elaborate endeavors, particularly genetic engineering and the rampant misuse of antibiotics (chapter 7). Please understand, though, that I do not deny the necessity to monitor the dynamics of human-microbe interactions—it is essential. However, by practicing healthy habits, we stand the greatest chance of living symbiotically with all other life-forms, which is crucial, as we should not allow them the opportunity to eradicate us either.

Along with ever-evolving microorganisms, we will also have to deal with our fair share of natural disasters in the future—like Hurricane Katrina, which devastated New Orleans in the autumn of 2005. What stood out the most for me from this tragedy was the overwhelmingly large number of sick and infirm people who were incapable of withdrawing from the city. Even though this scenario is a harsh reality of any type of emergency evacuation, I cannot help but feel that as a population, we *can* consciously change the number of people needing ambulatory assistance. Let me repeat a statistic that we mentioned back in chapter 1:

> Approximately 50 percent of *all* deaths in this country are due to faulty lifestyle choices (smoking, drinking, poor diet, etc.).

If we could reduce this number by even 10 percent, disasters like Katrina might claim a few less lives.

Not only that, but in today's political environment where the threat of terrorism and war looms constantly overhead, we will likely see the earth's natural resources—particularly freshwater—become even scarcer commodities. We cannot be sure of where the human evolutionary path might lead us, so doesn't it seem wise to prepare ourselves physically for any scenario that might eventually surface?

The best preparation would be to adopt the healthy, life-enhancing habits we have been discussing in this book. The six key principles we have outlined are the only things you need to strengthen and boost your body completely. With optimal health, you will not only have a greater chance of surviving a major catastrophe if one happens, but more importantly, you will find that great health gives you a large degree of personal fulfillment and enhances your life significantly.

One final point I would like to make before moving on is if we wish to keep our views on health in proper perspective, as well as the ways in which health serves us, then we must acknowledge a plain and simple fact that we are mortal beings! Although everyone is aware of the inevitability of death, many of us tend to see death as "bad" or undesirable. Death, however, is as important to life as life itself. Without it, we would not be able to support new life, human or other, as our vital resources would become exhausted from the uncontrolled growth in populations. The truth is that to defy death, we would have to defy the laws of the universe—particularly those that relate to the movement of energy, polarity, and rhythm, and, in fact, the law of evolution itself.

Remember that the first law of thermodynamics states that energy can be neither created nor destroyed; it can only change forms. Further, according to the law of polarity, one thing cannot exist without its exact opposite. Birth and death, then, represent the two poles of one type of energetic formation: our physical bodies. We cannot escape this fundamental progression. As energetic life-forms, we must naturally submit to these universal forces. Birth, life, and death occur together as one single process; they are, shall we say, inseparable. As this process unfolds, it does so in a very distinct rhythmic pattern—seventy to ninety years in the human perception of time—yet nothing more than a brief moment, a spark, in the grander scale of the infinite universe.

We must accept death, then, as a natural process. Although the physical body seems to appear and then disappear rapidly in a short wisp of time, we can rest assured that our energy remains in the universe forever. Major religions call this immortality. Yes, we are mortal beings, dependent on the physical laws of our physical world; however, we are immortal too—that is, immortal in spirit. So embrace it; don't fear death. Living your life in fear is not living at all. Not only will fearing death prevent you from experiencing all the richness life has to offer, but it will also lead you to make poor decisions with regard to your health and well-being.

## Prepare Yourself: The Paradigm Shift

By having a deeper understanding of the evolutionary process that governs all life and by acknowledging the inevitability and—perhaps even more importantly—the necessity of death, it will be easier for us to develop an appreciation for new and more useful ways in which to approach our health. The prevailing view among modern and, of course, predominantly Western societies is that health is but a fleeting asset. We believe that health depends heavily on genetics, socioeconomic status, and the quality of medical care. However, there is much more to the story than that.

It has been my goal with this book to expose the many weaknesses inherent in the current yet outdated health paradigm. Our existing views have, without a doubt, been useful; but now is the time to move forward—to progress or, shall we say, evolve to the next level of understanding. No longer is it adequate for us to wait and fall ill before we invest time and attention to our health. That is the *old* way.

The new paradigm for health is that of a life of *wellness*. This concept is much broader than what we use today and definitely serves us more completely and in a more fulfilling way. Wellness is not just about *feeling* well physically, but also about *doing* well—in mind, in body, and in spirit. We can also experience wellness beyond our individual selves, like socially or economically. We can also experience it collectively with our family or our community. It can extend to our relationship with the environment or with any of the various ecosystems that exist all around us. It can even extend to the planet as a whole. Wellness, then, is the most rational and logical paradigm for the modern age. It clearly defines the direction we need to move if we are to take our health to the next level.

Although a number of health professionals and everyday people already understand the necessity of making a paradigm shift, there are still a few obstacles to overcome before we make the final leap into a new way of thinking. These obstacles are in effect very deep-rooted beliefs that have developed for nearly a century, many of which have been built on the strength of past experiences. However, what we have only begun to realize is that these beliefs may be predicated on faulty assumptions, including our current culture of fear, our irrational belief in magic bullets, and the unconditional trust we place in large institutions and corporations to watch over and care for our health.

The first obstacle, the *culture of fear*, in which we find ourselves today, is a very subtle yet powerful phenomenon. Essentially, it is the distribution of information meant to scare us, cause worry, or create a sense of uneasiness within society. When enough fear has been spread throughout a culture, it can be used as a tool to influence the way people think. This influence can be exerted socially or politically as a way to shape public opinion or even to shape consumer spending. Either way, it is an enormously effective means of directing the consciousness of a large group of people so that they may act, or react, in a very specific manner.

Although it would be tempting for us to weave any number of fantastic conspiracy theories here, the truth is that almost every one of us—not just individuals but also groups, businesses, and governments alike—uses this tactic to gain an advantage. Fear is an effective motivator, and any group wishing maximal conformity will use it as they see fit. However, when we have the ability to recognize where fear-based information is being used, we will not feel *obligated* to concede to it when making decisions. And if, in fact, we truly have something to fear, then we can use all the information available to us in the ways which we see fit. By understanding the use of fear in the dissemination of information, we are better able to scrutinize the information and determine if it is unsubstantiated or weak.

One example we can use to see the effective application of fear is with governmental propaganda. This type of fear-based information is used to create the idea of a threat in the collective minds of a particular culture. This tactic has been used during wartime by practically every civilization in history. It was used in World War II to establish the Axis forces as an American enemy and even led to the internment of thousands of Japanese Americans. This could have only happened by creating a real fear in the minds of the American people. Fear was also used effectively throughout the Cold War and was helping to perpetuate it for over forty years. This should illustrate how powerful the use of fear is when wanting to influence large groups of people.

The way fear is used today is not much different than the way it has been used in the past. What is relevant to our discussions here, though, is the way it is used to influence our health decisions. The fear of illness, the fear of getting old, and the fear of death are all used effectively to sell us products, programs, and, of course, pharmaceuticals as the most desirable solutions to these threats. There are two deeply ingrained beliefs that allow these fears to hold such power over us. The first is the idea that human health is forever at peril, constantly threatened by various outside forces. In medical science, the most imminent threat to our health has historically been believed to be microorganisms—that is, germs or bugs. The second belief is that the only way to effectively maintain our health is by relying on external agents, like drugs or surgical procedures. As we have discussed several times throughout this book, these beliefs have developed over several decades, understandably as result of the discovery of the existence of microorganisms but also as a result of the many successes that modern medicine has realized (chapter 7).

Unfortunately, the information used to perpetuate these myths is only part of the truth. The other part is that our health also depends on lifestyle behaviors. Lifestyle behaviors may play an even greater role than we have yet to imagine, at least as far as our ability to withstand outside forces in maintaining health is concerned. Even so, the fear-based beliefs that I have previously mentioned have been used to perpetuate our current health paradigm. They have also been employed to establish the large majority of treatment protocols used today—drugs, surgeries, and, now, genetic engineering. Just notice the multitude of television commercials dedicated to prescription drugs. At one time, remember, advertising prescription drugs was considered unethical and off-limits; yet today, it is used with increasing regularity and has certainly helped to develop a greater reliance on pharmaceuticals by an ever-growing number of people.

The fear tactic continues to be used with regularity by the media for their own self-serving motives. Just notice the amount of press we receive on the possibility of a mass health crisis due to diseases like bird flu or bioterrorism. All this "frightening" news merely perpetuates a reliance on drugs or vaccines and is exploited quite readily by the pharmaceutical industry and the government. This occurs not as a conspiracy, but because we as a society still cling to the idea that health is mainly the result of forces outside our immediate control. I am not suggesting that we ignore these real threats; however, living in fear of them only serves to keep us dependent on a paradigm that rejects individual responsibility and control over our own health. And as a major plus to the trillion-dollar medical, pharmaceutical, and insurance industries, it keeps us reliant on them to care for our health since we couldn't possibly care for ourselves, now could we?

The second obstacle we must overcome before a shift in thinking takes place is our irrational belief in magic bullets. We have discussed this extensively in chapter 7, so we need not go over it further here. But please understand that this erroneous belief is flawed in many ways. There is just no such thing as a panacea or a slam dunk answer to our health woes. This has been proven repeatedly, and the chance of us ever finding one in the future is unlikely. The longer we keep the hopes alive of finding a magic bullet, the longer it will take us to bring our health to the next level.

The third obstacle we face is our dogmatic trust and dependency on the medical, pharmaceutical, and insurance industries to care for our health. I have mentioned before that the practice of medicine is, without a doubt, both necessary and advantageous to our health and well-being. However, far too many people look to medicine as their sole source of health care, even to the point of neglecting their own responsibility. They do so in the hope that modern medicine might save them if they perchance fall ill.

The reality is that the power of medical care is in its ability to handle crises or emergency situations. Rarely should it be used as an alternative to the meticulous, personal care necessary to maintain proper health. It should instead be used as a last resort—that is, when no better option is available. Nothing can supercede medical care in its ability to address immediate and potentially life-threatening situations. I wouldn't want any other type of care if a loved one or I were faced with a life-or-death situation or a severe loss of function (loss of a limb, fracture, appendicitis, etc.). When we finally appreciate the true utility of the practice of medicine, then will we be one step closer to completing our paradigm shift. Adopting this one simple habit, knowing when and when *not* to use the medical system, can alleviate many of the problems we see in health care today.

This goes for our worship of pharmaceutical substances too. Medicines have very valuable uses, and I firmly advocate the continued research and development of newer and more effective drugs. However, we must be able to place these commodities in their proper perspectives. Knowing when to turn to drugs is as crucial as knowing when to seek medical care. Pharmaceutical substances are meant to treat us when all else fails or, otherwise, during a life-or-death situation. When used repeatedly as a first line of defense, pharmaceuticals can cause as many problems as they were meant to handle. The indiscriminate use of medication at the first sign of a sniffle, a skin blemish, or simply when we can't "wait out" a cold or flu is not only useless, but can be downright dangerous. There are numerous accounts of adverse drug reactions causing sickness or death, and we have already discussed the dangers of antibiotic-resistant microorganisms. Drugs are indeed useful; they are not, however, factors that improve our health.

The fourth and, in my opinion, most detrimental obstacle we face in making a full paradigm shift is our reliance on the health insurance industry. I am not the lone voice of discontent here. Many groups and individuals such as doctors, politicians, and consumer advocates are aware of this unstoppable juggernaut in the health and medical industries.

The health insurance industry is the quintessential beneficiary of the *culture of fear* that we have been discussing. It is a business whose sole existence is based on the fear that injury and infirmity are inevitable for most people, and that sooner or later, extensive medical care will be necessary. Inherent in this belief is the concept that medical costs will continue to rise at a rate outside of what the average American family can afford. Armed with this weaponry, the insurance industry has succeeded in assuring itself a firm footing in the American culture while making itself one of the wealthiest and most powerful institutions in history.

While I might concede that the belief regarding the future costs of health care is well founded, the fear of the inevitability of illness and infirmity is what I take grave exception to. The truth is that this belief is completely unsubstantiated. True, there are hordes of Americans falling ill every day; however, as we pointed out numerous times before, most of today's chronic illnesses are due to faulty lifestyle choices. If we can adopt habits that are health enhancing while reducing those that are health diminishing, our need for overpriced and, quite frankly, inadequate insurance coverage will decrease dramatically. It is as simple as that.

How will the insurance industry convince us to purchase their plans if we no longer need them in the same way we do today? They won't be able to. As we witness a swing in today's health care coverage from the traditional employer-provided benefits to the newer individual-responsibility class, it will be harder for insurers to retain a hold on their customer base unless they can find a way to make coverage more affordable.[293] I could go on for pages discussing the viability of health insurance reform, but I will save that for another book. Suffice it to say that reform will be impossible if we continue to neglect our health and, in turn, indiscriminately use the medical system as our first and, often, sole line of defense.

The reality is that a paradigm shift is happening already. It is not a question of "if" and "how," but "when will it be complete?" The answer to this question is truly up to you and me. The sooner we accept wellness as a superior approach, the sooner this shift will be fulfilled. Fortunately, the wheels have already started to turn. Our old paradigm has definitely served us and has, in fact, been instrumental in our evolution; however, we know its flaws and have the understanding necessary to take it to the next level.

As a testament to the inevitability of this shift, one need only pay attention to the multitude of articles published in newspapers and magazines every day. New books on health and wellness are cropping up daily, and television commercials also reflect these changes; they all seem to be jumping on the wellness bandwagon. Hooray! This is the hippest bandwagon to be on. Just ask Kaiser Permanente. They have fabulous commercials on television expressing their commitment to wellness and endorsing the same life-enhancing activities we have outlined in this book. Kaiser Permanente? Hey, hats off to them. That's what I would call responsible health advertising.

Even grocery chains seem to be getting into the act. A local Southern California chain uses a glowing and healthy-looking doctor on their television commercials to discuss wellness tips as they relate to food. Bravo! That's exactly what we need. Add to that the numerous "health food" chains popping up everywhere, the increased memberships at gyms and yoga studios, and the growth of the vitamin and bottled water industries, and what we have are the makings of a true paradigm shift. Even Coca-Cola and Pepsi are getting into the act. Why? Because trend forecasters on these megacorporations' payrolls have been correctly predicting the direction in which society has been moving over the last couple of years. This has become so apparent that *BusinessWeek* has labeled baby boomers the most health-conscious generation in history. The magazine perceptively points out that boomers are more likely to be educated on matters of health, and they are more likely to take their health into their own hands.[294] I couldn't be more proud. We have certainly come a long way, haven't we?

## Integrating the Six Keys: Each Key Affects the Others

OK, we know that striving for health is a worthwhile endeavor. And we also know that changing the way we think about health is imperative. So by looking at health in a different way—that is, by having a deeper understanding of health and how it works—we have the foundation to change how we care for it, and our health will certainly flourish as a result.

Individuals are not the only ones taking heed of these changes: Corporate America, commercial agriculture, mainstream medicine, and small businesses are all following suit and entering the wellness arena. Wellness is now big business, precisely because it is what people want; they want to be in control of their own destiny and not leave something as precious as their health in the hands of others. Presumably, you want to be in control of your health too. That is why you are reading this book.

You have received numerous pointers within these pages, probably just enough to seem slightly overwhelming. But since it is better to actually incorporate these practices than to be weighed down by them, we will take the time to tie all six keys to optimal health together.

The six keys are interdependent. Just as we are not isolated beings acting separately from one another, the six keys to optimal health work best when done collectively. Each key has an enormous impact on the others and should, therefore, be carried out together as much as possible.

Although powerful in their own right, the keys are further strengthened when practiced simultaneously. This concept is known as *synergy* and is one of the most fundamental and advantageous aspects of all health-enhancing behaviors. Synergy is a combined interaction of forces that enhances the individual effects of each separate component. The six keys work in exactly this way—that is, they work synergistically.

Each key provides its own benefits to your health. As you begin to add subsequent keys to your routine, your health will benefit more than if the effects were simply additive—they will be exponentially enhanced. A great way to illustrate this point is with a basic mathematical analogy. If we were to add ten plus ten, we would have twenty. This is an *additive effect*. You would probably agree that it's not too shabby since we have doubled the result. In fact, most people would be pretty happy if they could double their health.*

Now let's multiply ten times ten. What we now end up with is one hundred. This is called a *multiple effect* and is clearly superior to a simple additive one. In this instance, we receive five times more benefit than in the previous example. Can we all agree that, as far as our health is concerned, a multiple level of enhancement would be highly advantageous?

Well, if that notion excites you, then you'll be ecstatic to hear how healthy behaviors actually work to enhance one another—they do so in an exponential fashion. This is best illustrated by taking ten to the tenth power, or $10^{10}$. This equals one with ten zeros behind it, or in other words, ten billion. Ten billion! This is exponential growth, and is exactly how the six keys work in tandem. Add to this that each key makes its own exponential contribution, and the implications to our physical health are astronomical.

We can easily see the ways in which each key affects the others. Take diet for example; a healthy diet provides the energy and nutrients necessary for

---

\*     Please note that our purpose is to demonstrate a principle only, not suggest that health
      can be measured numerically

basic daily functioning. When we embark on a regular exercise program, our dietary needs actually change. We, in fact, need more calories, more protein, more vitamins, and, subsequently, more water. When we meticulously adhere to a supportive nutritional regimen, we are able to increase the results we receive from our workouts considerably.

Nutrition also plays a vital role in our ability to respond to bodywork. Joint health, muscle elasticity, neurotransmitter production, and the healing process all improve with a sound, healthy diet. This is no less true for our mental health or even our capability to handle, process, and detoxify the poisons we are exposed to on a daily basis. Good nutrition is essential for the many reparative and restorative processes that occur while we sleep as well. Without a supportive nutritional regimen, then, all the aforementioned functions become hampered. The body will continue to carry out its processes in the absence of sound nutrition; however, it will do so at a much reduced rate. In other words, the body will do what it can with the materials it is given; but when it receives all the necessary resources, it actually flourishes.

What about exercise, then? How does it enhance the other five keys? Regular exercise improves our blood circulation, thereby increasing the amount of nutrients our tissues and organs receive. It also helps to stabilize our spine, lubricate our joints, and increase our freedom of movement, which serves to support any bodywork we receive. Regular physical activity also improves our sleep patterns, our breathing, and our mental outlook. It even increases the chances that we hydrate properly as people who work out regularly tend to drink more water than those who do not.

And what about bodywork? How does it heighten the other keys? Regular bodywork, like chiropractic care and massage, improves blood flow, which, of course, improves the assimilation of vital nutrients and oxygen. Chiropractic care also frees up stuck joints, thereby increasing range of motion and, consequently, improving the results we get from each workout. Since the nervous system controls and coordinates all bodily functions, chiropractic enhances movement, digestion, elimination, and every other physiological process dependent on the nervous system (which means all of them) by removing subluxations that may interfere with proper neurological functioning. Chiropractic can also improve sleep by removing pain and rebalancing the neuroendocrine system (i.e., neurotransmitters and hormones), which is essential for maintaining healthy sleep patterns. Bodywork has positive effects on our mental health too as pain interferes with our brain's proper functioning and can lead to stress, anxiety, and depression. Furthermore, chiropractic's wide-reaching effects help restore homeostasis to the body, ensuring proper hormonal balance in the most natural way.

Sleep has its own wide-ranging effects on the other keys. As we have mentioned before, sleep is vital to our mental faculties. When we deprive ourselves of sleep, we interfere with our cognitive abilities, our memory storage, and our problem-solving capacity. Each is necessary for proper mental health. Since many restorative processes occur during sleep, depriving ourselves can hamper digestion and the assimilation of vital nutrients, which can ultimately lead to hindered tissue repair. Furthermore, sleep is necessary for the healing process, so getting a sufficient amount of rest allows us to respond better to bodywork. And obviously, sleep is the time we replenish our energy stores (ATP), which is vital for movement and exercise. Less obvious, however, may be that our muscles depend on sleep for their repair and growth processes; to get in shape, then, you need sleep—so get plenty of it.

Proper mental functioning, particularly the ability to put life circumstances into perspective, are vital to the health and wellness of the body. The ways in which our mind affects our total health are immeasurable, yet we know that it does to a very large degree. Our mental state affects our digestion, how much we eat, and even the types of foods we eat. It not only determines our eating patterns, but our exercise and sleep patterns as well. Our mental state also determines how much we will benefit from bodywork as impatience is often a factor in the discontinuation of care. And of course, our state of mind plays an enormous role in whether we will turn to drugs (prescription or recreational) and may even lead to an addiction—or an overdose.

Finally, toxin avoidance is a huge factor in how it affects every other key. Obviously, toxins weaken the body and interfere with the uptake and processing of nutrients. Toxins affect sleep patterns and mental health. They can also weaken our vital organs like the heart, lungs, and blood vessels, thereby diminishing our ability to exercise. This ultimately affects our ability to reap the rewards inherent in any exercise program. Toxins adversely affect the nervous system and make it difficult for our bodies to accept and maintain the numerous benefits that come along with bodywork.

As you can see, each key has an enormous impact on the others—we just can't separate one key from the next. Many of us fail to recognize the synergistic effects of our behaviors simply because we have not been taught this concept. Instead, we have been raised on a paradigm that teaches us that the human body is made up of systems. We have consequently separated these systems—the cardiopulmonary system, the vascular system, the hepatic system, etc.—and have treated them as separate units. How else could we justify the removal of an organ unless we see it as a separate and independently functioning entity? Yet the truth is that the human body, and all of its systems, is an amazingly integrated whole. All systems work together interdependently: an activity or behavior that enhances one also enhances the others and has positive effects on the entire body.

You see, we have been conditioned to believe that each system in the body has its own unique needs as well as separate and distinct ways to strengthen it. Almost anybody will tell you that aerobic exercise is for cardiovascular health and that chiropractic care is for back pain, just as most people will be able tell you that vitamin A is necessary for proper eyesight and that excessive alcohol consumption can cause cirrhosis of the liver. What we have a harder time seeing, though, is the bigger picture—like how aerobic exercise may affect mood, or how vitamin A is an important antioxidant, or how chiropractic care can improve circulation. More precisely, people will usually know the most basic benefits each key has to offer, yet they are unaware of the magnitude of each key in the optimization of health. Even worse, most people do not know how severely their health can be compromised if they *do not practice* the six keys together. I hope this book has been adequate in providing you with sufficient reason to embark on this remarkable and invigorating program.

## The Health Line: What We Can Expect on the Road to Optimal Health

When thinking of the six keys, it helps to visualize a pie chart with six equal slices, each slice representing an individual key (figure 1). By envisioning it in this way, you'll understand how each key contributes to the health of the whole being. More importantly, though, you'll be able to appreciate that you do not necessarily have to practice each key at every moment to enjoy great health, although doing so will certainly give you the greatest chance of experiencing *optimal health* and *well-being*.

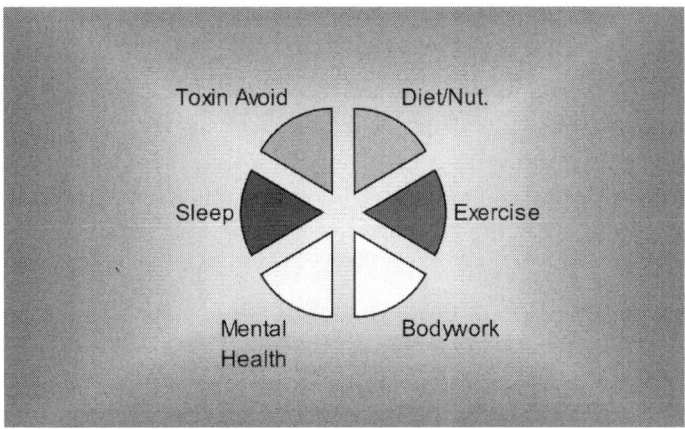

**Figure 1: Six Keys to Optimal Health**

Let's say you practice five of the six keys regularly but neglect exercise. You can see that only one piece of the pie is missing from your regimen. Not too bad since you will obtain enormous benefits from attending to the other five keys. It is important to understand, though, that due to the synergistic effects of each key, the deficiency is even greater than the 17 percent of the pie that this slice inhabits because exercising actually increases the effects of all other keys. More importantly, if you were to neglect a few more keys, your health would eventually suffer. The take home lesson here is the more keys you practice, the more your health will flourish.

We can illustrate this concept even further by looking at another chart (figure 2):

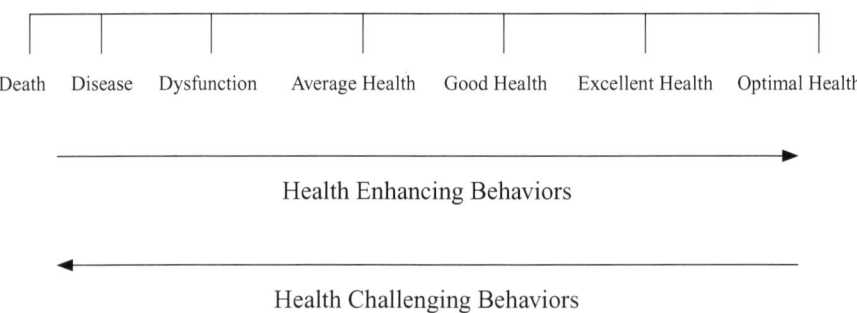

**Figure 2: Health Line**

This chart shows how we can improve our health by simply doing the right things. We can further enhance it by avoiding, or at least minimizing, some of the more detrimental behaviors that we might engage in. Health-enhancing behaviors include all of those outlined in this book (nutrition, exercise, bodywork, sleep, etc.); whereas health-challenging behaviors include exposure to toxins (smoking, excessive alcohol, pollution, etc.), engaging in reckless behaviors (driving under the influence of alcohol, unprotected sex with multiple partners, wearing a Giants hat at Dodger Stadium, etc.), and, of course, neglecting those behaviors that promote health.

When we engage regularly in health-enhancing behaviors, we move further down the scale to the right, or closer toward optimal health. When, instead, we neglect these activities (i.e., lack of exercise, poor diet, repeated sleep deprivation, etc.), we have the tendency to move to the left, or closer toward dysfunction or disease.

It is important to understand that reaching the farthest end of the scale on the right, perhaps it might be called *perfect health*, is not possible—actually, there is no such thing. We can definitely approximate perfect health, we call it optimal health, but there isn't exactly an end point for us to reach in this regard. Saying it in a different way, one does not simply reach the top of the "health mountain" and then all is complete. Since we can almost always improve our health, there will always be another level for us to reach. Instead, we actually fluctuate between two points on the health scale, usually on either side of the area labeled Average Health.

This brings up an important point: just as there is no such thing as perfect health, there is no such thing as *permanent health* either. As living organisms, we must experience dysfunction, or stress, at various times in our lives. The frequency with which we do so really depends on each individual; however, rest assured that this fluctuation between health and dysfunction is normal. Only by experiencing dysfunction can our adaptive processes take over, allowing us to get ever stronger and better able to withstand the constant stresses that present themselves in life. This is precisely how we are able to take our health to the next level. Remember that everything changes and everything evolves. In order to survive as a species, we must always have new challenges to adapt to. These might include new or previously undiscovered microorganisms, environmental pollutants, natural disasters, or even wars. It might also include injuries, accidents, or even, perhaps, violent experiences. In any case, illness is a natural part of life. It is how we adapt to illness that really determines our survivability as living creatures. Our ability to adapt is what, in fact, determines *wellness*.

We can certainly control how far we fluctuate on the left side of the scale, though, toward dysfunction or disease. As I have said before, most of us experience dysfunction to one degree or another  be it physical, chemical, hormonal, or whatever; nevertheless, entering into a state of full-fledged disease is not inevitable. The dysfunction we experience can be something as simple as a cold or sports injury. It might even be a weakened state of health caused by chronic insomnia or drug addiction. Either way, these dysfunctional states can be reversed. And the duration of dysfunction is controllable too. How do we control it? By practicing the six keys to optimal health, that's how. Basically, there is no other way.

Yes, medical care is definitely necessary, especially when we fall far to the left on the health scale. Disease states often need medical intervention as do some of the more chronic states of dysfunction. But even under these circumstances, the six keys must be practiced purposefully because they are behaviors that facilitate the natural healing process. To move toward the right, or into the area of health, is only possible through the body's own innate healing ability. No drug or surgical procedure can cause healing—only the body can heal itself. Outside interventions—like medications, surgery, ice, heat, herbal remedies, acupuncture, and even vitamins—only serve to remove obstacles to the healing process or at least enhance the process in some way. They do not actually carry out the healing. Healing can only be accomplished by the body itself, which must go through its own physiological processes to bring about homeostasis.

The bottom line is that the more keys you focus on and practice, the further up the scale of health you will go. The closer you move toward excellent or optimal health, the more you will experience the rewards that accompany it. Keep focusing on the six key habits and try not to fall into the trap of thinking you should never get ill. Challenges to your health are a necessary component of your development and will ultimately lead to wellness. If you keep these principles in mind and also apply them, I assure you that the results will definitely be worth the effort.

## Some Useful Tips on Incorporating the Six Keys

In chapter 1, we discussed America's poor ranking in the world in terms of the health of its population. One reason this ranking is so low has to do with some detrimental behaviors we have adopted in this country like the overconsumption of fast foods, our addiction to sodas, and the abuse of prescription and recreational drugs to name just a few. Another reason is that a large number of people still consistently neglect some of the more life-enhancing behaviors like exercise, sleep, or bodywork. We know that good health is not possible when faulty behaviors become a way of life.

On the other end of the spectrum, many people are already practicing the six keys to one extent or another, and they are experiencing great results. They may not be addressing every slice of the pie, but they are doing enough to enjoy fantastic health. Remember, even practicing half the keys on a regular basis enhances your health significantly.

Whether you engage in healthy behavior regularly or have not yet incorporated them into your lifestyle, you will definitely find this next section useful. We will discuss a few of the obstacles you may encounter while embarking on this endeavor of health. The three we touch upon here have to do with what I typically find to be the greatest barrier for most people to overcome—their own perspective.

### 1.  It's not about being perfect

Some people, when first setting out to adopt healthy habits, have a tendency to become obsessive. Fanaticism is perhaps the most difficult obstacle to overcome because people with this predisposition also tend to be highly motivated. These people may develop an intense enthusiasm, which will only increase as they experience continued results. On the surface, hyperenthusiasm might seem desirable, but it can actually present a couple of major problems.

Problem number 1 is that an unbalanced enthusiasm can easily lead to *burnout*. What this means is that when approaching an endeavor with such great intensity, it might be difficult, if not impossible, to maintain the same passion over a significant amount of time. One might then discontinue the entire effort since one may have the erroneous belief that this program can only be effective if one's intensity is maintained continuously. For people like this, balance between discipline and relaxation is hard to find; yet for healthy behaviors to become lifestyle habits, balance is essential.

The second major problem is that "life just happens." Whether one becomes busy at work, has a new child, gets sick, or goes on vacation, things arise that may interfere with the ability to observe one's health regimen. Sometimes the only food available is . . . junk food. Sometimes people have to work late to meet a deadline . . . so they lose sleep. Sometimes people have injuries that prevent them from exercising. Sometimes they just feel lazy. And guess what? It's all OK.

There is no rule that says you have to be perfect. This is true even if you have a choice in the matter. Perhaps you enjoy a cigar now and again. Perhaps you like Ben & Jerry's. Perhaps you *"feel like* staying out all night." It's still OK.

The biggest mistake is in trying to always be perfect. There will be times and circumstances where you won't be able to adhere to your regimen. And when this is the case, acknowledge your incredible ability to be flexible and just roll with the punches.

Appreciate that you *mostly* eat well, *mostly* exercise, and *mostly* scc your chiropractor; but on occasion, you just don't. Guilt trips are basically neutralized when you adopt this manner of thinking. When you make it firm in your mind that the six keys are lifestyle habits, you won't have to worry about missing a day or two, a week, or even a couple of weeks at the gym—you'll be back because it's what you do. Don't worry about periodically abstaining from any of the other keys, either. Make them a natural part of your lifestyle, and you will be assured of picking them up again. It's only a matter of time.

You will only be able to overcome the desire to be perfect if you fully understand the importance of making these behaviors lifestyle habits. The six keys to optimal health are not meant to be just intellectual exercises, but behaviors to be acted upon with regularity. The only way to enjoy permanence of these habits is by having a balanced perspective and by putting as much effort into the six keys as you do with all your other activities including work, hobbies, and relationships. They are that important.

## 2. Integrate one key at a time

We have pointed out that the biggest problem self-motivated perfectionists face when embarking on a new health regimen is their unrealistic desire for . . . well, perfection. Most people, though, have a much different problem—just getting started in the first place.

There are many reasons that keep people from beginning a regimen of any kind, but feeling overwhelmed is usually the most common. I admit that for newcomers, the voluminous information contained within *The Six Keys to Optimal Health* may seem intimidating at first. I assure you, though, there is an easy way to do all the six keys without feeling defeated from the start. The secret is to incorporate the six keys into your life one by one.

The best way to initiate the first step of action is to identify whether you are practicing any of the six keys *regularly* at this time. The number of keys you practice can now be designated a number (activity level 1 if you currently do one key, activity level 2 if you do two, etc). As we have discussed throughout this book, consistency is crucial. If you cannot realistically say you do any of the keys regularly, then the number you designate should be zero. If you are still unsure about where you stand in this regard, I offer you some useful criteria by which to evaluate. Regarding healthy behaviors—exercising, receiving bodywork, eating at home, taking vitamins, etc.—consider anything you do less than one time per week as "not regular." On the other hand, consider any behaviors that should be avoided—smoking, eating fast foods, recreational drug use, sleep deprivation, etc.—that you do more than one time per week as also "not regular." For each key, if more than 50 percent of that category is not done with regularity (use the checklist at the end of each chapter), then consider it zero.

The best way to approach this game plan is to first address it from a perspective of someone who does not practice any of the six keys regularly, that is, the ones whose activity level is zero. If this is the case, then determine which behavior is easiest for you to adopt; most likely, this will differ from person to person. From my experience, I know that quitting habits are much harder than taking on new ones. So trying to quit smoking, or drinking liquor, or sodas, will probably not be the best place to start. In fact, that is probably the surest way to becoming frustrated and simply quitting your efforts altogether. Start instead with something simple, like eating at home regularly. This is an easier behavior to change than, say, giving up cigarettes. You might also want to start with something that will give you the most rapidly tangible results, like exercising or receiving regular bodywork. The advantage here is that you will see immediate changes take place, which will then increase your enthusiasm and motivation. Continue to add behaviors in each category over time—let's say, one or two every couple of weeks. If you start with diet, keep adding dietary habits as we addressed in chapter 2 until you bring them above 50 percent. You can, at this point, continue to master all the dietary behaviors or, if you wish, move on to the next key and come back to diet later.

Once you have mastered more than 50 percent of the actions in any one category, the next step would be to pick another key that you find easy to do. You can also choose to address a key that works in tight conjunction with the first. Therefore, if you started with exercise, you may want to take on diet next or perhaps bodywork. I have found that for some people, especially those who have pain, starting with bodywork is a great idea. Generally, when people suffer from chronic pain, they have a much harder time focusing on anything else—be it diet, exercise, or sleeping well. When you choose the next key you wish to master, embark on it the same way you did the first—just make sure you continue to practice the habits you previously adopted in addition to the new ones. Again, add new behaviors systematically over time.

If you are somebody who addresses one or several of the six keys already, then you can add some of the other ones in the same way. You may even incorporate more at a time although this is certainly not a must. Whichever way you decide to go, start slowly and enjoy. Try to get your activity number up to 4 or 5, and you'll be doing pretty well. Of course, when you reach 6, you'll realize the best results of all.

### 3.   Achieving health is dynamic: It's a never-ending process

We have already touched upon this concept briefly, but it is important enough for us to discuss again here. Achieving health is a dynamic process; in other words, it never ends. What this means is that if you want to enjoy all the benefits associated with great health, you will have to work at it continuously. You will never reach the top of the mountain because its height is infinite. How high you climb up the mountain of health is up to you, and it depends on how far you wish to go. Amazing, I know; but just like life, the possibilities are endless.

Also important is to remember that health fluctuates. Getting ill is vital to gaining health. Illness serves a vital function by adding occasional stress to our bodies. This, in turn, allows us to adapt, bringing us to ever-new levels of wellness.

Something else to consider is that our cells die and are reborn constantly. This is called *cell turnover*, and although it happens at differing rates for different tissues, almost every cell goes through this process. What this means is that our bodies are changing repeatedly—new cells replace old ones—so that we are not exactly the same person we were even last year.

Why does this information matter? It does because it will help keep you thinking with the proper perspective. Life and death go together, and both take place repeatedly during your lifetime—around you and even within your own body. By understanding this concept, you will not have the unrealistic expectations that health is all you should experience. Therefore, even though your health will fluctuate, you can in fact experience great health most of the time.

## The Determinants of Health

We have spent all this time discussing health—how to achieve it and why we should strive for it at all. Yet an important question is still remaining: how do we know if our efforts are actually getting results? This is a valid question and one we have to answer if we ever wish to continue on this journey. If we can determine the criteria by which to evaluate our progress, then perhaps this would help us to maintain a continued desire and commitment conducive toward achieving our goal of great health.

The most common methods used today to measure health are actually tests that determine sickness. We call them *objective measures*, and they are based on observable information we gather through testing. We compare this information to a set of averages that we consider "normal" and then determine whether the values fall into the range of what we would call "healthy." Some of these tests assess blood pressure, some heart rate, and others blood composition. We evaluate them by comparing the results to values we consider "normal"; however, the term "normal" is a misnomer since what we really mean is "average." The difference between "normal" and "average" is that "average" is a *range* that we typically observe in otherwise healthy people. Whether one falls toward the top of the range or the bottom matters somewhat, but measurements on either end of the range are still considered "normal." Values falling just slightly out of range are not necessarily abnormal, mind you; they are merely not the average.

Objective measures are very useful, especially in cases where a large discrepancy exists between the measured value and the average range. Their greatest significance is their ability to alert us to potential or actual disease states in people. As useful as these tests are in this regard, they are not necessarily the best indicators of health as a whole. In fact, in the past, they were mostly used to determine the onset or progression of a particular illness. This fell right in line with the prevailing view that health is simply the absence of symptoms of disease. However, in today's climate where wellness is now recognized as more than just a symptom-free state, these types of tests are being used more and more to determine our level of health.

As I mentioned already, most objective tests used in health care today have a wide range that is considered "average" or "normal," but falling outside of this range does not necessarily mean "abnormal." One of the most often misinterpreted tests is the blood cholesterol analysis. Total cholesterol levels less than 200 mg/dL are considered "optimal." Anything above 240 mg/dL is considered "high" and a predisposing factor for the development of heart disease.

Cholesterol is a substance naturally produced by the body as it is a necessary component of cell membranes, bile, and many hormones. There are two main sources of this vital material: that which the body manufactures on its own (endogenous) and that which we get from our diet (exogenous). Since we need a constant supply of cholesterol at all times, levels remain fairly constant throughout our lifetime. The more we get in our diet, the less we produce endogenously; and the less we eat, the more we produce. This is the body's simple way of maintaining homeostasis.

The reason this is important is because when a cholesterol test indicates high levels of cholesterol in some people and these people then reduce their dietary intake to bring down their cholesterol level, they still may end up testing high. The usual medical recommendation for this type of scenario is to start these people on a regimen of cholesterol-lowering drugs, the *statins*. The problem here is that this protocol is predicated on the assumption that the human body is incapable of determining its own cholesterol needs. Although there is indeed a medical disorder called *familial hypercholesterolemia* (FH) in which the body overproduces cholesterol to its own disadvantage, it actually is a pretty rare genetic disorder.

What may be more likely is that some people just happen to run a bit higher on the cholesterol range than the average. It is really not that big of a deal. In light of this, it is most daunting that statin drugs are routinely prescribed to people who may have readings between 200 to 240 mg/dL (for instance, at 230), which should, by all accounts, be considered "normal," not "high." Why, then, are these people given drugs? The rationale is that they are "borderline high," and so they *need* the drugs to prevent their cholesterol from getting any higher; that is, they need them prophylactically. But what this really does is blur the lines even further or, in other words, ignores what we consider "normal" in the first place. By the way, this is a perfect example of the health paradigm in which we currently live. Anyone else think it's time for a change?

My main point here is that objective measures are useful but not absolute. This holds especially true when we use them to evaluate normal functions like cholesterol levels instead of what they should be used for—to detect potential disease states. High blood pressure is not a disease nor is high cholesterol; they are both merely indicators of possible disease states. As such, measuring them is enormously useful; however, they are not true indicators of health (inasmuch as if you're without either, you're probably dead).

I would like to propose an even better way to evaluate health, one that does not rely on "expert" opinion from an outside source. Instead, I propose that you rely on the opinion and observation of the expert in the best position to make that determination, the person most likely to know your needs and what does and doesn't agree with you, the person most in touch with your habits and your lifestyle—and that person is you!

Not only do you know intuitively what's best for your health, but you also know which way to care for it. You have the best ability to interpret the many messages your body sends to you at any given time. I am not suggesting that you forgo doctors—heavens no! Doctors are in the best position to evaluate dysfunction, illness, and disease. And when you do not feel right, you'd better get their expert opinion right away. However, there isn't a doctor in the world who knows your body and your health better than you do, especially when you adopt healthy habits and are in tune with your body. So as far as evaluating your level of health is concerned, no one can even come close to you.

This point is very important to understand: if you do not regularly practice the healthy habits outlined in this book or if you simply do not focus on maintaining good health, then by all means, you should be under the watchful eye of a doctor. On the other hand, if you are diligent in caring for your health, you will pretty much know how you are functioning most of the time. The truth is that your body has many ways to let you know when something is physically wrong, and you will certainly be able to recognize these moments when they come; and, of course, you should then act accordingly. But if you are someone who does not take the time to develop this connection to your body, then you will need to be checked for potential illness with some sort of regularity.

So what are the criteria you can use to evaluate your health? I believe that you can do it most effectively by simply observing three things: how you look, how you feel, and, especially, how you function. The first criterion, determining how you look, is the simplest of the three. It holds the distinction of being neither the most objective nor the most subjective category to evaluate. True, there is no standard or normal way one should look; however, we all have a personal reference point that we can use to determine where we want to be.

Every person can remember a time (could be the present) when they have looked their best. We all look our best when we are healthy. Unfortunately, many have come to believe that the only way to look their best is through surgical or chemical enhancement (plastic surgery and/or steroids, hormones, or diet pills), yet there is no comparison to looking good through natural and healthy means. Beauty, vigor, and vitality naturally radiate when embarking on a regimen of good health because, in essence, it is the way all living things respond when given what they need to fully express life. Take a plant, for example. Fail to provide it with sunlight and water, and how will it appear? It will look limp, lifeless, and discolored. Now take that same plant and give it sufficient water and sunlight, and what happens? It will take a turn for the better. It will stand firm and upright, and it will naturally thrive. The same is true for human beings—neglect to give a person basic life-enhancing substances, like water or food, or allow them to ignore some very essential activities, like exercise or sleep, and they too will appear less than lively. On the other hand, people who have all the raw material they need to maintain life and who also engage in health-enhancing behaviors will naturally give off the glow of a thriving and flourishing life-form.

Some of the physical enhancements you can expect to receive from practicing the six keys to optimal health are the following:

- *Clear eyes*: This comes from being well rested, well nourished, and having optimal blood flow and optimal nerve function. Quite the opposite of the bloodshot and clouded look of one who is exhausted, malnourished, or regularly abusing drugs or alcohol.
- *Clear, healthy skin*: This also comes from being well nourished and well rested. Exercise and bodywork stimulate blood circulation, giving a rosy appearance while regular movements increase tone and prevent sagging. Proper hydration, adequate fats in the diet, and abstaining from toxic substances (cigarettes, drugs, and alcohol) can also prevent premature wrinkling.
- *Toned muscles and slim body*: Exercise tones muscles and helps burn fat, leading to the development of one's most natural body shape and size.
- *Clean white teeth and rosy pink gums*: Eating whole, natural foods helps clean teeth naturally and keeps the gums stimulated while avoidance of toxins prevents premature yellowing, bleeding gums, and bad breath (halitosis).
- *Great posture*: Regular bodywork, flexibility exercises, and strength training improve posture—giving a firm, erect, and confident appearance.

These are the most obvious signs you will see when embarking on the six keys to optimal health. You may also notice other physical enhancements that are unique to you. In my opinion, these are the most tangible assets you will attain to evaluate your health; and yes, in my vanity, I find them the most fun too. Give it time, and you will soon know exactly what I'm talking about.

The next criterion to use when determining your state of health is how you feel. This is definitely the most subjective of the three, simply because it takes time to develop a strong connection to all the signals your body uses to communicate to you. However, once you become in tune with your body's signals, it will be the most powerful tool you have by far. The key here is to try to always listen to your body. If you feel bloated following a meal—that's a sign. If you feel pain—that's a sign too. If you feel exhausted, run-down, and on the verge of catching cold—that's a huge sign. Listen to your body. Slow down, get some rest, avoid offending foods, get a chiropractic adjustment, get a massage—whatever you do, listen to those signs. They are your body's way of telling you something is wrong. We are energetic beings, and when our natural flow of energy is disrupted, we feel it. Don't ignore these signals. Ignoring them may not only lead to things like colds, flu, and exhaustion, but also to more serious situations, like heart attacks, nervous breakdowns, or dehydration. Trust me when I say this: it's not worth ignoring these signs. Listen to your body—it will never lie to you.

The third and final criterion you can use to evaluate your health is to determine how your body is functioning. This is definitely the most objective of the three criteria as there are factors you can use to compare your current state of function to the standard. The presence of pain is the most obvious measure available to you. Pain has the very vital function of acting as a warning signal; basically, it lets you know that something is amiss. The simplest example we can provide is what happens when you touch a hot object. The burning sensation you feel makes you remove your hand from the object immediately. Without this type of protective mechanism, we would have no way to ensure our safety. More importantly, though, we might not be able to ensure our own survival. Fortunately, we have a built-in pain mechanism for most of our organs and tissues. When they become compromised—either through dysfunction or disease—pain kicks in, telling us that there may be an impending danger. Think about all the different types of pain people experience (chest pain, warning of potential heart disease; low back pain, warning of biomechanical dysfunction; cramping, warning of possible dehydration; etc.). We are blessed that, as a result of our evolution, we have developed such an intricate and precise system as this. What a tragedy that many people choose to mask or ignore these warning signals with powerful pain medications until the underlying problem gets worse. Pain should never be ignored—when it persists for an extended period, immediate professional attention is warranted.

Another way we can evaluate function is through a physical or mental performance evaluation. This may relate to strength, cardiovascular endurance, flexibility, sexual endurance, or mental function. If you periodically measure and log your results in various activities, you can always compare future performances to previous ones. For instance, you can record how much weight you lift; how far you can stretch; or how far and how long you can walk, run, or swim. For the most part, you should be able to exceed your past performances; at the very least, you should be able to maintain the same level. True, as you age, your performance may decline a bit but not dramatically. If you are returning to a particular activity after some time off, expect your performance to decline a little. In fact, it is important not to try to match your last performance as I guarantee, it won't come easily; and worse, you may end up hurting yourself. As far as your sexual capability is concerned, you may experience a slight decline in desire and performance over the years; but it should not be to the degree that sex becomes impossible to engage in, at least not for physical reasons anyway. Mental function can be evaluated through various methods like memory games, mathematical problem solving, or puzzles relating to logic. A great book and one that I highly recommend for its protocol in assessing mental function is *Age-Proof Your Mind* by Dr. Zaldy Tan. You can find the information on this book in the suggested reading list in back.

In essence, there are ways to effectively evaluate your health. When you start to care for your health as one of your greatest assets, these methods will become invaluable to you. Even if you do not end up practicing the six keys consistently, you can still use the methods I have just discussed to analyze your state of health at any given time. Without a doubt, your body will give off the same warning signals—perhaps even more so—if you become sick. When people fall ill—especially when entering a disease state—how they look, feel, and function will be highly reflective of their condition. So once again, don't ignore the warning signs—they can be a matter of life or death. Seek medical intervention immediately. Western medicine is the greatest and most advanced crisis care system there is. If you are in a state of disease, don't hesitate; you will get the best care possible with medical intervention. Even so, continue to practice the six keys to optimal health at all times. By combining Western medicine with the health-enhancing behaviors of the six keys, you will stand the greatest chance of recovery and survival.

## A Bit Philosophical

I have just spent significant time discussing how to determine if one's efforts toward better health have actually been worthwhile. For the most part, I have put forth purely physical measures, but other methods are available to help one make these evaluations.

For the last three hundred to four hundred years, people have looked primarily to science for answers regarding questions on the universe, on man, and on man's health. In fact, the scientific method has been so effective in providing answers that people in general tend to think of science as infallible. Science is a valuable asset indeed—without it, we would not realize the great advances we have made so far. But science has its limitations—most significantly, human error.

The concept of human error is taught in every introductory science course there is. Basically, all experiments conducted by man have human fallibility inherent in them. Put simply: human beings make mistakes. And since humans both design studies and collect data, then human error is certainly possible in their conclusions as well. Add to this that we have a limited knowledge of the workings of a vast and infinite universe, we are only able to analyze the information we gather with our present knowledge. This too may bring us to some erroneous conclusions.

It is therefore important to recognize that science cannot answer all of man's unanswered questions, including matters of human health. For example, there was a time when the Newtonian laws of physics were seen as absolute. They appeared to be true under every imaginable circumstance, and they were testable as well. These laws held up under the rigorous scrutiny of science, further cementing their certainty in the human consciousness. At about the turn of the twentieth century, though, physicists like Albert Einstein theorized and proved that the Newtonian laws did not hold up under certain conditions. This opened up the possibility that the universe was far greater and more complex than we had previously imagined.

A more recent example of human fallibility in the face of science involved the use of the drug thalidomide during the 1950s and 1960s. This drug was given to pregnant women all around the world to combat morning sickness. It was hailed as a wonder drug, which provided a "safe, sound sleep."[295] Tragically, thalidomide caused horrifying birth defects in babies born to mothers who took the drug. Once again, we did not have all the answers despite rigorous scientific evaluation.

Stories like these are all too numerous, and surely, you get the point without my delving into them any further. The main point here is that science is not, and perhaps may never be, the only means to answering all our burning questions.

So what methods should we use, then, *in addition* to science to provide us with the answers we are looking for? Why not use the same methods man has used before he had science, some of which he still uses today—philosophy and spirituality? Whoa! I can hear the discontented outcries as I write this. Today's powerful and vocal fundamentalist movement, the secular movement known as *scientism*, will surely be objecting loudly. This dogmatic belief system sees the scientific method as the only viable means of providing answers to questions of the universe. If you feel this way, please, hear me out. I assure you that I will not bore you with an illogical argument.

Since we know, through quantum physics, that the universe is constantly created and expanded by the collective consciousness of all people on the planet (and likely every energetic life-form in the universe), doesn't it make sense that we can never "know it all"? We simply have no way of knowing all there is to know—where we are going as people, as a species, as a planet. We may never even be able to approximately know it all, as the universe is expanding and contracting at all times, beyond our very comprehension. Therefore, many roads are available to lead us to the truth, including some that may not be so popular in Western society but may very well be making a comeback. The truth is that although our current way of thinking has allowed us to answer many questions and solve numerous problems—and, indeed, has even perpetuated our evolution as a species—we may need a new or different way to address many of today's difficult issues. Science has been great, and it will likely continue to surprise and fascinate us; however, we should also use a philosophical and spiritual approach to answer complex questions of the universe.

We find ourselves in an era where society is so heavily influenced by the latest scientific research that most people don't realize the extent to which our knowledge is growing, and as a result, we just cannot view the latest research findings as absolute. Today, green tea may be "in" (understood to have anticancerous properties), but based on what we learn tomorrow, it may be "out" (no longer be as accurate as we once believed). However, if we can adhere to philosophical principles, those which we deduce from our already-existing knowledge, then we will not need to worry about whether today's scientific truth is tomorrow's miscalculation. By approaching life in this way, we need not be confused by the latest research on diet, exercise, hydration, sleep, drug use, or any other issue pertaining to health because, philosophically speaking, the principles on health remain the same. Put sufficient energy into the six key areas of health, and wellness will be yours. Understand that, in essence, all people are the same—we are energetic beings—and as such, these principles are true for all of us.

The only thing that differentiates people is the expression of their life experiences. This includes their experiences regarding health and wellness. By understanding and acknowledging this point, you will be better able to understand the following concept. As I mentioned earlier, we all go through a process of evolution. If we can look at this fact from a spiritual perspective, we can then use our imagination to speculate that, perhaps, all of life's challenges, including those revolving around health, may serve as a function to stimulate our personal growth and evolution.

Every individual on this planet has challenges he or she must overcome. These challenges may pertain to finances, relationships, family, or even matters of health. I propose, then, that all major health challenges facing people may be spiritual in nature. In other words, challenges present themselves to teach us something important. What these lessons are can only be uncovered by the individual involved. It may be something as simple as giving attention to one's body, slowing down one's hectic pace, or learning to love oneself. Whatever illnesses you are experiencing, please attempt to find the lesson within. The lesson may be of a physical, mental, emotional, or spiritual nature; whichever avenue you need to investigate, never give up and please seek help. Sometimes the solution can be found through a collaborative effort. There are countless stories of people undergoing miraculous recoveries from terminal illnesses. Without a doubt, these people found a way to uncover the spiritual lesson inherent in their illness. Once again, I want to emphasize that any illness should be comanaged by you and a qualified health professional. However, approaching it from a spiritual perspective can be very empowering and may actually help you through the experience. Before you brush this off as an unsubstantiated or backward notion, I'd like to point out that the Association of American Medical Colleges (AAMC) recognizes the value of spirituality in the healing process; in fact, more than two-thirds of the country's medical schools teach courses in spirituality and medicine.[296] They wouldn't do so if there were no validity in the concept. Think about that for a while.

## The Proof Is in the Pudding

The time has finally come for us to end our journey together. Now is the time for you to embark upon your own journey. Hopefully, you have been inspired to take the journey of wellness; and in your quest, I hope that you will use the six keys to optimal health to get there. Through my extensive research and through the observation and treatment of numerous patients, I know the power inherent in practicing the principles outlined in this book. More importantly, though, I have experienced the many wonderful benefits of these habits personally, as I have been on my own journey for nearly twenty years. I can fully attest that by taking on each of the six keys one by one, the health benefits you can enjoy will be astounding. I have yet to reach a plateau in my efforts, and every day, my journey takes me to new and undiscovered strata of health and well-being.

Simply reading this book will not be enough. To truly appreciate all that health has to offer, you must embark on this journey in more than just an intellectual manner—you must practice these principles regularly and give them time to take hold. As they say, the proof is in the pudding. You will never know what the six keys have to offer if you do not try them yourself. As one of my teachers says, "To know and not do is to not know."[297]

You may have found yourself questioning, and even discounting, many of the principles in this book. That's OK—it means you're thinking. Critical analysis is very important when taking on any endeavor; in fact, I encourage you to always question what you hear and never take anything for granted. Dogmatism serves no one, and this is equally true for what I have presented to you in this book. Do the research yourself if you have any further questions. There are always two sides to a story, and balance is essential. Never stop learning about health, and you will discover that there is always something more to learn.

Whichever way you decide to proceed, please give it adequate time. All processes take time, especially when it comes to your health and well-being. Most importantly, though, have fun with your practice. Achieving and maintaining great health should be enjoyable, and I am quite certain that you will agree with me once you get started.

If nothing else, I wish you to walk away from this reading with the knowledge of four important points:

- You are in complete control of your health.
- Make caring for your health a regular part of your lifestyle.
- Get in tune with your body and always listen to its messages.
- And finally, teach your children these principles.

If you can accept and do these four things, then you will succeed.

I want to leave you with my final words of absolute gratitude for giving me the opportunity to share this information with you. I realize that this manuscript is as much a gift to me as it is to you. By having the opportunity to write it, I have had the chance to learn this material to an even deeper degree than I ever thought possible. Thank you for giving me your valuable time. Good luck with your endeavors, and may you experience life to your absolute fullest capacity and contentment.

# APPENDIX

1. Pfizer's Lipitor: a cholesterol-lowering drug

   Side effects include liver damage, abdominal pain, allergic reaction, back pain, changes in eyesight, cold, constipation, diarrhea, dry eyes, dry skin, flu symptoms, gas, hair loss, headache, heartburn, indigestion, inflammation of sinus and nasal passages, itching, joint pain, leg cramps, muscle aching or weakness, purple or red spots on the skin, rash, sore throat, urinary problems, vomiting, and weakness.

2. Merck's Zocor: another cholesterol-lowering drug

   Minor side effects include constipation, diarrhea, fatigue, gas, heartburn, and headache.

   Major side effects include abdominal pain or cramps, blurred vision, dizziness, easy bruising or bleeding, itching, muscle pain or cramps, rash, and yellowing of the skin or eyes.

3. TAP Pharmaceutical's Prevacid: an antacid

   Side effects include allergic reaction (difficulty in breathing; closing of the throat; swelling of the lips, tongue, or face; or hives)

   Less serious side effects may be more likely to occur, including diarrhea, nausea, and abdominal pain

   Side effects other than those listed here may also occur. Talk to your doctor about any side effect that seems unusual or that is especially bothersome (http://www.drugs.com/Prevacid)

4. Johnson & Johnson's Procrit: treats chemotherapy-related anemia. Procrit is not for patients with uncontrolled high blood pressure. High blood pressure has been noted rarely in cancer patients treated with Procrit and blood pressure should be monitored carefully. Drugs like Procrit may increase the risk of blood clots. In studies, the most common side effects included fever, diarrhea, nausea, vomiting, edema, shortness of breath, tingling, and upper respiratory infection.

5. Eli Lilly and Company's Zyprexa: an antipsychotic

   Contact your doctor immediately or seek medical attention if you experience side effects including uncontrollable movements of the mouth, tongue, cheeks, jaw, arms, or legs.

   Contact your doctor immediately or seek medical attention if you experience fever, sweating, severe muscle stiffness (rigidity), confusion, or fast or irregular heartbeats. These could be symptoms of a potentially fatal side effect called *neuroleptic malignant syndrome* (NMS).

Use caution when driving, operating machinery, or performing other hazardous activities. Olanzapine may cause dizziness or drowsiness. If you experience dizziness or drowsiness, avoid these activities.

Dizziness may be more likely to occur when you rise from a sitting or a lying position. Rise slowly to prevent dizziness and a possible fall.

Use alcohol cautiously. Alcohol may increase drowsiness and dizziness while taking olanzapine.

Maintain adequate fluid intake and use caution in hot weather and during exercise to avoid becoming overheated during treatment with olanzapine. It is easier to become dangerously overheated while taking olanzapine.

6.  Amgen's Epogen: another anemia drug

If you experience any of the following serious side effects, stop using epoetin alfa and seek emergency medical treatment: an allergic reaction (difficulty in breathing; closing of your throat; hives; or swelling of your lips, tongue, or face) or seizures.

Other less serious side effects may be more likely to occur. Continue to use epoetin alfa and talk to your doctor if you experience increased blood pressure, headache, a "flulike" feeling, increased heart rate, nausea, vomiting, diarrhea, numbness or tingling, tiredness, muscle aches, or a rash (*http://epogen.drugs.com*).

7.  AstraZeneca's Nexium: another antacid

If you experience an allergic reaction (difficulty in breathing; closing of your throat; hives; or swelling of your lips, tongue, or face), stop taking esomeprazole and seek emergency medical attention.

Other less serious side effects may be more likely to occur. Continue to take esomeprazole and talk to your doctor if you experience headache, diarrhea, nausea, flatulence, abdominal pain, constipation, or dry mouth.

Side effects other than those listed here may also occur. Talk to your doctor about any side effect that seems unusual or that is especially bothersome. (*http://nexium.drugs.com*).

8.  Pfizer's Zoloft: an antidepressant

While you are taking sertraline, you may need to be monitored for worsening symptoms of depression and/or suicidal thoughts, especially at the start of therapy or when doses are changed. Your doctor may want you to monitor for the following symptoms: anxiety, panic attacks, difficulty in sleeping, irritability, hostility, impulsivity, severe restlessness, and mania (mental and/or physical hyperactivity). These symptoms may be associated with development of worsening symptoms of depression and/or suicidal thoughts or actions. Contact your health care provider if you develop any new or worsening mental health symptoms during treatment with sertraline. Do not stop taking sertraline without first talking to your health care provider.

If you experience any of the following serious side effects, stop taking sertraline and contact your doctor immediately or seek emergency medical treatment: an allergic reaction (difficulty in breathing; closing of the throat; hives; or swelling of the lips, tongue, or face), an irregular heartbeat or pulse, low blood pressure (dizziness, weakness), high blood pressure (severe headache, blurred vision), or chills or fever.

If you experience any of the following less serious side effects, continue taking sertraline and talk to your doctor: headache, tremor, nervousness, anxiety, nausea, diarrhea, dry mouth, changes in appetite or weight, sleepiness or insomnia, decreased sex drive, impotence, or difficulty having an orgasm.

Side effects other than those listed here may also occur. Talk to your doctor about any side effect that seems unusual or that is especially bothersome.

9. Pfizer's Celebrex: an anti-inflammatory

Notify your doctor immediately if you develop side effects including abdominal pain, tenderness, or discomfort; nausea; bloody vomit; bloody, black, or tarry stools; unexplained weight gain; swelling or water retention; fatigue or lethargy; a skin rash; itching; yellowing of the skin or eyes; "flulike" symptoms; or unusual bruising or bleeding. These symptoms could be early signs of dangerous side effects.

Also from *http://www.adrugrecall.com/celebrex/effects.html*:

"Celebrex side effects are serious and life threatening, with reports of death, cardiovascular problems, kidney and liver damages, and ulcers. The Celebrex side effects experienced were the source of criticism by many people that felt the company did its best to minimize the appearance of Celebrex side effects in order to gain an upper hand with competing arthritis drug Vioxx. Within months of its entrance to the U.S. market, Celebrex side effects were reported, accounting for 10 deaths and 11 instances of gastrointestinal hemorrhages.

"The pharmaceutical company pushed for the removal of certain Celebrex side effects warning labels to be removed in order to gain marketing advantages. Celebrex patients immediately responded to Celebrex advertisements that showed the great benefits of the arthritis drug but did not seem to adequately warn of Celebrex side effects. The FDA sent Celebrex maker a letter due to the misrepresentation the agency felt the company was making about Celebrex in its attempts to deter attention away from Celebrex side effects."

10. Pfizer's Neurotonin: treats epilepsy

Side effects include blurred vision or double vision; decreased coordination (clumsiness, unsteadiness, dizziness); continuous, uncontrolled back and forth and/or rolling eye movements; unusual tiredness or weakness (fatigue, drowsiness); persistent sore throat or fever; swelling of hands, ankles, or feet; mental or mood changes (anger, depression, irritability); memory loss; trembling or shaking; severe anxiety; joint pain; difficulty in breathing; or potential links to suicidal behavior. (*http://neurontincase.com/neurontin.htm*)

Author's Note: Any of these symptoms may and often are treated with other medication, possibly leading to, well . . . further side effects.

# SUGGESTED READING

Aeschliman, Michael D. *The Restitution of Man: C. S. Lewis and the Case Against Scientism*. Wm. B. Eerdmans Publishing Company, Grand Rapids, MI: 1998.

Angell, Marcia. *The Truth about the Drug Companies* Reprint edition. New York: Random House Trade Paperbacks, 2005.

Baptiste, Baron. *Journey Into Power: How to Sculpt Your Ideal Body, Free your True Self and Transform your Life with Baptiste Power Vinyasa Yoga*. Cambridge, MA: Baptiste Power Yoga Institute Inc. 2002.

Barge, Fred H. *One Cause, One Cure: The Health & Life Philosophy of Chiropractic*. IA: Barge Chiropractic Publishing, Incorporated, 1996.

Breggin, Peter R. *The Anti-Depressant Fact Book*. New York: Perseus Publishing, 2001.

Brennan, Barbara Ann. *Hands of Light: A Guide to Healing Through the Human Energy Field* Reissue edition. New York: Bantam, 1988.

Bryson, Christopher. *The Fluoride Deception* New Ed edition. New York: Seven Stories Press, 2006.

Capra, Fritjof. *The Hidden Connections*. New York: DoubleDay, 2002.

———. *The Turning Point*. Reissue edition. New York: Bantam, 1984.

Carrington, Patricia. *Learn to Meditate Kit: The Complete Course in Modern Meditation* Bk&Cassett edition. Element Books, 1998.

Chopra, Deepak. *Ageless Body, Timeless Mind* Reissue edition. New York: Harmony, 1994.

———. *Perfect Health*. New York: Three Rivers Press, 2000

———. *Quantum Healing: Exploring the Frontiers of Mind/Body Medicine* Reprint edition. New York: Bantam, 1990.

———. *Restful Sleep*. New York, NY: Three Rivers Press, 1996

Clerc, Olivier. *Modern Medicine: The New World Religion*. Fawnskin, CA: Personhood Press, 2004.

Cohen, Jay S. and Jeremy P. *Over Dose*. New York: Tarcher/Penguin, 2001.

Cohen, Jay S. *What You Must Know About Statin Drugs & Their Natural Alternatives*. Garden City Park, NY: Square One Publishers, 2004.

Corning Creager, Caroline. *Therapeutic exercise Using the Swiss Ball* Reprint edition. Berthoud, CO: Executive Physical Therapy, 1994.

Coulter, H. David. *Anatomy of Hatha Yoga: A Manual for Students, Teachers, and Practitioners*. Honesdale, PA: Body and Breath, 2002.

Demartini, John F. *Count Your Blessings* 1st edition. Carlsbad, California: Hay House, 2006.

———. *The Breakthrough Experience*. Carlsbad, California: Hay House, 2002.

———. *Wisdom of the Oracle*. Authorhouse, 2001.

———. *You Can Have an Amazing Life In Just 60 Days*. Carlsbad, California: Hay House, 2005.

Dement, W.C. and C. Vaughn. *The Promise of Sleep*. New York: Dell, 2000)

Dyer, Wayne W. *Manifest Your Destiny* Reprint edition. New York: HarperTorch, 1999.

———. *Meditations for Manifesting* Audio CD. Carlsbad, California: Hay House Audio Books,

Epstein, Donald M. *The Twelve Stages of Healing*. San Rafael, CA: Amber-Allen Publishing, 1994

Fontana, David. *Learn to Meditate: A Practical Guide to Self-Discovery and Fulfillment*. San Francisco, CA: Chronicle Books, 1999.

Grant-Williams, Renee. *Voice Power: Using Your Voice to Captivate, Persuade, and Command Attention* 1st edition. New York: AMACOM/American Management Association, 2002.

Hauri, Peter and Linde, Shirley. *No More Sleepless Nights* 2nd edition. Hoboken, NJ: John Wiley and Sons, Inc., 1996

Hawkins, David R. *Power vs. Force: The Hidden Determinants of Human Behavior*. Carlsbad, California: Hay House, 2002.

Hay, Louise. *Heal Your Body* 4th edition. Carlsbad, California: Hay House, 1984.

———. *You Can Heal Your Life* Gift edition. Carlsbad, California: Hay House, 1999.

Hill, Napoleon. *Think and Grow Rich* Reissue edition. New York: Ballantine Books, 1987.

Holmes, Ernest. *The Science of Mind* Reprint edition. New York: Tarcher, 1998.

Institute of Medicine. *To Err is Human*. Washington, DC: National Academies Press; 1st edition, 2000.

Kaufman, Francine. *Diabesity* Reprint edition. New York: Bantam, 2006.

Le Fanu, James. *The Rise and Fall of Modern Medicine* Reprint edition. New York: Carroll & Graf Publishers, 2002.

Lewis, Thomas. *The Medusa and the Snail*. New York: Penguin Books, 1995

Margolis, Joeseph. *The Unraveling of Scientism: American Philosophy at the End of the 20th Century*. Ithaca, NY: Cornell university press, 2003.

Matzer Rose, Marla. *Muscle Beach: Where the best Bodies in the World started a fitness revolution*. Los Angeles: L.A. Weekly Books, 2001.

Mayer, Ernst. *What Evolution Is* Reprint edition. Jackson, TN: Basic Books, 2002.

McArdle, William D. *Exercise Physiology: Energy, Nutrition, and Human Performance* 5th edition. New York: Lippincott Williams & Wilkin, 2001.

McGee, Charles T. *Heart Frauds: Uncovering the Biggest Health Scam in History*. Colorado Springs, CO: Piccadilly Books, 2001.

Mercola, Dr. Joeseph. *Dr. Mercola's Total Health Program*. Schaumburg, IL: Mercola.com, 2003.

Murphy, Joeseph and McMahon. *The Power of the Subconscious Mind* Revised edition. New York: Bantam, 2001.

Nat Hanh, Thich. *The Miracle of Mindfulness*. Boston, MA: Beacon Press, 1999.

Pierpaoli, Walter. *The Melatonin Miracle*, Reprint edition. New York: Pocket Books, 1996

Pilzer, Paul Zane. *The Wellness Revolution*. Hoboken, NJ: Wiley; New edition, 2003.

Ram Dass. *Paths to God* Reprint edition. New York: Three Rivers Press, 2005.

Rav Berg. *Kabbalah To the Power of One* English edition. Richmond Hill, NY: Research Centre of Kabbalah, 1991.

Ravnskov, Uffe. *The Cholesterol Myths*. Winona Lake, IN: New Trends Publishing, Inc., 2000.

Reiter, Russel J. and Jo Robinson. *Your Body's Natural Wonder Drug—Melatonin*. New York: Bantam, 1995.

Rinpoche, Sogyal. *The Tibetan Book of Living and Dying* Reprint edition. San Francisco: Harper, 1994.

Rondberg, Terry A. *Chiropractic First*. Chandler, AZ: Chiropractic Journal, 1996.

———. *Under the Influence of Modern Medicine*. Chandler, AZ: Chiropractic Journal, 1998.

Rosen, Richard. *The Yoga of Breath* 1st edition. Boston, MA: Shambhala, 2002.

Rosencwaig, R. and Hasnain Walji. *The Melatonin and Aging Source Book*. Hohm Press, 1997.

Rosenthal, Marilyn M. and Kathleen M. Sutcliffe. *Medical Error: What Do We Know? What Do We Do?* 1st edition. San Francisco, CA: Jossey-Bass, 2002.

Rovell, Darren. *First in Thirst: How Gatorade Turned the Science of Sweat into a Cultural Phenomenon*. New York: AMACOM, 2005.

Sagan, Carl. *Billions and Billions: Thoughts on Life and Death at the Brink of the Millennium* Reprint edition. New York: Ballantine Books, 1998.

Schlosser, Eric. *Fast Food Nation*. New York: Harper Perennial; Reprint edition, 2002.

Smolensky, M. and L. Lamberg. *The Body Clock Guide to Better Health* 2nd Rep edition. New York: Owl Books, 2001.

Strauss, Joeseph B. *Chiropractic Philosophy* 3rd edition. Levittown, PA: Foundation for the Advancement of Chiropractic Education,1994.

        . *Enhance Your Life Experience*. Levittown, PA: F.A.C.E, 1996.

Tan, Zaldy. *Age Proof Your Mind*. New York: Grand Central Publishing, 2005.

Tarnas, Richard. *The Passion of the Western Mind* 1st Ballantine Books ed. New York: Ballantine Books, 1993.

Tolle, Eckhart. *The Power of Now* Reprint edition. Novato, CA: New World Library, 2004.

Vella, Mark. *Anatomy for Strength and Fitness Training* 1st edition. New York: McGraw-Hill, 2006.

Weil, Andrew. *Healthy Aging*. New York: Knopf Publishing Group, 2005.

Wilk, Chester A. *Medicine, Monopolies, and Malice*. New Hyde Park, NY: Avery Publishing Group, 1996.

Yogi Ramacharaka. *The Science of Breath*. Chicago, IL: Yoga Publication Society, 1940.

Zukav, Gary. *The Dancing Wu Li Masters: An Overview of the New Physics*. New York: Harper Perennial Modern Classics, 2001.

        . *The Seat of the Soul* Reprint edition. Old Tappan, NJ: Free Press, 1990.

# ABOUT THE AUTHOR

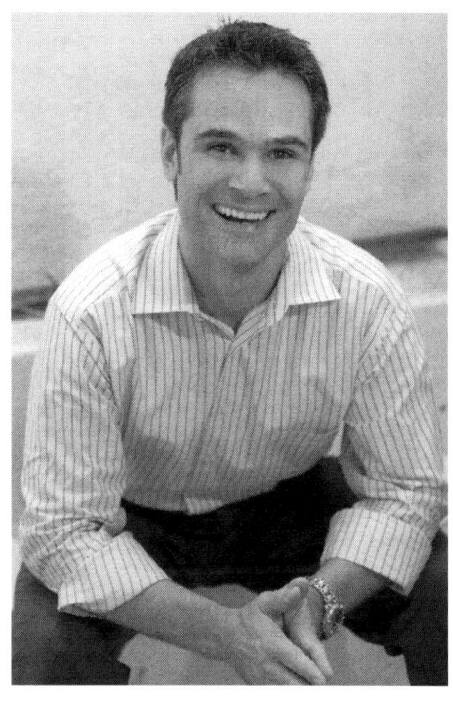

DR. NICOLAS CAMPOS is a noted health expert, researcher, clinical chiropractic sports physician, molecular biologist, devoted yogi, and health lecturer. He was born in San Francisco on December 26, 1967. Maybe it was the influence of the city's various countercultures, or maybe San Francisco just had a way of producing people who are different, but Dr. Campos could never be called a conformist. This is especially true regarding his philosophy on health. His views on health have been shaped by Western and Eastern philosophies, scientific thought, yogic principles, new age spiritualism, and modern-day mind-body theories.

Nicolas was fortunate to have a mother whose enthusiasm for health was readily passed on to her children. They watched Jack LaLanne, enjoyed "health foods", took daily doses of vitamins, and had regular chiropractic care. Nicolas was shocked years later when he discovered that these practices were not common to everyone but instead considered "on the fringe".

Always rebellious, Nicolas turned away from the healthy lifestyle of his family and entered into the world of drugs and alcohol. What started out as a kick and an attempt to forge an identity eventually became a full-fledged disorder. Alcohol and narcotic addiction, trouble with the law, and a twenty-year cigarette habit were all sitting on top of his list of early accomplishments. It took a near brush with death to snap Nicolas out of his self-destructive behaviors. As it turned out, it was precisely what he needed to turn his life around.

A high school dropout, Nicolas returned to school to receive his bachelor of arts degree from the University of California-Berkeley in molecular and cell biology. Nicolas completed the program with an emphasis in the rapidly developing field of immunology. It was during this period, particularly as he studied premedical courses, that he first became aware of the inconsistency between the modern medical paradigm and health.

Nicolas earned his doctorate degree in chiropractic in 2000. The field of chiropractic was a perfect fit for him as it allowed him to pursue his continued interest in human health while remaining consistent with his philosophy that health is a birthright, and only through meticulous care may it flourish. He was also able to incorporate his love of athletics by earning a postgraduate degree in sports chiropractic from the American Chiropractic Board of Sports Physicians in 2002.

Dr. Campos practices in West Hollywood, California, bringing a unique approach to caring for his clientele. He encourages all his patients to embark on a regimen of good health by following the principles outlined in his book *The Six Keys to Optimal Health*. Understanding the need to act as a role model, Dr. Campos practices what he preaches, making the *six keys* an integral part of his lifestyle. He feels fortunate to have the opportunity to influence and guide so many people through his work, and he is especially thrilled to be the chiropractor of choice for a large number of professional dancers—his absolute favorite athletes.

The doctor's current projects include an interactive Web site, http://*www. drnickcampos.com*, monthly health articles, podcasts, and a fun and informative blog, *http://6keysoptimalhealth.blogspot.com/*. A dynamic speaker, Dr. Campos, spends his time speaking to audiences about health, wellness, and personal empowerment; tools that allow people to reach their highest potential.

Dr. Campos spends his spare time reading and writing—that is, when he is not playing with his family, practicing yoga, working out at the gym, playing basketball, or running with his dogs. His interests range from sports to history to business; but his real passions are science, philosophy, spirituality, and the mysteries of the universe. His favorite authors and two greatest influences are Dr. John F. Demartini and Dr. Fritjof Capra—both having inspired the philosophy that is the basis for his current book.

Dr. Campos uses his work to motivate and educate people from all over the world. He is dedicated to promoting a new planetary wellness paradigm, which he calls the Personal Responsibility in Health Movement. Dr. Campos uses ancient wisdom and modern-day perspectives to inspire and motivate people to adopt the healthy behaviors that will lead them to make wellness one of their highest priority values.

# ENDNOTES

## Chapter 1

[1] The World Health Report 2000—Health systems: Improving performance. Published by the World Health Organization, Geneva, Switzerland (http://www.who.int/whr/2000/en/whr00_en.pdf) Site visited: March 17, 2006.

[2] Preamble to the Constitution of the World Health Organization as adopted by the International Health Conference, New York, 19-22 June, 1946; signed on 22 July 1946 by the representatives of 61 States (Official Records of the World Health Organization, no. 2, p. 100) and entered into force on 7 April 1948.

[3] The American Association for the Advancement of Science Web site, AAAS News Archives, Experts at AAAS Briefing Mull the Outer Limits of the Human Lifespan, February 18, 2006, (http://www.aaas.org/news/releases/2006/0218ageing.shtml), Site visited: March 24, 2006

[4] Capra, F. *The Turning Point* Reissue edition. New York: Bantam, 1984

[5] Strauss, J. Chiropractic Philosophy, Foundation for the Advancement of Chiropractic Education, 3rd Edition, 1994

[6] Tarnas, R, The Passion of the Western Mind, Ballantine Publishing Group, 1991

[7] Mes, D., Wharton Journal, Published Monday, October 4, 2004 (http://www.whartonjournal.com/news/2004/10/04/Perspectives/The-Best.Healthcare.System.In.The.World-740101.shtml), Site visited 1-24-05.

[8] Starfield, B., Is US Health Really The Best In The World?, JAMA. 2000 Jul 26;284(4):483-5.

[9] Health Grades Quality Study, Patient Safety in American Hospitals, July 2004, article can be found at: (http://www.healthgrades.com/media/english/pdf/HG_Patient_Safety_Study_Final.pdf), Site visited: April 16, 2006.

[10] Dr. Joseph Mercola's Web site, (.http://www.mercola.com/2004/jul/7/healthcare_death.htm) site visited: April 9, 2007. This article was provided free from www.mercola.com, subscribe now for the free eHealthy News You Can Use.

[11] Starfield, B., Is US Health Really The Best In The World?, JAMA. 2000 Jul 26;284(4):483-5.

[12] Starfield, B. Is US health really best in the world?, JAMA. 2000 Jul 26;284(4):483-5

[13] U.S. Department of Justice Web site, Press Release, Two Doctors Indicted In 'Rent-A-Patient' Scheme That Billed Insurance Companies For Unnecessary Surgeries,

Los Angeles, CA, October 12, 2005, (http://www.usdoj.gov/usao/cac/pr2005/143.html), Site visited: April 7, 2006.

[14]  Protocare Sciences, Prepared for California Health Care Foundation, Addressing Medication Errors in Hospitals, article can be found at: http://www.chcf.org/documents/hospitals/addressingmederrorsframework.pdf), Site visited: January 24, 2005.

[15]  WrongDiagnosis.com, Unknown Author, Statistics About Nosocomial Infections, Information compiled from CDC/NNIS 1992, (http://www.wrongdiagnosis.com/n/nosocomial_infections/stats.htm), Site visited: April 16, 2006.

[16]  Starfield, B., Is US Health Really The Best In The World?, JAMA. 2000 Jul 26;284(4):483-5.

[17]  Washington Monthly Web site, Longman, PJ, The Health of Nations, April 2003 (http://www.washingtonmonthly.com/features/2003/0304.longman.html), Site updated: April 2003, Site visited: March 24, 2006.

[18]  The National Academies Press Web site, Curry, SJ, et al, Fulfilling the Potential of Cancer Prevention and Early Detection, National Cancer Policy Board, Institute of Medicine, National Academies Press, 2003, (http://darwin.nap.edu/books/0309082544/html/R1.html), Site visited: March 24, 2006.

[19]  Harvard School of Public Health Web site, Sacks, F., The Worldwide Obesity Epidemic, (http://www.hsph.harvard.edu/symposium/sacks_files/v3_document.htm), Site visited: April 7, 2006.

[20]  Center for Disease Control Web site, Ogden, C.L., et al., Mean Body Weight, Height, and Body Mass Index, United States1960-2002, Advance Data From Vital Health Statistics, Number 347, October 27, 2004,(http://usgovinfo.about.com/gi/dynamic/offsite.htm?zi=1/XJ&sdn=usgovinfo&zu=http%3A%2F%2Fwww.cdc.gov%2Fnchs%2Fdata%2Fad%2Fad347.pdf), Site visited 1/24/05.

[21]  Centers for Disease Control Web site, National Center for Health Statistics, Prevalence of Overweight and Obesity Among Adults: United States, 1999-2002, (http://www.cdc.gov/nchs/products/pubs/pubd/hestats/obese/obse99.htm), Site update: 12/16/04 Site visited: 1/24/05.

[22]  Plastic Surgery Research.info Web site, Cosmetic Plastic Surgery Research Statistics and Trends for 2001, 2002 and 2003, (http://www.cosmeticplasticsurgerystatistics.com/statistics.html), Site visited 1/25/05.

## Chapter 2

[23]  Beyond Vegetarianism Web site (http://www.beyondveg.com/nicholson-w/hb/hb-interview1c.shtml#anatomically%20modern) Site Visited: February 28, 2005

[24]  Centers for Disease Control Web site, (http://www.cdc.gov/nccdphp/dnpa/obesity/defining.htm), Site updated: 6/25/04, Site visited: 3/12/05

[25]  McDonald's Web site, (http://www.mcdonalds.com/), Site updated: 3/11/05, Site visited:3/12/05

[26]  McDonald's Web site, (http://www.mcdonalds.com/app_controller.nutrition.index1. html), Site updated: 3/11/05, Site visited: 3/12/05

[27]  CNN Web site, (http://www.cnn.com/2004/US/03/02/mcdonalds.supersize. ap/), Wednesday, March 3, 2004 Posted: 2:15 AM EST (0715 GMT), Site visited:3/12/05

[28]  McDonald's Web site, (http://www.mcdonalds.com/app_controller.nutrition.index1. html), Site updated: 3/21/05, Site visited: 3/21/05

[29]  BusinessWeek online, (http://businessweek.com/magazine/content/04_20/b3883099. htm), Posted: May 17, 2004, Site visited: 3/12/05

[30]  The Beverage Network Web site for the beverage industry, (http://www.bevnet. com/news/2002/03-01-2002-softdrink.asp), Posted: 3/1/2002, Site visited: 3/12/05

[31]  Bray, G.A., Nielsen, S.J., and Popkin, B.M., Consumption of high-fructose corn syrup in beverages may play a role in the epidemic of obesity, American Journal of Clinical Nutrition, Vol. 79, No. 4, 537-543, April 2004

[32]  wasingtonpost.com, Sweet but Not So Innocent, (http://www.washingtonpost. com/ac2/wp-dyn/A8003-2003Mar10?language=printer), Posted: March 11, 2003, Site visited: 3/12/05

[33]  The Beverage Network Web site for the beverage industry, (http://www.bevnet. com/news/2002/03-01-2002-softdrink.asp), Posted: 3/1/2002, Site visited: 3/12/05

[34]  Bray, G.A., Nielsen, S.J., and Popkin, B.M., Consumption of high-fructose corn syrup in beverages may play a role in the epidemic of obesity, American Journal of Clinical Nutrition, Vol. 79, No. 4, 537-543, April 2004

[35]  Hollenbeck, C.B., Dietary fructose effects on lipoprotein metabolism and risk for coronary artery disease, American Journal of Clinical Nutrition, Vol 58, 800S-809S Copyright © 1993 by The American Society for Clinical Nutrition, Inc

[36]  Bray, G.A., Nielsen, S.J., and Popkin, B.M., Consumption of high-fructose corn syrup in beverages may play a role in the epidemic of obesity, American Journal of Clinical Nutrition, Vol. 79, No. 4, 537-543, April 2004

[37]  Mathematica Policy Research, Inc. Web site, (http://www.mathematica-mpr. com/nutrition/FITS-January%202004.ppt#14), Site visited: 3/12/05

[38]  Schlosser, E. Fast Food Nation, HarperCollins, 2002.

[39]  Findarticles.com, US trade surplus in processed foods expected to continue, Food Review, May-Aug 1996, (http://www.findarticles.com/p/articles/mi_m3765/ is_n2_v18/ai_18509722) Site visited: 3/26/05

[40]  University of Sydney Web site, (http://www.econ.usyd.edu.au/drawingboard/ digest/0406/mcilwain.html) McIlwain, D., Can the Science of Love Catch up with Common Sense?, 14 June 2004, Site Visited: 3/28/05,

41   Center for Science in the Public Interest Web site, Public Health Reports, January/ February 2000, Vol. 115, (http://www.cspinet.org/reports/obesity.pdf) Site visited: 3/13/05

42   Purdue University Web site, Better Soil, Better Yields, Conservation Technology Information Center 2001, (http://www.ctic.purdue.edu/CTIC/Better%20Soil%20B etter%20Yields.pdf) 2001, Site visited: 4/10/05

43   Mahan, L.K. and Escott-Stump, S., Krause's Food, Nutrition, and Diet Therapy, 9th Ed., p. 50, W.B. Saunders Co. 1996

44   University of Maryland Medical Center Web site, (http://www.umm.edu/altmed/ ConsSupplements/Omega3FattyAcidscs.html) site updated: April 2002, site visited: May 6, 2005.

45   Dr. Joseph Mercola's Web site, (http://www.mercola.com/2001/sep/8/omega_3.htm) site visited: May 9, 2005. This article was provided free from www.mercola.com, subscribe now for the free eHealthy News You Can Use.

46   English, J., Do Your Antioxidants Suppress Enough Free Radicals?, Life Extension magazine, Feb. 2005, p. 22.

47   National Institute of Health Web site, Office of Dietary Supplements, (http://ods. od.nih.gov/factsheets/selenium.asp) Site visited: May 20, 2005.

48   English, J., R-Dihydro-Lipoic Acid, Life Extension magazine, Feb. 2005, p. 66.

49   English, J., R-Dihydro-Lipoic Acid, Life Extension magazine, Feb. 2005, p. 68.

50   English, J., R-Dihydro-Lipoic Acid, Life Extension magazine, Feb. 2005, pp. 69-70.

51   BBC news Web site, ( http://news.bbc.co.uk/1/hi/health/1484659.stm), Aug. 12, 2001, Site visited:5/21/05

52   Guyton, A.C., Hall, J.E. Textbook of Medical Physiology, pp. 892-893, W B Saunders Co; 9th edition January 15, 1996

53   American Federation for Aging Research Web site, (http://www.infoaging.org/b-cal-home.html), published: November 1, 2000, updated and reviewed: July 8, 2003, update reviewed by: Charles Mobbs, Ph.D., Site visited: May 22, 2005.

54   Society for Neuroscience Web site, (http://apu.sfn.org/content/Publications/Brain Briefings/caloricrestriction.html), published: July 2001, Site visited: May 22, 2005.

55   Dr. Joseph Mercola's Web site, ( http://www.mercola.com/article/sugar/dangers_ of_sugar.htm) site visited: May 22, 2005. This article was provided free from www. mercola.com, subscribe now for the free eHealthy News You Can Use.

56   Diabetes Health Magazine Web site, Hypoglycemia—What Every Person on Insulin Should Know, July 1997, (http://www.diabeteshealth.com/read,1023,878.html) Site visited: May 22, 2005.

57   The Anaesthesia Education Web site, Fluid Physiology, Ch. 2—Fluid Compartments, (http://www.anaesthesiamcq.com/FluidBook/fl2_1.php), Site visited: May 27, 2005.

[58] Mayo Clinic Web site, Dehydration, ( http://www.mayoclinic.com/invoke. cfm?id=DS00561) site updated: January 31, 2005, site visited: May 27, 2005.

[59] Andersen, G.D., Nutrition, Basic Sports Injuries, SCU Postgraduate Division, p. 96

[60] Andersen, G.D. Understanding Fluid, Electrolyte, And Carbohydrate Replacement During Activity, Natural Medicine Journal, Vol. 1, Number 9, November 1998, p. 18.

[61] 7online.com, Study: One in Five Americans Now 'Extremely Obese', (http://abclocal. go.com/wabc/news/health/wabc_101403_obesity.html) New York-WABC, October 14, 2003, Site visited: May 28, 2005.

# Chapter 3

[62] Tipton, CM, Contemporary exercise physiology: fifty years after the closure of Harvard Fatigue Laboratory, Exerc Sport Sci Rev. 1998;26:315-39.

[63] Northern Arizona University Web site, History of Exercise Science, Dr. Pauline Entin Department of Exercise Science and Athletic Training, (http://jan.ucc.nau. edu/~pe/exs190web/exs190history.htm), Site updated: Spring 2005, Site visited: June 20, 2005.

[64] University of New Mexico Web site, The History of Fitness, Lance C. Dalleck, M.S. and Len Kravitz, Ph.D., (http://www.unm.edu/~lkravitz/Article%20folder/history. html), Site visited: June 20, 2005.

[65] University of New Mexico Web site, The History of Fitness, Lance C. Dalleck, M.S. and Len Kravitz, Ph.D., (http://www.unm.edu/~lkravitz/Article%20folder/history. html), Site visited: June 20, 2005.

[66] Ariel Dynamics Worldwide Web site, Optimization of Human Performance for All Ages, (http://www.arielnet.com/Main/adw-26.html), Site visited: June 20, 2005.

[67] International Health, Racquet, and Sportsclub Association Web site, U.S. Health Club Numbers Continue To Climb (http://www.ihrsa.org/pressinfo/pressreleases/02_01_ 22.html) Site visited: June 24, 2005

[68] Healthy People 2010 Web site, ( http://www.healthypeople.gov/) Site visited: June 24, 2005.

[69] Maritz Research Web site, Let's Get Physical: More Than Half Of Americans Claim To Exercise Regularly, Maritz Poll, ( http://www.maritzresearch.com/release. asp?rc=189&p=1&T=P) Site updated: February 2000, Site visited: June 24, 2005.

[70] Olivardia, R., et al, Muscle dysmorphia in male weightlifters: a case-control study. Am J Psychiatry. 2000 Aug;157(8):1291-6

[71] Masters Athlete Physiology and Performance Web site, Training Adaptations in Skeletal Muscle, (http://home.hia.no/~stephens/mustrn.htm), Site updated: 2005, Site visited: June 26, 2005.

72    Guyton, A.C., Hall, J.E., Textbook of Medical Physiology, 9th Ed. W.B. Saunders Co., 1996, p. 1061

73    Masters Athlete Physiology and Performance Web site, Strength Training and Endurance Performance, (http://home.hia.no/~stephens/str&end.htm), Site updated: 2005, Site visited: June 30, 2005.

74    Obgyn.net, Death is more likely to occur sooner than later after osteoporotic fracture, Osteoporosis, March 4, 2004, ( http://www.obgyn.net/newsheadlines/womens_health-Osteoporosis-20040304-126.asp), Site visited: June 30, 2005.

75    American Academy of Orthopedic Surgeon's Web site, Deep Vein Thrombosis, (http://orthoinfo.aaos.org/fact/thr_report.cfm?Thread_ID=264&topcategory=Knee), Site updated: June 2001, Site visited: July 3, 2005.

76    Christopher, S.D., et. al., Hyponatremia among Runners in the Boston Marathon, New England Journal of Medicine, Vol. 352:1550-1556, Num 15, April 14, 2005.

77    Guyton, A.C., Hall, J.E., Textbook of Medical Physiology, 9th Ed. W.B. Saunders Co., 1996, p. 84

78    Dr Nick Campos' Web site, Investigating Yoga—The Truths Behind an Ancient Practice—An Interview with Arun Deva, ( http://www.drnickcampos.com/health-newsletter/investigating-yoga.html), July 2004. Site visited: July 4, 2005.

79    Yoga Journal Web site, Lee, C., FAQ page, Site updated: 2002, Site visited: July 3, 2005

80    Dr Nick Campos' Web site, Investigating Yoga—The Truths Behind an Ancient Practice—An Interview with Arun Deva, ( http://www.drnickcampos.com/health-newsletter/investigating-yoga.html), July 2004. Site visited: July 4, 2005.

81    Life Extension Foundation Web site, Kahn, C., The Growing Impact of Growth Hormone, (http://search.lef.org/src-cgi-bin/MsmGo.exe?grab_id=21&EXTRA_ARG=&CFGNAME=MssFind%2Ecfg&host_id=42&page_id=9700096&query=%22hgh%22&hiword=GROWTH+HORMONE+hgh+GROWTH+HORMONE+), Site visited: July 4, 2005.

82    Khansari, D.N. and Gustad, T., Effects of long-term, low-dose growth hormone therapy on immune function and life expectancy of mice, Mechanisms of Ageing and Development 1991;57:87-100.

83    Weintraub, A., Selling the Promise of Youth, BusinessWeek, March 20, 2006

84    Mayo Clinic Web site, How to Keep Your Mind Sharp: Preventive Action, Site updated: April 29, 2005, Site visited: July 8, 2005.

85    The President's Council on Physical Fitness and Sports Web site, Landers, D.M., The Influence of Exercise on Mental Health, (http://fitness.gov/mentalhealth.htm), Series 2, Number 12, Dec. 1997, Site visited: July 9, 2005.

86    The President's Council on Physical Fitness and Sports Web site, Landers, D.M., The Influence of Exercise on Mental Health, (http://fitness.gov/mentalhealth.htm), Series 2, Number 12, Dec. 1997, Site visited: July 9, 2005.

[87]    The President's Council on Physical Fitness and Sports Web site, Landers, D.M., The Influence of Exercise on Mental Health, (http://fitness.gov/mentalhealth.htm), Series 2, Number 12, Dec. 1997, Site visited: July 9, 2005.

[88]    University of Bristol Web site, School of Chemistry, Millward, J., A Chocolate Composition, Phenylethylamine, (http://www.chm.bris.ac.uk/webprojects2001/millward/phenylethylamine.htm) Site visited: July 9, 2005.

[89]    Sabelli, H., et al, Sustained antidepressant effect of PEA replacement, *Neuropsychiatry Clin Neurosci*, 1996 Spr, 8:2, 168-71.

[90]    University of Bristol Web site, School of Chemistry, Millward, J., A Chocolate Composition, Phenylethylamine, (http://www.chm.bris.ac.uk/webprojects2001/millward/phenylethylamine.htm) Site visited: July 9, 2005.

[91]    Szabo, A., et al, Phenylethylamine, a possible link to the antidepressant effects of exercise?, *Br J Sports Med* 2001 Oct;35(5):342-3

# Chapter 4

[92]    Capra, F. *The Turning Point* Reissue edition. New York: Bantam, 1984.

[93]    The University of Cambridge Web site, The History of Massage, C.U Massage Society, (http://www.cam.ac.uk/societies/cumass/html/history.htm), Site visited: May 22, 2006.

[94]    National Center for Complimentary and Alternative Medicine Web site (http://nccam.nih.gov/health/chiropractic/index.htm) National Institute of Health, Last Updated: Feb 05, 2004, Site visited: February 8, 2005.

[95]    Apkarian, A.V., Sosa, Y., Sonty, S., Levy, R., Harden, R., Parrish, T. and Gitelman, D. Chronic Back Pain Is Associated with Decreased Prefrontal and Thalamic Gray Matter Density, The Journal of Neuroscience, November 17, 2004, 24(46):10410-10415; doi:10.1523/JNEUROSCI.2541-04.2004

[96]    The Orthoteers Orthopaedic Education Resource Web site (http://www.orthoteers.co.uk/Nrujp~ij33lm/Orthartcartlub.htm) Last updated: Nov 1, 2004, Site visited: February 9, 2005

[97]    A. J. Lipowitz and C. D. Newton, Degenerative Joint Disease and Traumatic Arthritis, International Veterinary Information Service Web site, 1985; B0088.0685 (http://www.ivis.org/special_books/ortho/chapter_87/87mast.asp#refs ) Last updated: 1/1/85, Site visited: 2/9/05

[98]    Nordin, M., Frankel, V. Basic Biomechanics of the Musculoskeletal System, Lea & Febiger, 2nd edition, 1989

[99]    Spine-health.com (http://www.spine-health.com/topics/cd/depression/depression01.html) Last updated: 2/9/05, Site visited: 2/9/05

[100]   Leach, R.A. The Chiropractic Theories, 3rd Edition (p. 111), Williams and /Wilkins, 1994

[101]   Guyton, A.C., Hall, J.E. Textbook of Medical Physiology, W B Saunders Co; 9th edition January 15, 1996

[102]   American Chiropractic Association Web site, History of Chiropractic Care, (http://www.acatoday.com/level2_css.cfm?T1ID=13&T2ID=62), Site visited: May 28, 2006.

[103]   Wardwell, W.I., Chiropractic: History and Evolution of a New Profession, Mosby, Inc. 1992

[104]   Wilk, C.A., Medicine, Monopolies, and Malice: How the Medical Establishment Tried to Destroy Chiropractic in the U.S., Avery Publishing, June 1996.

[105]   Inadvertent clavicular fractures caused by "chiropractic" manipulations in an infant: an unusual form of pseudoabuse. Sperry K, Pfalzgraf R., J Forensic Sci. 1990 Sep; 35(5):1211-6.

[106]   The appropriateness of manipulation and mobilization of the cervical spine. Santa Monica, CA: RAND Corporation 1996: xiv

[107]   Dynamic Chiropractic Web site, (http://www.chiroweb.com/archives/12/06/25.html) Site updated: January 31, 2005, Site visited: February 14, 2005.

[108]   Foundation for Chiropractic Education and Research (FCER) Web site, (http://www.fcer.org/html/Research/institutions.htm) Site visited 2/14/05

[109]   Meade TW; Dyer S; Browne W; Townsend J; Frank AO, Low back pain of mechanical origin: randomized comparison of chiropractic and hospital outpatient treatment, British Medical Journal 1990 Jun 2;300(6737):1431-7

[110]   Meade TW; Dyer S; Browne W; Frank AO, Randomised comparison of chiropractic and hospital outpatient management for low back pain: results from extended follow up, British Medical Journal 1995 Aug 5;311(7001):349-51

[111]   Cherkin DC; MacCornack FA, Patient evaluations of low back pain care from family physicians and chiropractors, Western Journal of Medicine 1989 Mar;150(3):351-5

[112]   Stano M; Smith M, Chiropractic and medical costs of low back care, Medical Care 1996 Mar;34(3):191-204

[113]   Wilk, C.A., Medicine, Monopolies, and Malice, Published by Chester A. Wilk, 1996.

[114]   Dynamic Chiropractic Web site, Taken from Schwarzenegger speeches to International Chiropractic Association Symposium, (http://www.chiroweb.com/arnold/schwarzenegger.html), Site updated: February 1, 2005, Site visited: February 14, 2005

[115]   Planet Chiropractic, ( http://www.planetc1.com/cgi-bin/n/v.cgi?id=964447489) Site visited: February 14, 2005

[116]   Dr. Phil Show, aired Wednesday, February 11, 2004

[117]   CNN.com ( http://www.cnn.com/CNN/Programs/people/shows/madonna/profile.html) 2004 Cable News Network LP, LLLP., Site visited: February 14, 2005

118    Dynamic Chiropractic Web site, Taken from interview with Emmitt Smith in Dallas Morning News, ( http://www.chiroweb.com/archives/21/01/15.html), Site updated: February 14, 2005, Site visited: February 14, 2005

119    Dynamic Chiropractic Web site, ( http://www.chiroweb.com/archives/13/02/11.html), Site updated: February 14, 2005, Site visited: February 14, 2005

120    Spineguys Web site, (http://www.spineguys.com/newsletter/05142003.asp), Site visited: February 14, 2005.

# Chapter 5

121    MayoClinic.com, Author unknown, Sleep: Your body's means of rejuvenation, July 6, 2004, (http://www.mayoclinic.com/health/sleep/SL00002), Site visited: April 16, 2006.

122    Serendipity Web site, Miller, R.M., Sleep, 1998, Site visited: April 16, 2006.

123    National Naval Medical Center Web site, Molinaro, LCDR J.D., DC, USN, Sleep Disturbances and Its Effect on Stress and Healing, February, 2001, (http://www. bethesda.med.navy.mil/careers/postgraduate_dental_school/comprehensive_ dentistry/pearls/Pearlsd9.htm), Site visited: April 16, 2006

124    BBCco.uk Web site, Tighe, J., Sleep Deprivation, June 2000, (http://www.bbc. co.uk/health/conditions/mental_health/coping_sleep.shtml), Site updated: Oct. 2005, Site visited: April 16, 2006.

125    National Space Biomedical Research Institute Web site, Mullington, J.M., Sustained Partial Sleep Deprivation: Effects on Immune Modulation and Growth Factors, Harvard Medical School, 1997-1998, (http://www.nsbri.org/Research/Projects/ viewsummary.epl?pid=94), Site visited: April 16, 2006.

126    National Institute of Neurological Disorders and Stroke, Author Unknown, Brain Basics, Understanding Sleep, What Does Sleep Do For Us?, (http://www.ninds.nih. gov/disorders/brain_basics/understanding_sleep_brain_basic_pr.htm) Site updated: December, 8, 2005, Site visited: April 16, 2006.

127    Born, J., Memory Formation in Sleep: Giving a Wave to Dreams, Department of Clinical Neuroendocrinology, University of Lübeck, Germany, Neuropsychobiology 2001;44:212-214 (DOI: 10.1159/000054944)

128    Mednick S, Nakayama K, and Stickgold R., Sleep-dependent learning: a nap is as good as a night. Nat Neurosci. 2003 Jul;6(7):697-8.

129    National Institute of Neurological Disorders and Stroke, Author Unknown, Brain Basics, Understanding Sleep, Sleep Disorders, ( http://www.ninds.nih.gov/disorders/ sleep_apnea/detail_sleep_apnea.htm) Site updated: January 25, 2006, Site visited: April 16, 2006.

[130] National Sleep Foundation Web site, Insomnia, (http://www.sleepfoundation.
org/sleeptionary/index.php?id=19) Site updated: March 28, 2005, Site visited: July
6, 2005.

[131] WebMD.com, Breus, M., MD, Sleep: More Important Than You Think, Chronic
Sleep Deprivation May Harm Health, May 2003, (http://my.webmd.com/content/
article/64/72426.htm), Site updated: March 15, 2006, Site visited: April 16, 2006.

[132] WebMD Health Web site, DeNoon, D., Ambien Linked to Sleep Eating, March 15,
2006, Site visited: April 21, 2006.

[133] Kirn, W., Sleep Is For Sissies, Time Magazine, December 20, 2004

[134] Duke University Web site, News and Communications, Lawrence K., The 'Scheduling'
Story That Became a 'Sleep Deprivation' Story, April 20, 2004, (http://www.
dukenews.duke.edu/news/story_0404.html), Site visited: April 16, 2006.

[135] National Review Online, Cheaney, J.B., Literary Malaise Jimmy Carter's leadership
inabilities between novel covers, December 8, 2003, (http://www.nationalreview.
com/comment/cheaney200312080932.asp), Site visited: April 16, 2006.

# Chapter 6

[136] University of North Texas Web site, Kennerly, R.C., A Brief History of the Origins
of Behavioral Medicine, (http://www.unt.edu/bmed/abrief.htm#top%20of%20inde
x%20page), Site updated: 2002, Site visited: August 4, 2005.

[137] University of North Texas Web site, Kennerly, R.C., A Brief History of the Origins
of Behavioral Medicine, (http://www.unt.edu/bmed/abrief.htm#top%20of%20inde
x%20page), Site updated: 2002, Site visited: August 4, 2005.

[138] Tarnas, R. The Passion of the Western Mind, Ballantine Books, 1991, p. 302

[139] Tarnas, R. The Passion of the Western Mind, Ballantine Books, 1991, p. 267

[140] University of North Texas Web site, Kennerly, R.C., A Brief History of the Origins
of Behavioral Medicine, (http://www.unt.edu/bmed/abrief.htm#top%20of%20inde
x%20page), Site updated: 2002, Site visited: August 4, 2005.

[141] Engel, G.L. The need for a new medical model: a challenge for biomedicine 1977,
Science 196:129-36.

[142] Collinge, W., PhD. The American Holistic Health Association Complete Guide to
Alternative Medicine, Warner Books, 1997.

[143] National Center for Complimentary and Alternative Medicine Web site, (http://nccam.
nih.gov/about/aboutnccam/index.htm), Site updated: June 9, 2005, Site visited:
August 8, 2005.

[144] Breggin, M.D., PR, The Anti-Depressant Fact Book, Perseus Publishing, 2001

[145] National Institute of Mental Health Web site, Depression, (http://www.nimh.nih.
gov/publicat/depression.cfm#ptdep1), Site updated:9/02/05, Site visited: 9/02/05.

[146] World Health Organization Web site, Mental Health, Depression, (http://www.google.com/search?hl=en&q=Depression%2Bdefinition) Site visited: 9/02/05.

[147] Antipsychiatry.org Web site, Stevens, L., J.D., The Myth of Biological Depression, (http://www.antipsychiatry.org/depressi.htm), Site updated: 2001, Site visited: September 2, 2005.

[148] The Biology of Mental Disorders, Congress of the United States, Office of Technology Assessment, U.S. Gov't Printing Office, 1992, p. 84

[149] Breggin, M.D., PR, The Anti-Depressant Fact Book, Perseus Publishing, 2001, p. 22

[150] *Diagnostic and Statistical Manual of Mental Disorders—Fourth Edition* (DSM-IV), published by the American Psychiatric Association

[151] Royal College of Psychiatrists Web site, Alcohol and Depression, (http://www.rcpsych.ac.uk/info/help/alcohol/index.asp), Site visited: 9/23/05

[152] EurekaAlert! Web site, (http://www.eurekalert.org/pub_releases/2003-04/aaos-tea042503.php) Conner, K.R. et. al., The elderly, alcohol dependence and risk factors for suicide, American Association of Suicidology, April 25, 2003, Site visited: 9/23/05

[153] Cleveland Clinic Health Systems Web site, Medicines that can cause mood disorders, (http://www.cchs.net/health/health-info/docs/2200/2284.asp?index=9287), Site updated: 10/15/2001, Site visited: 9/23/05.

[154] Breggin, M.D., PR, The Anti-Depressant Fact Book, Perseus Publishing, 2001, p. 22

[155] RxList.com, The Top 300 Prescriptions for 2004 by Number of US Prescriptions Dispensed, ( http://www.rxlist.com/top200.htm), Site visited: October 2, 2005.

[156] Fischer, S. and Greenberg, R.P., Prescriptions for happiness?—effectiveness of antidepressants. Psychology Today, Sept-Oct 1995.

[157] Kirsch, I. et al, The Emperor's New Drugs: An Analysis of Antidepressant Medication Data Submitted to the U.S. Food and Drug Administration. *Prevention & Treatment*, Volume 5, Article 23.

[158] Breggin, P.R., The Anti-Depressant Fact Book, Perseus Publishing, 2001, p. 35

[159] Biopsychiatry.com, The Rebranding of a Disease, Jerome Burne, New Statesman, March 11, 2002, (http://www.biopsychiatry.com/bigpharma/index.html), Site visited: October 3, 2005.

[160] Psychiatric Times Web site, Levy, N., Smith, N.K., Lactation and Psychotropic Medications: Treatment Considerations, Psychiatric Times, May 2000, Vol. XVII, Issue 5, (http://www.psychiatrictimes.com/p000562.html), Site visited: October 9, 2005.

[161] Gilbert et al (2000), Decrease in Thalamic Volumes of Pediatric Patients With Obsessive-compulsive Disorder Who Are Taking Paroxetine, *Arch Gen Psychiatry.* 2000;57:449-456.

[162] Breggin, P.R., The Anti-Depressant Fact Book, Perseus Publishing, 2001, p. 74

[163] National Cancer Institute Web site, Sexuality and Reproductive Issues (PDQ®), Health Professional Version, Pharmacological Effects of Supportive Care Medications on

Sexual Function, ( http://www.cancer.gov/cancertopics/pdq/supportivecare/sexuality/HealthProfessional/page4/print), site updated: July 17, 2006, Site visited: August 4, 2006.

[164] U.S. Food and Drug Administration Web site, FDA Launches a Multi-Pronged Strategy to Strengthen Safeguards for Children Treated With Antidepressant Medications, (http://www.fda.gov/bbs/topics/news/2004/NEW01124.html), October 15, 2004, Site visited:

[165] Biomedcetral.com, Aursnes, I. et al (2005), Suicide attempts in clinical trials with paroxetine randomized against placebo, *BMC Medicine* 2005, **3**:14 , doi:10.1186/1741-7015-3-14, Site visited: October 10, 2005

[166] Breggin.com, Breggin, P.R., Eric Harris was taking Luvox (a Prozac-like drug) at the time of the Littleton murders, April 30, 1999, ( http://www.breggin.com/luvox.html), Site visited: October 10, 2005.

[167] Dr. Demartini.com, (http://www.drdemartini.com)

[168] Dr. Ronald H. Matson's Web site, Professor of Biology and Chair, Kennesaw State University, Scientific Laws and Theories, (http://science.kennesaw.edu/~rmatson/Biol%203380/3380theory.html), Site updated: August 2, 2005, Site visited: October 21, 2005.

[169] Alzheimer's Association Web site, Statistics about Alzheimer's disease, (http://www.alz.org/AboutAD/statistics.asp#3), Site visited: October 28, 2005.

[170] Tan, Z., M.D., Age-Proof Your Mind, Warner Books, 2005, p 114.

[171] Andell, R., Crowe M., Pedersen, N. L., Mortimer, J., Crimmins, E., Johansson, B. and Gatz, M., Complexity of Work and Risk of Alzheimer's Disease: A Population-Based Study of Swedish Twins, *The Journals of Gerontology Series B: Psychological Sciences and Social Sciences* 60:P251-P258 (2005)

[172] Tan, Z., M.D., Age-Proof Your Mind, Warner Books, 2005, p 130.

[173] British Medical Journal Web site, (http://bmj.bmjjournals.com/cgi/content/full/317/7168/1272), Berger, A., Brain cells can regenerate, *BMJ* 1998;317:1272 (7 November), Site visited: October 28, 2005.

[174] Science Daily Web site, (http://www.sciencedaily.com/releases/2005/10/051012231439.htm), Long-term Tobacco Use Associated With Dulled Thinking And Lower IQ, Study Finds, October 12, 2005. Site visited: October 28, 2005.

[175] Official Tiger Woods Web site, Tiger's Tips, Stick to Your Routine, 7/20/05, (http://www.tigerwoods.com/news/fullstory.sps?iNewsid=201832&itype=6273), Site visited: October 30, 2005.

[176] Banquet, J.P., Spectral Analysis of the EEG in Meditation, Electroencephalography and Clinical Neurophysiology. 1973, *35:143-151.*

[177] Delmonte, M.M., Physiological responses during meditation and rest, Applied Psychophysiology and Biofeedback (Historical Archive), Volume: 9, Number: 2, June 1984, pp. 181-200.

[178] Delmonte, M.M., Physiological responses during meditation and rest, Applied Psychophysiology and Biofeedback (Historical Archive), Volume: 9, Number: 2, June 1984, pp. 181-200.

[179] The Institute of Noetic Sciences Web site, Murphy, M., and Donovan, S., The Physical and Psychological Effects of Meditation, (http://www.noetic.org/research/medbiblio/ch3_1.htm), Ch 3: Behavioral Effects, Site visited: October 30, 2005.

# Chapter 7

[180] U.S. Environmental Protection Agency Web site, The Love Canal Tragedy, EPA Journal 1979, (http://www.epa.gov/history/topics/lovecanal/01.htm), Site visited: March 9, 2006.

[181] Commission on Life Sciences, Monitoring Human Tissues for Toxic Substances, Committee on National Monitoring of Human Tissues, p21, Board on Environmental Studies and Toxicology, National Academy Press, Washington, D.C. 1991

[182] Environmental Protection Agency Web site, EPA History, Publications, Douglas M. Costle: Oral History Interview, (http://www.epa.gov/history/publications/costle/23.htm), Site updated: February 17, 2006, Site visited: March 31, 2006.

[183] Scorecard (The Pollution Information Site) Web site, Pollution Locator, Toxic Chemical Releases, (http://www.scorecard.org/env-releases/us-map.tcl), Site updated: September 2004, Site visited: March 31, 2006.

[184] Commission on Life Sciences, Monitoring Human Tissues for Toxic Substances, Committee on National Monitoring of Human Tissues, p21, Board on Environmental Studies and Toxicology, National Academy Press, Washington, D.C. 1991

[185] Crinnion, W.J., Environmental Medicine, Part 1: The Human Burden of Environmental Toxins and Their Common Health Effects, Altern Med Rev 2000;5(1):52-63

[186] American Heart Association Web site, Statistical Fact Sheet, Leading Causes of Death Statistics, U.S. 2002, (http://www.americanheart.org/downloadable/heart/1103834819155FS23LCD5.pdf) Site updated: 2004, Site visited: March 31, 2006.

[187] U.S. Food and Drug Administration, Center for Food Safety and Applied Nutrition Web site, Pesticides, Metals, Chemical Contaminants & Natural Toxins, (http://www.cfsan.fda.gov/~lrd/pestadd.html), Site visited: March 31, 2006.

[188] Environmental Protection Agency Web site, About Pesticides, (http://www.epa.gov/pesticides/about/), Site updated: Tuesday, June 21, 2005, Site visited: March 31, 2006.

[189] The United Kingdom Parliament Web site, Organophosphates, Post 122, December 1998, (http://www.parliament.uk/post/pn122.pdf) Site visited: March 31, 2006.

[190] Environmental Protection Agency Web site, Pesticides: Organophosphates, Organophosphate Pesticides in Food—A Primer on Reassessment of Residue Limits,

May 1999, (http://www.epa.gov/pesticides/op/primer.htm), Site updated: Tuesday, October 11, 2005, Site visited: March 31, 2006.

[191] Environmental Protection Agency Web site, 2000-2001 Pesticide Market Estimates: Usage (Page 3), (http://www.epa.gov/oppbead1/pestsales/01pestsales/usage2001_3.html#table3_8), Site updated: Tuesday, May 2nd, 2006, Site visited: July 31, 2006.

[192] The U.S. Department of Agriculture Web site, Agricultural Marketing Service, Consumer Brochure, April 2002, (http://www.ams.usda.gov/nop/Consumers/brochure.html), Site visited: March 31, 2006.

[193] Alliance of Bio-Integrity Web site, Why The Venture To Genetically Engineer Our Food Offends Science, Religion, And The Bill Of Rights, (www.biointegrity.org/Overview.html), Site updated: 1998-2001, Site visited: March 31, 2006.

[194] Green Left Weekly Web site, Smith J.M., Exposing government lies about GM foods, 2004, (http://www.greenleft.org.au/back/2004/585/585p21.htm), Site visited: March 31, 2006.

[195] The Campaign to Label Genetically Engineered Foods, 2003, (www.thecampaign.org), Site visited: March 31, 2006.

[196] Alliance of Bio-Integrity Web site, Why The Venture To Genetically Engineer Our Food Offends Science, Religion, And The Bill Of Rights, (www.biointegrity.org/Overview.html), Site updated: 1998-2001, Site visited: March 31, 2006.

[197] The Campaign to Label Genetically Engineered Foods, 2003, (www.thecampaign.org), Site visited: March 31, 2006.

[198] BioEd Online Web site, Giles, J., Organic Food Contaminated with GM, Feb 6, 2004, (http://www.bioedonline.org/news/news.cfm?art=766), Site visited: March 31, 2006.

[199] Losey J, et al. (1999) "Transgenic Pollen Harms Monarch Larvae." Nature 399(6733): 214.

[200] Author unknown, Famine and the GM Debate, BBC News, Nov. 14, 2002, (http://news.bbc.co.uk/2/hi/africa/2459903.stm) Site visited 6/16/04

[201] Sexton, S., The world is hungry for justice, not genetics, Health Matters, Spring 1999, Issue 36

[202] World Food Programme Web site, What is Hunger?, Unknown author, Hunger, Humanity's Oldest Enemy, (http://www.wfp.org/aboutwfp/introduction/hunger_what.asp?section=1&sub_section=1) Site visited 1/23/05

[203] BSEInfo Web site, Beef Industry Facts, (www.bseinfo.org/beeffacts.htm), Site updated: March 29, 2005, Site visited: March 31, 2006

[204] Eat Wild Web site, Robinson, J., Grass-fed Basics, (www.eatwild.com/basics.html), Site visited: January 23, 2005.

[205] Raloff, J., Hormones, Here's the Beef, Science News, Jan. 5, 2002, Vol. 161, No.1, p. 10

206  Newsweek online, Cowley, G., Cannibals to Cows: The Path of a Deadly Disease, (http://www.msnbc.msn.com/id/3069552/site/newsweek/), Site updated: March 3, 2001, Site visited: March 31, 2006

207  The Coloradoan Web site, Mook, B., Complexity defines beef industry, January 18, 2004, (www.coloradoan.com/news/stories/20040118/business/249662.html), Site visited: January 23, 2005.

208  French, P. et al, Fatty acid composition, including conjugated linoleic acid, of intramuscular fat from steers offered grazed grass, grass silage, or concentrate-based diets, J. Anim. Sci. 2000. 78:2849-2855

209  Clancy, K., Greener Pastures, How grass-fed beef and milk contribute to healthy eating, Union of Concerned Scientists, March 2006, The full text of this report is available online at *www.ucsusa.org* or may be obtained from: UCS Publications, Two Brattle Square, Cambridge, MA 02238-9105

210  Neufeld, L. "Consumer Preference for Organic/Free Range Chicken," Department of Agricultural Economics, Kansas State University, Thesis, August 2002.

211  The United States Environmental Protection Agency, Water On Tap, What You Need to Know, Office of Water (4601), EPA 816-K-03-007, www.epa.gov/safewater, October 2003.

212  National Defense Resource League Web site, Author unknown, Study Finds Safety of Drinking Water in U.S. Cities at Risk, (http://www.nrdc.org/water/drinking/uscities.asp), Site updated: June 10, 2003, Site visited: April 1, 2006.

213  National Defense Resource League Web site, What's On Tap? Grading Drinking Water in U.S. Cities., (http://www2.nrdc.org/water/drinking/uscities/pdf/chap02.pdf), June 2003, Site visited: March 22, 2006.

214  American Dental Association Web site, Fluoridation Facts 2005, (http://www.ada.org/public/topics/fluoride/facts/fluoridation_facts.pdf), Site visited: April 1, 2006.

215  National Defense Resource League Web site, On Earth Magazine, Fall 2004, Reviews, (http://www.nrdc.org/onearth/04fal/reviews2.asp), Site visited: April 1, 2006.

216  American Dental Association Web site, Fluoridation Facts 2005, (http://www.ada.org/public/topics/fluoride/facts/fluoridation_facts.pdf), Site visited: April 1, 2006.

217  Hellwig E, Lennon AM, Caries Res. 2004 May-Jun;38(3):258-62 )

218  Yiamouyiannis, J.A., Ph.D., Fluoride: Journal of the International Society for Fluoride Research, April 1990 (Volume 23, Issue 2, Pages 55-67).

219  Fluoride Action Network Web site, Health Effects: Tooth Decay Trends In Fluoridated Vs. Unfluoridated Countries, (http://www.fluorideaction.org/health/teeth/caries/who-dmft.html), Site visited: April 1, 2006.

220  Masters, R., and Coplan, M., Adverse Health and Behavior from Silicofluorides, Summary of Research, (http://www.dartmouth.edu/~rmasters/AHABS/SiFSummary.pdf) Site visited: April 1, 2006

[221]  Dr. Joseph Mercola's Web site, Is Fluoride Really As Safe As You Are Told?, February 9, 2002, (http://www.mercola.com/2002/feb/9/fluoride_safety3.htm), this article was provided free from www.Mercola.com, subscribe now for the free eHealthy News You Can Use, Site visited: January 23, 2005.

[222]  Masters, R., and Coplan, M., Adverse Health and Behavior from Silicofluorides, Summary of Research, (http://www.dartmouth.edu/~rmasters/AHABS/SiFSummary.pdf) Site visited: April 1, 2006

[223]   Dr. Joseph Mercola's Web site, Is Fluoride Really As Safe As You Are Told?, February 9, 2002, (http://www.mercola.com/2002/feb/9/fluoride_safety3.htm), Site visited: January 23, 2005.

[224]  Begley, S., Don't Drink the Water?, Newsweek, February 5, 1990. Article can be found at: (http://www.fluoridealert.org/health/cancer/ntp/news2.html) Site visited: April 1, 2006.

[225]  National Research Council (1993). Health Effects of Ingested Fluoride. National Academy Press, Washington DC

[226]  Chemical & Engineering News, August 1, 1998

[227]  National Institute of Arthritis and Musculoskeletal and Skin Diseases Web site, Raab, C. and Fleming, R., Arthritis Prevalence Rising as Baby Boomers Grow Older, May 5, 1998, (http://www.niams.nih.gov/ne/press/1998/05_05.htm), Site visited: April 1, 2006.

[228]  Mullenix, P. et al (1995). Neurotoxicity of sodium fluoride in rats. *Neurotoxicology &Teratology*, 17, 169-77

[229]  Fluoride Action Network Web site, Statement from Dr. Phyllis Mullenix on the Neurotoxicity of Fluoride, September 14, 1998, (http://www.fluoridealert.org/pmullenix2.htm), Site visited: April 1, 2006.

[230]  Fluoride Action Network Web site, Greater Boston Physicians For Social Responsibility, Toxic Threats to Child Development—Fluoride, May 2000, (http://www.fluoridealert.org/psr.htm), Site visited: April 1, 2006.

[231]  Luke J, Fluoride Deposition in the Aged Human Pineal Gland. *Caries Res 2001;35:125-128 (DOI: 10.1159/000047443).*

[232]  American Dental Association Web site, Fluoridation Facts 2005, (http://www.ada.org/public/topics/fluoride/facts/fluoridation_facts.pdf), Site visited: April 1, 2006.

[233]  Pierre, M. Galletti, M.D., PH.D and Gustave Joyet, D.Sc. *The Department of Medicine and Radiology, Kantonspital, Zurich, Switzerland*, Effect Of Fluorine On Thyroidal Iodine Metabolism In Hyperthyroidism, Journal of Clinical Endocrinology, Year 1958, Volume 18, Pages 1102-1110)

[234]  Rx list.com, The Top 300 Prescriptions for 2004 by Number of US Prescriptions Dispensed, NDC PHAST Retail Audit, (http://www.rxlist.com/top200.htm), Site visited: January 23, 2005.

235  Fluoride Action Network Web site, Vice President of EPA's Scientist Union Testifies Against Fluoridation, Statement of Dr. J. William Hirzy National Treasury Employees Union Chapter 280 Before The Subcommittee On Wildlife, Fisheries And Drinking Water, United States Senate, (http://www.fluorideaction.org/hirzytestimony.pdf) Site visited: April 1, 2006.

236  Fluoride Action Network Web site, Facts about Fluoridation, Fluoride Action Network March 2002, (http://www.fluoridealert.org/fluoride-facts.htm), Site visited: April 1, 2006.

237  BBC News Web site, Author Unknown, Fluoride plan goes down the drain, Thursday, 18 November, 2004 (http://news.bbc.co.uk/2/hi/uk_news/scotland/4022833.stm) Site visited: April 1, 2006.

238  Fluoride Action Network Web site, Facts about Fluoridation, Fluoride Action Network March 2002, (http://www.fluoridealert.org/fluoride-facts.htm), Site visited: April 1, 2006.

239  National Resources Defense Council Web site, Author Unknown, Bottled Water, Pure Drink or Pure Hype?, (http://www.nrdc.org/water/drinking/bw/chap2.asp), Site visited: April 1, 2006.

240  Beverage Marketing Corp. Web site, Rodwan Jr., J.G., Bottled Water 2004: U.S. and International Statistics and Developments, (http://www.beveragemarketing.com/news3e.htm), Site visited: April 1, 2006.

241  International Bottled Water Association Web site, Hemphill, G.A., Bottled Water Now Number-Two Commercial Beverage In U.S., Says Beverage Marketing Corporation, (http://www.bottledwater.org/public/downloads/Bev_Marketing_2004_Release_04082004.doc) Site visited: April 1, 2006.

242  Hartford Advocate Web site, Howard, B., What's in your Bottled Water?, August 28, 2003, (http://www.hartfordadvocate.com/gbase/News/content?oid=oid:30865), Site visited: April 1, 2006.

243  ABC News Web site, Baumgartner, M., Study: Bottled Water No Safer Than Tap Water, (http://abcnews.go.com/Business/story?id=87558&page=1), Site visited: April 1, 2006.

244  Hartford Advocate Web site, Howard, B., What's in your Bottled Water?, August 28, 2003, (http://www.hartfordadvocate.com/gbase/News/content?oid=oid:30865), Site visited: April 1, 2006.

245  National Resources Defense Council Web site, Bottled Water: Pure Drink Or Pure Hype, Exploding Sales: Marketing A Perception of Purity. (http://www.nrdc.org/water/drinking/bw/chap2.asp), Site visited: April 14, 2006.

246  National Resources Defense Council Web site, Bottled Water: Pure Drink Or Pure Hype, While bottled water marketing conveys images of purity, inadequate regulations

offer no assurance. (http://www.nrdc.org/water/drinking/nbw.asp), Site updated: 4/29/99, Site visited: April 14, 2006.

[247] National Resources Defense Council Web site, Bottled Water: Pure Drink Or Pure Hype, Exploding Sales: Marketing A Perception of Purity. (http://www.nrdc. org/water/drinking/bw/chap2.asp), Site visited: April 14, 2006.

[248] brandchannel.com, Bottled Water Floods the Market, Karolefski, J. (http://www. brandchannel.com/features_effect.asp?pf_id=88) Site visited: April 14, 2006

[249] National Resources Defense Council Web site, Bottled Water: Pure Drink Or Pure Hype, Exploding Sales: Marketing A Perception of Purity. (http://www.nrdc. org/water/drinking/bw/chap2.asp), Site visited: April 14, 2006.

[250] National Resources Defense Council Web site, Bottled Water: FAQ, (http://www. nrdc.org/water/drinking/qbw.asp), Site visited: April 14, 2006.

[251] International Bottled Water Association Web site (http://www.bottledwater. org/public/whatis_main.htm), Site visited: April 14, 2006.

[252] United States Environmental Protection Agency Web site, What You Need to Know about Mercury in Fish and Shellfish, (www.epa.gov/waterscience/fishadvice/advice. html), Site updated: February 27, 2006, Site visited: April 15, 2006.

[253] University of Minnesota Web site, Allchin D, The Poisoning of Minamata, (http:// www1.umn.edu/ships/ethics/minamata.htm), Site visited: April 15, 2006.

[254] PBS.org, Author unknown, The Mercury Story, January 21, 2005, (www.pbs. org/now/science/mercuryinfish.html), Site visited: April 15, 2006.

[255] U.S. Tuna Foundation Web site, Tuna Industry Renews Its Call to Revise the Risk Assessment for Mercury in Fish, (www.tunafacts.com/press/2004/aug11.cfm), Site updated: August 11, 2004, Site visited: April 15, 2006.

[256] Pope III C. A., PhD; Burnett R. T., PhD; Thun, M. J., MD; Calle E. E., PhD; Krewski, D., PhD; Ito, K., PhD; Thurston, G. D., ScD, Lung Cancer, Cardiopulmonary Mortality, and Long-term Exposure to Fine Particulate Air Pollution, *JAMA*. 2002;287:1132-1141.

[257] Pope, CA 3rd, Epidemiology of fine particulate air pollution and human health: biologic mechanisms and who's at risk?, Environ Health Perspect. 2000 Aug;108 Suppl 4:713-23. (http://www.ehponline.org/members/2000/suppl-4/713-723pope/pope-full. html), Site visited: March 23, 2006.

[258] Centers for Disease Control Web site, National Institute for Occupational Safety and Health, Approaches to Safe Nanotechnology: An Information Exchange with NIOSH, (http://www.air-purifiers-cleaners.com/hepa-filters.htm), Site visited: April 15, 2006.

[259] American Lung Association Web site, Author Unknown, Air Cleaning Devices, (http://www.lungusa.org/site/pp.asp?c=dvLUK9O0E&b=35696), Site updated: February 2000, Site visited: April 15, 2006.

[260] CNN.com, from MayoClinic.com, Teens and smoking: What parents can do, July 1, 2005, (http://www.cnn.com/HEALTH/library/HQ/00139.html), Site visited: April 15, 2006.

[261] This process is a derivative of a technique developed by Dr. John F. Demartini

[262] University of Missouri, St. Louis Web site, Keele, R.O., Drug classifications, from *Drugs in American Society*, 5th and 6th editions, Erich Goode, McGraw-Hill, 1999/2005. Chapter 1, (http://www.umsl.edu/~rkeel/180/classify.html), Site updated: January 19, 2006, Site visited: April 15, 2006.

[263] Ecstasy.org, Jansen, K.L.R. (1997) Adverse Psychological Effects Associated With The Use Of Ecstasy (MDMA) And Their Treatment. In: Ecstasy Reconsidered (Saunders, N. ed.) pp112-128. Nicholas Saunders, 14 Neal's Yard, London WC2 9DP, United Kingdom, article found at: (http://ecstasy.org/info/karl.html), Site visited: April 15, 2006.

[264] Mittleman M. A., MD, DrPH; Mintzer D.; Maclure M., ScD; Tofler G. H., MB; Sherwood J. B., RN;. Muller J. E, Triggering of Myocardial Infarction by Cocaine, 1999, *Circulation.* 1999;99:2737-2741.

[265] National Institute on Drug Abuse Web site, U.S. Department of Health and Human Services, Mind Over Matter Teaching Guide, Opiates Mechanism of Action, (http://teens.drugabuse.gov/mom/tg_opi2.asp), Site visited: April 15, 2006.

[266] National Institute on Alcohol Abuse and Alcoholism Web site, U.S. Department of Health and Human Services, (http://pubs.niaaa.nih.gov/publications/GettheFacts_HTML/facts.htm), Site visited: April 16, 2006.

[267] E-medicine.com, Cohagan, A., DO, Alcohol and Substance Abuse Evaluation, (http://www.emedicine.com/emerg/topic20.htm), Site updated: March 16, 2005, Site visited: April 16, 2006.

[268] National Institute on Alcohol Abuse and Alcoholism Web site, U.S. Department of Health and Human Services, Alcohol and Aging, Alcohol Alert, No. 40, April, 1998, article can be found at: (http://alcoholism.about.com/cs/alerts/l/blnaa40.htm), Site updated: October, 2000, Site visited: April 16, 2006.

[269] MedicalOnline.com, Author unknown, Drugs and Drug Abuse, Heroin, (http://www.medicalonline.com.au/wwwroot/medical/drugs/heroin.htm), Site visited: April 16, 2006.

[270] American Heart Association Web site, Statistics you need to know, Source for Medication Statistics: The National Council on Patient Information, (http://www.americanheart.org/presenter.jhtml?identifier=107), Site visited: April 16, 2006.

[271] U.S. Department of Health and Human Services, Merlis, M. Explaining the Growth in Prescription Drug Spending: A Review of Recent Studies, article can be found at: (http://aspe.hhs.gov/health/Reports/Drug-papers/merlis/Merlis-Final.htm), Site visited: April 16, 2006.

[272]   University of Michigan Web site, Human Resources and Affirmative Action, Benefits Office, Kellog, K., There's Good News, Bad News In New Drug Development, University Record, September 18, 2000, article can be found at: (http://www. newyorker.com/printable/?critics/041025crat_atlarge), Site visited: April 16, 2006.

[273]   American Chemical Society Web site, Lesney, M.S., Patents and Potions, Entering the Pharmaceutical Century, article can be found at: (http://pubs.acs.org/journals/ pharmcent/Ch1.html), Site visited: April 16, 2006.

[274]   American Chemical Society Web site, Lesney, M.S., Patents and Potions, Entering the Pharmaceutical Century, article can be found at: (http://pubs.acs.org/journals/ pharmcent/Ch1.html), Site visited: April 16, 2006.

[275]   Lazarou J, Pomeranz BH, Corey PN, Incidence of adverse drug reactions in hospitalized patients: a meta-analysis of prospective studies. JAMA. 1998 Apr 15;279(15):1200-5.

[276]   The American Iatrogenic Association Web site, Antibiotic overuse and microbial resistance, (http://www.iatrogenic.org/library/antibioticlib.html), Site visited: March 28, 2006

[277]   Deacon, J. University of Edinburgh, Institute of Cell and Molecular Biology, The Microbial World, Microorganisms and Microbial Activities, article can be found at: (http://helios.bto.ed.ac.uk/bto/microbes/penicill.htm), Site visited: April 16, 2006.

[278]   U.S. Department of Homeland Security Web site, Metropolitan Medical Response System, Super Bug Invading Health Clubs: MRSA Spreads Through Dirty Equipment, Towels, Oct. 26, 2004. article can be found at (http://mmrs.fema. gov/News/PublicHealth/2004/oct/nph2004-10-26a.aspx), Site visited: April 16, 2006.

[279]   Jeffords, J.M., Direct-To-Consumer Drug Advertising: You Get What You Pay For, Health Affairs, April 28, 2004, article can be found at: (http://www.healthmatters. org.uk/stories/medawar.html), Site visited: April 16, 2006.

[280]   MedicationSense.com, Cohen, J.S., Prescription Drug Use in America: The Startling Numbers And Their Implications, 2003 (http://www.medicationsense. com/articles/july_sept_03/prescript_drug_use.html), Site visited: April 16, 2006.

[281]   Almanac of Policy Issues Web site, Baker, C., Congressional Budget Office, April 24, 2004, Would Prescription Drug Reimportation Reduce U.S. Drug Spending?,(http:// www.policyalmanac.org/health/archive/prescription_drug_reimportation.shtml), Site visited: April 16, 2006.

[282]   Sherer, R.A., Does DTC Advertising Benefit Patients?, *Psychiatric Times*, May 2002, Vol. XIX, Issue 5.

[283]   New York times.com, Tuller, D. Experts Fear a Risky Recipe: Viagra, Drugs and H.I.V., October 16, 2001,(http://query.nytimes.com/gst/fullpage.html?sec=health&r es=9806EEDD1E3FF935A25753C1A9679C8B63), Site visited: March 29, 2006.

284  New Mexico State University Web site, Graham, J. & Higgins, M., Prescription drug abuse on the rise, 11.27/03, (http://www.roundupnews.com/news/2003/11/27/News/Prescription.Drug.Abuse.On.The.Rise-539464.shtml), Site visited: March 29, 2006.

285  Thomas, L., The Medusa and the Snail, Penguin Books USA Inc., New York, NY, 1979.

286  Simoni-Wastila, L., and Strickler, G. Risk Factors Associated With Problem Use of Prescription Drugs, Am J Public Health, Feb 2004; 94: 266—268.

287  U.S. Drug Enforcement Agency Web site, News Release, October 20, 1995, (http://www.dea.gov/pubs/pressrel/pr951020.htm), Site visited: March 29, 2006.

288  2004 Monitoring the Future Survey, funded by the National Institute on Drug Abuse, National Institutes of Health, DHHS, and conducted by the University of Michigan's Institute for Social Research

289  Lambert, N. (1998). Stimulant treatment as a risk factor for nicotine use and substance abuse. Program and Abstracts, pp. 191-8. NIH Consensus Development Conference Diagnosis and Treatment of Attention Deficit Hyperactivity Disorder. November 16-18, 1998. William H. Natcher Conference Center. National Institutes of Health. Bethesda, Maryland. Full paper can be found at: (http://psychrights.org/Research/Digest/ADHD/LambertinJensenandCooper(2002).pdf), Site visited: March 29, 2006.

## Chapter 8

290  Nhat Hahn, Thich, *The Miracle of Mindfulness*, Beacon Press, Boston, Mass 1987

291  *The American Heritage® Stedman's Medical Dictionary Copyright © 2002, 2001, 1995 by Houghton Mifflin Company. Published by Houghton Mifflin Company.*

292  *The American Heritage® Stedman's Medical Dictionary Copyright © 2002, 2001, 1995 by Houghton Mifflin Company. Published by Houghton Mifflin Company.*

293  University of Alabama Web site, Health Insurance and "Personal Responsibility": Shifting the Bill from the Employer to the Worker, Feb. 2005, (http://main.uab.edu/show.asp?durki=78031), Site visited: November 25, 2005.

294  BusinessWeek, Lee, L. and Kiley, D., Love Those Boomers, October 24, 2005 (http://www.businessweek.com/magazine/content/05_43/b3956201.htm), Site visited: November 25, 2005

295  Thalidomide Victims Association of Canada Web site, (http://www.thalidomide.ca/en/information/what_is_thalidomide.html), Site visited: December 2, 2005.

296  Hempel, J., The Devout Donor, BusinessWeek, November 28, 2005, p. 64

297  Demartini, J.F., You Can Have an Amazing Life . . . in just 60 days!, Hay House, 2005, p. 147.

# INDEX

## T

# Y

4684337R00166

Printed in Great Britain
by Amazon.co.uk, Ltd.,
Marston Gate.